The
HERBAL
HOME
COMPANION

The
HERBAL
HOME
COMPANION

Theresa Loe

Gramercy Books
New York

This 2000 edition is published by Gramercy Books™,
an imprint of Random House Value Publishing, Inc.,
201 East 50th Street, New York, New York 10022,
by arrangment with Kensington Publishing Corporation.

Gramercy Books™ and colophon are trademarks of Random House Value Publishing, Inc.

Random House
New York • Toronto • London • Sydney •Auckland
http://www.randomhouse.com/

Printed and bound in the United States of America

Library of Congress Cataloging-in-Publication Data

Loe, Theresa.
    The herbal home companion / Theresa Loe.
        p. cm.
    Originally published: New York : Kensington Books, c1996.
    Includes bibliographical references (p.) and index.
    ISBN 0-517-20554-8
        1. Herb gardening. 2. Herbs–Utilization. 3. Cookery (Herbs) 4. Herbs–Therapeutic use.
    I. Title.

SB 351.H5 L66 2000
635'.7–dc21

99-047732

8 7 6 5 4 3 2

To my parents,
who have always given me strength and encouragement.
And to my husband, Rick,
who offers his love and support in everything I do.

A very special 'thank you' goes out to:

My husband, Rick, who kept me "fed and watered" through the long, grueling hours at the computer and who was always willing to try my next culinary creation (especially the lemon ones). My mother, Betty Neff, not only for her support and enthusiasm, but for opening my eyes to the joys of cooking and crafting at a young age. My father, George Neff, for always having faith in my abilities and encouraging me to see my inner strength. My grandmother, Nada Grosshans, for being my gardening confidant. My sister, Carrie Christine, not only for being one of my recipe testers, but for diligently keeping the recipes "top secret." My brothers, Jimmie and Gary Neff, for their loving support and their willingness to taste recipes with "green things in them." My dear friend, Renee Mustard, who not only tested more than her share of recipes, but who acted as my personal cheering section from the very beginning. Another dear friend, Lisa Shaddox, who diligently used her gardening knowledge to proof numerous chapters and help research many of the botanical names. Betsy Amster, for her insightful guidance and faith in my abilities. Beth Lieberman, for her professionalism and assistance. Monica Harris, for her meticulous work and herbal enthusiasm. Linda Chlup, for her artistic expertise. Wendel Withrow, for his ardent proof reading and editing. Dr. Art Tucker, for his unequaled botanical nomenclature expertise. And last but not least, to my other wonderful recipe testers who made and subsequently ate everything edible in this book: Demitra Christine, Leslie Loe, Pattie Mucciolo, Brian Mustard and Lauren Mustard.

Contents

Introduction

More than any other type of plant, herbs awaken our senses. Their foliage and flowers offer unequaled fragrance, texture, flavor, and beauty. What's more, they have unlimited usefulness for the home, body, and spirit.

From the ancient Egyptians with their ointments and perfumes, to the Victorians with their herbal fragrances and floral displays, people have utilized these plants for centuries. Herbs are rich in history and tradition. The folklore and superstition associated with each herb is fascinating. Even some of their old-fashioned names reveal this folklore and conjure up all kinds of romantic images. Can't you just imagine a charming cottage landscape containing plants with names like apothecary's rose, carpenter's weed, dittany of Crete, ground apple, lad's love, lark's heel, lamb's ears, silver king, and sweet balm?

Since I was a child, I have been fascinated with both gardening and cooking. Herbs just naturally fit into my lifestyle from the very beginning. I became enchanted by these ancient plants and have been using them for quite some time to embellish my garden and decorate my home. I enjoy using them in everything from culinary endeavors to homemade cosmetics and decorations. I am constantly amazed by how much these plants have to offer.

When I walk through an herb garden, I am constantly touching and smelling the plants to see which ones are the most fragrant. Lemon verbena, with its bright green leaves, has a very striking, lemon peel scent that lingers for hours. A small sprig of this herb can be rubbed on the skin to create an instant cologne! Chamomile (aka ground apple) has a sweet green-apple fragrance that is released whenever the foliage is bruised or stepped upon. I grow it between stepping stones leading to my herb garden so that visitors will have fragrance even before they reach the herbs themselves. Rosemary, with its rich, pine-like scent, has long been considered the symbol for remembrance, and I sometimes place a sprig of this herb inside a card or letter so that the fragrance will remind friends of their last visit.

All herbs have something to offer. Their usefulness in and around the home is truly unlimited. In this book, I explore many ways to preserve the flavors, capture the scents, and showcase the beauty of these wonderful plants. You will learn how herbs can be grown in the garden, utilized in the kitchen, and added to the home in a decorative manner. I hope you will use these ideas and develop a few of your own, because herbs are meant to be celebrated!

What Is an Herb?

That is a question that has plagued herbalists, historians, and garden writers for a long time. Hundreds of years ago, the answer was easier. Herbs were medicines and "pot herbs" were flavorings and vegetables. But today, the term "herb" encompasses more than just a plant with medicinal value.

By one definition, herbs are herbaceous plants that do not develop persistent woody stems. But if that were true, how would lavender, rosemary, and thyme be classified? Another definition states that an herb is a plant whose leaves, stems, roots, or flowers are used for their culinary, cosmetic, aromatic, and/or medicinal properties. This seems to be the most popular definition today and is the one used for this book. But even it has some problems. By that definition, most vegetables could be included as herbs also!

And what about spices? Some say that spices are the seeds, roots, or barks of woody plants that are native to the tropics. But where does that leave a plant like *Coriandrum sativum?* The seed of this plant is called "coriander" and is used as a spice. However, the foliage, called cilantro, is used as an herb!

Clearly, there are no easy, black-and-white answers. Herbs are many things to many people. It really doesn't matter how or why a plant is considered an herb or a spice. What is important is the usefulness, history, and charm of these valuable plants.

Herbs in the Garden

Having your own herb garden can be a wonderful adventure for the senses and will allow you to experience herbs firsthand. With the snip of your clippers, you'll have an endless variety of flavor combinations to be added to your next meal. You'll discover that colorful blossoms from herbs such as borage, nasturtium and calendula are just as comfortable and beautiful in your dinner salad as they are in a vase. As you touch, clip, or tread upon some of these extremely fragrant plants, you'll release the lovely perfume of their essential oils. You'll experience the spicy scent of sweet basil and the romantic fragrances of lavender and rose-scented geranium.

In order to fully enjoy these wonderful plants, you will definitely want to grow some yourself! If you don't already have an herb garden, Chapter 1, "35 Herbs to Grow," gives you a head start toward an herbal green thumb. It covers all the growing information you need. Even if you already have an herb garden, you will find many interesting bits of herbal history, lore, and uses in this chapter. As you read through the herb profiles, be sure to keep in mind that you don't have to have a large garden area in order to enjoy the advantages of home grown herbs. Chapter 2, "Getting Started," details how you can grow herbs just about anywhere! In Chapter 3, "The Basics," you will learn how to keep your garden healthy and happy once it's established.

Chapter 1

꙳꙳꙳

35 Herbs to Grow

Botanical Names

Although the Latin or botanical names of a plant can be hard to remember and difficult to pronounce, they are extremely important in distinguishing one herb from another. Common names vary from region to region and can be used to identify several different plants. Some plants have many relatives which all go by the same common name. For example, the name "oregano" has come to mean many different plants. Some have wonderful culinary flavors and others either taste rancid or have no flavor at all! As you can see, it would be very important to a cook to grow and use the culinary variety of oregano. Without botanical names, the task of finding the correct oregano would be tedious at best. That is why I have included the botanical names of each herb mentioned in this chapter. It should help you identify the precise species you are interested in growing and using.

Sometimes, a plant has been renamed (or reclassified) recently. The old botanical name may appear in some seed catalogs and older herbals. This can cause some confusion. Where known, I have included some of the other names a particular variety may be listed under.

Annuals/Biennials/Perennials

You will notice that each herb is classified as either an annual, a biennial, a perennial, or a tender perennial. An annual is a plant that completes an entire life cycle in one year. It grows, flowers, sets seed, and dies. It must be replanted each spring. A biennial will usually flourish the first season, but will set seed and die during the second year. A perennial is a plant that should come back each year and can usually survive freezing temperatures. A tender perennial is a plant that will survive year after year only if it is brought indoors during the cold winter months. It will not survive freezing temperatures. If it does not survive, it must be replanted in the spring, just like an annual.

There are many herbs to grow and use. But these 35 herbs should provide a good beginning for any herb enthusiast. Every herb listed is used several times throughout the book in recipes, crafts, and fragrances.

Herb Profiles

Aloe Vera
Aloe barbadensis and *Aloe vera*

TENDER PERENNIAL

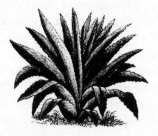

Description: Aloe vera plants look very tropical with their long, tapering leaves. These leaves are filled with a mucilaginous gel that soothes, heals, and moisturizes the skin. It is recorded in history as being used over 2,000 years ago as a healing herb for wounds. Even Cleopatra is believed to have rubbed fresh aloe gel on her skin every day to stay young-looking.

Originally from South Africa, aloe vera must be wintered indoors in areas with frost. But this is not a problem if aloe is kept in pots all year round. It only grows to 2 feet tall and does very well in containers, as long as it is not overwatered. Outdoors, it prefers full sun, but will tolerate some light shade. Propagate by severing the small offshoots it produces during the growing season and replanting them. (You will find aloe listed under two different botanical names: *Aloe barbadensis* and *Aloe vera*.)

Uses: The thick gel in the leaves is very soothing on any type of burn, chapped skin, insect bites, and poison ivy. Simply cut off a piece of the leaf and open it up to reveal the gel inside. Then, gently rub this gel on the affected area. Owing to its healing properties, aloe vera is a very common ingredient in cosmetics for dry, sensitive skin.

Recommended:
Aloe vera *(Aloe barbadensis)*

Artemisia
Artemisia spp.
TENDER PERENNIAL

Description: There are over 300 artemisias, but only a handful are popular in American herb gardens. The few described here have long medicinal histories, but today are primarily grown in home gardens for their ornamental and fragrant foliage.

Wormwood *(Artemisia absinthium)* was once hung on doors to keep away evil spirits. It was also used as a strewing herb, insect repellant, and liqueur flavoring. It is still used to flavor vermouth.

Wormwood is a beautiful plant with finely divided, silvery-gray leaves. In the mornings, the foliage can be covered with sparkling dew drops, which give it a surreal look. It stands about 3–4 feet tall and can grow in full sun to partial shade. Unfortunately, wormwood does not make a good companion plant. It contains a substance called absinthin, which washes off the leaves into the soil. It is toxic to other plants and can inhibit their growth if they are planted within 2 feet. But outside of this 2–3-feet perimeter, your plants will do fine. Therefore, it is best to give wormwood plenty of space or a special section of its own. It also does very well in containers. Propagate by root division or cuttings.

While Wormwood hath seed get a handful or twaine,
To save against March, to make flea to refraine;
Where chamber is sweeped and Wormwood is strowne
no flea for his life dar abide to be known.
What savour is better (if physic be true)
For places infected than Wormwood and Rue?"

—THOMAS TUSSER, FIVE HUNDRED POINTS, 1577

Southernwood *(A. abrotanum)* is also known as lover's plant, lad's love, and old man. It has feathery, gray-green foliage and stands about 3 feet tall. The leaves smell and taste bitter with a hint of lemon. The love-related names come from the old practice of putting sprigs into posies, which were then given to sweethearts. Southernwood was also used in aphrodisiac charms and perfumes. Like many other artemisias, southernwood is known for its insect-repelling qualities. Propagate by cuttings and layering.

Silver King Artemisia *(A. ludoviciana* 'Silver King') and Silver Queen Artemisia *(A. ludoviciana* 'Silver Queen') are grown in the same manner as the other artemisias. Both grow to 3 feet and are excellent wreath and craft herbs. Silver King has silvery, jagged leaves. Silver Queen has wider leaves and is more gray than silver. They are often confused for each other. (They are sometimes listed as *A. albula* 'Silver King' or 'Silver Queen'.)

Uses: All the abovementioned artemisias are so bitter tasting, they are seldom used in cooking. They are mainly grown for decorative and craft purposes. The leaves can be used in moth-repellant potpourri or hung in doorways and windows to repel flies. Their leaves are said to also repel beetles and mosquitos. Hang bundles wherever insects can be a problem.

The foliage of these plants is very useful in flower arranging. It can act as a filler or background to show off special flowers. Artemisias are also excellent for wreath and garland making. They hold their silver-green color well when dried.

Note: One artemisia *is* used extensively for cooking—*A. dracunculus,* better known as "French tarragon." *See* "Tarragon" in this chapter for more information.

Recommended:
Wormwood *(A. absinthium)*
Roman wormwood *(A. pontica)*
Southernwood *(A. abrotanum)*
Silver King *(A. lodoviciana* 'Silver King')

Basil
Ocimum basilicum

ANNUAL

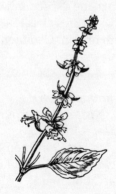

Description: Common basil, aka sweet basil, has strongly scented green leaves and white flowers. Native to Asia, Africa, and South and Central Americas, basil is probably most associated with Italian cooking. Basil did not reach Britain until the sixteenth century and then it was carried to North America with the early settlers.

There are over 150 different varieties of basil with very diverse flavors and leaf structures. (A few of the most popular varieties are listed below.) They all prefer full sun and are easily propagated by seed. Sow the seeds directly outdoors or into pots. Basil seedlings have long tap roots and do not like to be transplanted. Basil plants grow very well in pots outdoors or on a sunny windowsill.

In warm weather, basil tends to bolt and set seed. Once the plant has set seed, it begins to die. To prolong the growing season, constantly pinch back the flower heads and use the flavorful flowers in cooking. They can be sprinkled over salad, sliced tomatoes, spaghetti, or soup.

Uses: Basil is most commonly known as a culinary herb because of its rich, spicy flavor. It is the main ingredient in Italian pesto sauce and is a staple in all tomato sauces. Basil is usually considered a savory herb, but it can be a valuable ingredient in some sweet dishes as well.

Fresh basil has a very delicate flavor which will dissipate with long cooking times. It is best to add the herb at the end of the cooking process. (If you are making a sauce and wish to flavor it slowly, you should used dried basil.) Fresh basil should be chopped at the last minute or it will turn brown. Common basil can also be used as a mosquito repellent.

Recommended:
Common basil *(Ocimum basilicum)*
Opal or purple basil (*O. basilicum* 'Purpurascens')
Lemon basil (*O. basilicum* 'Citriodora')
Cinnamon basil (*O. basilicum* 'Cinnamon')
Green ruffles basil (*O. basilicum* 'Green Ruffles')
Bush basil (*O. basilicum* 'Minimum')

Bay, Sweet

Laurus nobilis

TENDER PERENNIAL

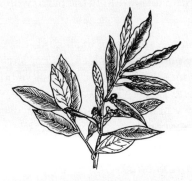

© Copyright Wheeler Arts

Description: Sweet bay is also known as bay laurel. It is an evergreen, Mediterranean tree with glossy, dark green leaves. Bay is known throughout history as the symbol of glory, victory, and honor. The Greeks and Romans anointed the heads of athletes and soldiers with wreaths made of bay.

Bay has an interesting history in Greek mythology. According to legend, the Greek Sun God, Apollo, was madly in love with a nymph named Daphne. Unfortunately, Daphne wasn't interested in Apollo at all. To hide herself from Apollo, Daphne changed into a bay tree. Apollo declared the bay tree sacred. From that day forward, Apollo wore a wreath of bay on his head in Daphne's memory.

Bay has many preservative and antiseptic qualities. Throughout history, the smoke from burning bay leaves was believed to protect against infection. It was commonly used during plagues. It is probably for this reason that bay has the reputation of being protective against all kinds of things, including witchcraft, evil, and lightning.

In mild climates, such as in Southern California, the bay tree can grow as tall as 20 feet. But normally, it is a very slow grower and rarely grows over 4 feet. It is an excellent container plant and is commonly grown as a topiary. Bay is difficult to grow from seed. Propagate from cuttings or layering. Although this perennial will survive frost in many areas, the leaves can get damaged. It is better to bring the plant inside during the harsh winter months. Grow bay in full sun.

Uses: Bay is a common flavoring in all kinds of cuisines. It can be used to season soup, stew, pickles, sauce, shellfish, game, and beef. It is sometimes used to infuse the milk of both sweet and savory puddings and sauces. The leaves of the bay tree hold their color very well when dried. They can be used in potpourri, wreaths, and other crafts.

Recommended:
Sweet bay *(Laurus nobilis)*

Borage
Borago officinalis
ANNUAL

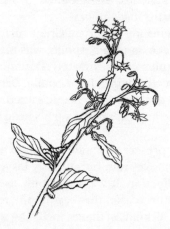

Description: Borage has a reputation for inducing courage and cheerfulness in those who partake in borage-flavored drinks (especially borage-flavored wine). Ancient Celtic warriors drank borage wine before going into battle. But no one knows for sure if it was the borage or the wine which eliminated their fears.

Borage is a highly ornamental plant that grows in full sun to 1 1/2–3 feet tall. Its leaves and stems are covered with tiny, stiff hairs. In midsummer, this herb is covered with bright blue, star-shaped flowers. The beautiful flowers have distinctive black anthers and are a favorite among the bees. Although borage is an annual, it usually self-seeds and comes up in the same area each spring. Borage grows quite easily from seed, but it has a long tap root and does not like to be transplanted. Sow seed directly in the garden in midspring.

Uses: Historically, borage has been used as a diuretic. More recently, the oil produced from borage seed has been found to contain high amounts of gamma linolenic acid (GLA) which has become a popular dietary supplement. Unfortunately, borage oil is very expensive because the seeds are extremely difficult to collect for processing. Some sources suggest that borage leaves and flowers should not be taken internally in large quantities or for long periods of time. However occasional consumption of young leaves and flowers pose no problems.

The young leaves have a cucumber flavor and can be used raw, steamed, or sautéed. They do not hold their flavor when dried or frozen, so they should only be used fresh. The flowers are commonly used to garnish candies, drinks, salads, and cakes. Borage is very ornamental and makes an unusual specimen plant. That alone makes it a good choice for any herb garden.

Recommended:
Borage *(Borago officinalis)*

Burnet, Salad

Poterium sanguisorba

PERENNIAL

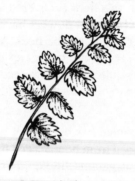

© Copyright Theresa Loe

Description: Salad burnet was very popular in Elizabethan England and was later a prevalent landscape plant in English cottage gardens. The Colonists brought burnet to America, where it is still treasured for its flavor and textured foliage. This delicate-looking herb has slender stems and dainty, fern-like leaves which have a distinctive cucumber flavor. (In the summer heat, the taste may change to sweet watermelon.) In midsummer it produces red-tipped, sphere-shaped flowers. It is commonly called burnet, salad burnet, or garden burnet. You may find it classified in older herb books as *Sanguisorba minor.* Today it is given the botanical name *Poterium sanguisorba.*

Salad burnet prefers full sun, but can tolerate partial shade. It is generally evergreen and can withstand most winters. It can be propagated by division or seeds. In fact, the plant is known to re-seed itself so well, it can become a slight nuisance.

Uses: Due to its delicious cucumber flavor, burnet is a popular salad herb. But it can also be added to salad dressings, cold soups, soft cheeses, delicate sauces, vegetable dishes, and chicken and fish recipes. It makes an excellent herb vinegar, which can be used for dressings and marinades. The leaves contain vitamin C and should be picked from the center of the plant, while young. The older leaves can be tough and bitter.

The leaves of salad burnet do not hold their flavor when dried. Therefore, only fresh leaves are recommended for culinary purposes.

Recommended:
Salad burnet *(Poterium sanguisorba)*

Calendula
Calendula officinalis
HARDY ANNUAL

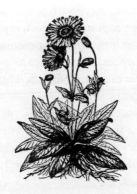

Description: Ancient herbalists called them marigolds. Today they are known by their botanical name, calendula, or their common name, pot marigold. Not to be confused with other marigolds (which are members of the genus *Tagetes*), calendulas are popular and useful bedding plants. They have oblong leaves with fine hairs and cheerful flowers, which range in color from pale yellow to deep orange. They flower almost continuously from early summer to late fall. Deadheading the spent flowers helps promote more blooms.

Grown for centuries in cottage gardens, calendulas are still popular as border and edging plants. They grow in neat, compact clumps which are about 1–2 feet tall. They prefer full sun, but in areas with very hot summers, they prefer some partial shade. They are easily propagated from fresh seed.

Calendulas are susceptible to powdery mildew and leaf spot, so they should be grown where there is good air circulation and drainage. They are sometimes attacked by leafhoppers, aphids, or whitefly. If this happens, dislodge the critters with a strong spray of water or use insecticidal soap for control.

Uses: Calendulas are most commonly used in culinary dishes. Sometimes called the poor man's saffron, the flowers can be dried and ground into a saffron substitute. They are added fresh to salads, sandwiches, soups, custards, butters, vegetables, rice, and cheese. They make excellent herbal vinegar and can be used as a festive garnish on just about anything.

Calendulas are said to have astringent, antiseptic, antifungal, and anti-inflammatory properties—which is probably why they are commonly used in commercial and homemade cosmetics. Calendula flowers have many ornamental uses as well. They can be used in fresh and dried flower arrangements. The dried petals make a colorful addition to potpourri too.

To use the fresh calendula blossoms, pick the flowers to use whole, or remove the individual petals. For dried petals, let the entire calendula blossom dry before removing the individual petals. The dried petals hold their color well and should be stored in an airtight container.

Recommended:
Pot marigold *(Calendula officinalis)*

Chamomile
Chamaemelum nobile
PERENNIAL

Description: *Chamaemelum nobile* (formerly known as *Anthemis nobilis*) is commonly called Roman or English chamomile.

There is some controversy about which *Chamaemelum* species is "the true" chamomile. But in most English-speaking countries, the perennial Roman chamomile is considered "true" chamomile. It grows to only about 8 inches tall when flowering and it has delicious apple-scented, feathery foliage. The flowers are small, daisy-like blossoms which stand on thin stems.

Another plant, with very similar characteristics, is also known as chamomile. Its botanic name is *Matricaria recutita* and its common name is German chamomile. German chamomile looks almost exactly like Roman chamomile except it grows taller and is an annual rather than a perennial. (The fragrance of Roman chamomile is a bit stronger.)

The name "chamomile" means "ground apple," and Roman chamomile makes an excellent ground cover, which releases the apple fragrance when stepped upon. Grow it between stepping stones or as a chamomile lawn. It prefers full sun to partial shade and does not do well in extreme heat. Southern gardeners may have to grow it as an annual. Propagate by division or seed. (The seeds should not be covered with soil because they need light to germinate.)

Uses: Chamomile has a long history as an herbal remedy, dating back to ancient Egypt and Greece. Even Peter Rabbit's mother knew the value of chamomile tea! Tea is made from dried chamomile blossoms and is used to aid indigestion and act as a mild sedative. And save those tea bags! Chamomile has anti-inflammatory properties, which make the tea bags excellent compresses for puffy eyes.

Chamomile is also a popular cosmetic ingredient. It is used in hair rinses to accentuate natural blond highlights and in lotions or creams to soothe and soften skin. The apple scent makes a nice addition to potpourri and flower arrangements as well.

Recommended:
Roman chamomile *(Chamaemelum nobile)*

Chives

Allium schoenoprasum

PERENNIAL

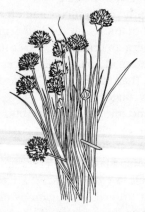

© Copyright Wheeler Arts

Description: There are over 400 species in the allium family including chives, garlic, leeks, and onions. The chive plant *(Allium schoenoprasum)* is the smallest member of this onion family and is sometimes called "onion chives." Owing to their beauty and versatility, chives are very popular in American herb gardens. They have dark green, reed-like leaves which are hollow and stand about 8–12 inches tall. They grow in clumps resembling small tufts of grass and have round, purple-pink blossoms that are actually made up of many tiny flowers. Chives grow in full to partial sun.

Onion chives are easy to grow from seed or division and do very well in pots and window boxes. They should be divided every 3–4 years. The leaves should be snipped from the base of the plant to encourage regrowth. They have a sweet, mild onion taste and are high in vitamins A and C.

There is another variety of chive called garlic or Chinese chives *(A. tuberosum),* which is useful to grow. It resembles onion chives but has flat (rather than hollow) leaves and white blossoms. The flavor of this slightly larger plant is similar to mild garlic and can actually be substituted for garlic in cooking. Garlic chives are slightly less vigorous than onion chives.

Uses: Onion chives are very popular in both American and French cooking. They are generally used fresh because they do not dry well at home. (The commercially dried chives found in the store are freeze-dried.) Chives should be added at the end of recipes, because long cooking times can dissipate their flavor. Use scissors or a very sharp knife to mince or chop the chives. A dull knife can pulverize them! Fresh chives can be added to salads, vegetables, cheese, butter, eggs, sauces, or chicken and fish recipes. The leaves are sometimes tied decoratively around julienned vegetables. The flowers are also flavorful in the abovementioned recipes and can add color to flower arrangements.

Recommended:
Onion chives *(Allium schoenoprasum)*
Garlic chives *(A. tuberosum)*

Coriander/Cilantro
Coriandrum sativum

ANNUAL

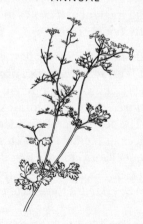

Description: This herb has an ancient history as a culinary herb and has been grown for thousands of years in India and China. It was popular in England up to the Tudor Era. The Colonists brought seed over from England to America. It is one of the few herbs which has a different name for the seed and the leaves of the same plant. The seeds of the plant are generally called coriander seeds. But when referring to the foliage, this plant is called cilantro or Chinese parsley. Although this can be confusing, all three names are correct.

Coriander/cilantro grows in full sun and has very strong smelling and tasting foliage. The lower leaves are fan-like and look very similar to Italian flat-leaf parsley. The upper leaves are lacy and feathery, like dill. This herb has delicate, pinkish-white flowers which appear in umbrella-shaped clusters. The delicate flower stems can snap in the wind, so some staking or protection may be necessary. If you live in an area with extremely hot summers, you may want to plant this herb in partial shade and keep it watered well.

Coriander/cilantro is very easy to grow from seed and it self-sows freely. It has a long tap root which makes it difficult to transplant, so you should sow the seeds directly in the garden or pots. Harvest the seeds in mid- to late summer right as they ripen. If you wait too long, they will fall off in the garden and scatter. This herb does very well in pots, but is not recommended for indoor growing owing to its strong fragrance. It grows to about 12–18 inches tall and makes a pretty border plant.

Uses: Many people do not care for the flavor or scent of cilantro leaves. Some claim it is an acquired taste. However, in the Southwestern United States, cilantro is as common as parsley in restaurants and grocery stores. It is used in Mexican, Chinese, and Vietnamese dishes. The leaves can be added to rice, chutneys, beans, and spicy sauces. It blends very well with tomato or lime flavorings. When using cilantro for the first time, use a very light hand. The flavor can easily overpower the dish. Cilantro is a delicate herb and should be added at the end of cooking or sprinkled raw over the dish.

Coriander seed is more familiar to people. The seed is popular in pastries, breads, pickles, and curries.

Recommended:
Coriander/cilantro *(Coriandrum sativum)*

Dill

Anethum graveolens

ANNUAL

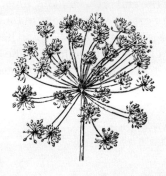

Description: Magicians and sorcerers used dill to cast spells. Old herbals boasted that it could cure hiccups. But dill is probably most noted for being a pickle herb (dill pickles). Growing in full sun, dill will reach a height of 2–4 feet. It has lacy blue-green foliage with large umbels of tiny yellow flowers. The flowers will produce brown, oval-shaped seeds. All parts are aromatic and flavorful, which is probably why dill has been so popular in herb gardens throughout history. Dill is very attractive to bees. Be careful not to disturb them when you are harvesting it.

Dill has a long tap root and does not transplant well. It should be propagated by seeds which are planted directly in the garden. They should only be lightly covered with soil because they need some light to germinate. For a continuous supply of seeds and leaves, dill should be planted in successive plantings from spring to midsummer. It is sensitive to wind damage and should be placed in the garden where it will receive some protection. The seeds should be harvested when the tips begin to turn light brown. (*See* "Harvesting and Drying Herbs" in Chapter 2 for more information.)

Uses: Dill has many other uses besides being the main flavoring in dill pickles. It can be added to potato salad, herb butter, bread, dip, cheese, vegetables, eggs, and fish recipes. It makes an excellent vinegar, which can be used to create salad dressings and marinades. The foliage has a lighter taste than the seeds and is called "dill weed" in many recipes. Snip some fresh dill leaves and toss them into foods at the end of the cooking time. Dill is delicate and cannot stand high heat for long periods of time.

The seeds are said to aid in digestion and have a calming, sedative effect. They can be chewed to freshen the breath. The flower umbels make excellent additions to flower arrangements, because their unusual shape adds a touch of lightness.

Recommended:
Dill *(Anethum graveolens)*

Fennel
Foeniculum vulgare
PERENNIAL

Description: Common fennel grows from 3 to 5 feet, depending upon the climate, and has filigreed leaves and umbels of flowers. It looks very similar to dill. It is said that dill and fennel should not be planted next to each other in the garden or they might cross-pollinate. Fennel has a very distinctive anise or licorice flavor and is much loved by bees and butterflies. It grows in full sun and is best propagated by seed which is sown directly into the garden.

There are also several annual varieties of fennel. The most popular for culinary purposes is Florence fennel *(Foeniculum vulgare* var. *azoricum)*. It has a shorter bulb and is also known as finocchio, sweet anise, or vegetable fennel. It is often confused with another annual, *F. vulgare* var. *dulce,* which has thinner leaves at the base. Both can be used in cooking.

SWALLOWTAIL BUTTERFLIES

Fennel plants are hosts to many swallowtail butterfly species. They might spend their entire lives living on or near a fennel plant. The colorful caterpillars have beautiful markings and will not overly damage the plant. If you find one, leave it alone and soon you may find its chrysalis hanging from a stem. In no time at all, a beautiful swallowtail butterfly will emerge and flutter around your garden!

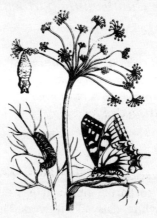

Uses: All parts of the fennel plant are edible and delicious. The seeds are commonly used in cakes, breads, cookies, sausage, liqueurs, butters, and fish recipes. The stalk, bulb, and leaves can be used to flavor salads, vegetables, rice, cheese, soup, and chicken and fish recipes. The Florence fennel bulb is commonly used as a vegetable. It can be steamed or sautéed with other root vegetables to create a delicious side dish.

The seeds are sometimes used to soothe a hungry stomach and to sweeten the breath. Mild fennel tea is sometimes consumed by nursing mothers to help relieve their baby's colic. Fennel is also used to dye wool a pretty yellow or brown color. The leaves are said to be astringent and are sometimes used in cosmetic recipes.

Recommended:
Common fennel *(Foeniculum vulgare)*
Florence fennel *(F. vulgare* var. *azoricum):* Annual.
Bronze leaf fennel *(F. vulgare* 'Rubrum'): This fennel has beautiful, coppery foliage.

Feverfew
Chrysanthemum parthenium
PERENNIAL

". . . Of joys that come to womankind
The loom of fate doth weave her few,
But here are summer joys entwined
And bound with golden feverfew."

—George R. Sims (1847–1922)

Description: Feverfew is a semi-evergreen perennial which grows in full sun to partial shade. It has divided yellow-green leaves and small, white, daisy-like flowers. There are both single- and double-blooming varieties.

Feverfew is easy to grow from seeds, division, or cuttings. The seeds should not be covered with soil when planting because they need light to germinate. To grow feverfew as a perennial, you must pinch off the flowers before they go to seed. If you don't, the plant may die after setting seed. However, if the flowers are removed, feverfew will stay bushy and continue to grow for another season. In some areas, feverfew is grown as a half-hardy annual. (Feverfew is sometimes listed as *Tanacetum parthenium.*)

Uses: Feverfew was once used as a cure for fevers (hence, the name). But today, it is more commonly thought of as a possible headache remedy. There are many studies being conducted on the benefits of eating feverfew leaves to cure migraines and arthritis pain. One problem with feverfew is that some people are allergic to it and many people get irritating sores in their mouths from eating it.

Feverfew should be grown for its many ornamental and decorative qualities. It is a lovely cottage garden plant and is very attractive in window boxes and perennial borders. It is an excellent flower arrangement plant because the flowers can hold up both in and out of water. When dried, feverfew is terrific in all kinds of craft projects.

Recommended:
Double flowering feverfew (*Tanacetum parthenium* 'Flore Pleno')
Golden feverfew *(T. parthenium* var. *aureum):* Light yellow-green leaves that are extremely ornamental in the garden and in craft projects.

Hyssop
Hyssopus officinalis
PERENNIAL

Description: Hyssop is a very beautiful, semi-evergreen shrub with bushy growth and narrow, aromatic leaves. Its flowers are very attractive to bees, butterflies, and humans! From June to late August, hyssop has spiked branches that are covered with whorls of deep blue blossoms. There are also pink and white blooming varieties. Bees are so attracted to this plant, that beekeepers used to rub the hives with hyssop leaves to keep the bees nearby. When bees frequently visit hyssop flowers, their honey develops a delicious flavor. Elizabethans loved to grow hyssop as a hedge in their knot gardens. The only disadvantage to a hyssop hedge is that the constant pruning never allows the plant to come into full flower.

Hyssop has a long history of being used as a cleaning and purifying herb. It was strewn over sickroom floors and used in the purifying rituals of temples. A distilled oil of hyssop has been used in perfumery for centuries and is mentioned in many of the old recipes for *eau-de-Cologne.* It was also used in soap recipes and as a flavoring for liqueur.

Hyssop grows to about 1–2 feet tall in full sun. It will accept some light shade. The leaves have a camphor-like odor, which may explain why it is seldom bothered by pests or disease. Hyssop can be propagated by seeds, cuttings, and division. The seeds are slow to germinate so they should be sown in early spring.

Uses: Hyssop's leaves have a bitter, slightly mint flavor. They can be used in salad, rice, cheese, and lamb or chicken recipes. But hyssop is probably most valued for its ornamental qualities. It not only is very colorful in the garden, but is an excellent flower-arranging herb. The dried flowers and leaves can be added to potpourri too.

Recommended:
Hyssop *(Hyssopus officinalis)*
White blooming hyssop *(H. officinalis* 'Alba')
Pink blooming hyssop *(H. officinalis* 'Rosea')

Lamb's Ears

Stachys byzantina

PERENNIAL

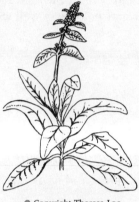

© Copyright Theresa Loe

Description: Lamb's ears (aka woolly betony and woundwort) has dense, woolen, silver-gray foliage. Each fuzzy leaf feels exactly like a soft lamb or bunny ear. The plant forms a spectacular carpet in the garden with silver rosettes of leaves that stand approximately 8 inches tall. The pink flowers form on thick, fuzzy stems that are 1–2 feet tall. Lamb's ears have an endearing quality. Everyone seems to love them, especially children. Once they touch the soft leaves, people just can't seem to stop petting them. Hummingbirds and bees are especially attracted to the blossoms of this ornamental plant.

Lamb's ears can be propagated by seeds or division. People in highly humid areas may have difficulty growing this herb. It does not do well with excessive moisture of any kind. It is extremely ornamental and makes an attractive specimen when grown under rosebushes. It is also perfect for a silver garden or a moon garden when combined with white blooming plants.

Uses: The leaves of lamb's ears are mildly astringent, and in the past, they were used to bandage wounds. The leaves have an absorbing quality, which helped stop mild bleeding. However, today this plant is grown purely as an ornamental. The gray foliage and fuzzy-stemmed blossoms are particularly attractive in fresh-cut flower arrangements because of their unusual texture. The Victorians used lamb's ears extensively in posies. The fresh leaves can be used to cover an entire wreath and then allowed to dry in place. The leaves hold their gray color very well when dried.

Recommended:
Lamb's ears *(Stachys byzantina)*

Lavender

Lavandula angustifolia

TENDER PERENNIAL

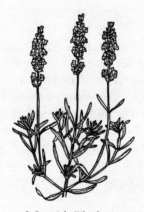

© Copyright Wheeler Arts

"And Lavender, whose spikes of azure bloom
Shall be erewhile, in arid bundles bound,
To lurk amidst her labours of the loom,
And crown her kerchiefs clean with mickle rare
perfume."

—William Shenstone

Description: There are many different species and varieties to choose from, but English lavender *(Lavandula angustifolia)* is probably one of the most well known. (It is sometimes listed as *L. vera.*) It grows in full sun to a height of 2–3 feet. It is a bushy shrub with gray-green leaves and purple spike flowers. (There are also white and pink blooming varieties available.)

Lavender can be propagated by seeds. However, cuttings or layering is recommended to ensure that the offspring is true to the mother plant. It makes a great potted plant and can even be trained into a topiary or bonsai shape. Lavender is traditionally planted in cottage gardens, along walkways, and in rock gardens. If planted outside a window, the sweet fragrance can waft in with a gentle breeze. In areas with cold winters, lavender should be potted up and brought indoors for the winter. Lavender does not tolerate humidity well.

Valued for centuries for its beauty, fragrance, flavor, and cosmetic properties, lavender has become a classic in the herb garden. The name *Lavandula* comes from the Latin *lavare,* which means "to wash." A standard ingredient in soaps, lavender has a long history as a cleaning and purifying herb. Linen was often dried on the blooming bushes of lavender to impart its fragrance. Lavender was also believed to protect against everything from witchcraft to the evil eye. Victorians believed that the fragrance was so powerful, they even used it in their smelling salts to revive swooning women.

Uses: Although lavender has gone out of fashion as a flavoring, it has a deliciously sweet flavor that should be more utilized. It can be used in jelly, custards, ice cream, cookies, and various other desserts and pastries.

Lavender is probably best known for its fragrant and cosmetic properties. It can be used to make soaps, toilet waters, perfumes, lotions, and many other aromatic cosmetics. The romance of lavender can also be captured in potpourri, sachets, and sleep pillows. Dried lavender is known for its moth-repelling virtues and makes a very refreshing alternative to moth balls. The blossoms of lavender hold their fragrance and color very well and should be used freely in dried crafts.

Recommended:
English lavender *(Lavandula angustifolia)*
Hidcote lavender *(L. angustifolia* 'Hidcote')
French lavender *(L. dentata)*
Pink blooming lavender *(L. angustifolia* 'Rosea')

Lemon Balm
Melissa officinalis
TENDER PERENNIAL

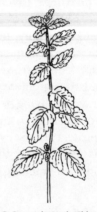

© Copyright Linda Chlup

Description: Lemon balm is also known as balm, sweet balm, and melissa. It is a loosely branched plant with lemon-scented and -flavored foliage. It reached its peak in popularity during the Elizabethan Era, where it was used to flavor food, wine, and tea. It was brought to America with the Colonists and was used as a tea to relieve melancholy. (Thomas Jefferson even grew lemon balm at Monticello.) Its lovely, lemon scent made it useful as a strewing herb and its leaves were rubbed on furniture to make the wood sweet-smelling. But lemon balm is probably best known throughout history as a bee herb. It was rubbed inside the bee hives to encourage bees to move in. It was also believed that the fragrance calmed the bees. In fact, "Melissa" is the Greek name for honeybee.

The leaves of lemon balm are light green and oval-shaped with scalloped edges. The flowers are tiny, white, and inconspicuous. Lemon balm grows to approximately 2 feet in full sun, but it will tolerate some shade. (In very hot climates, it prefers it.) It can be propagated by seeds, layering, or division. For quick propagation, division is the best choice. The seeds will germinate best if they are left uncovered. Although lemon balm is related to mint, it is much better behaved in the garden than ordinary mint. The roots spread but are easily torn out, which makes the plant very controllable. Lemon balm is deciduous. It should be mulched in cold areas through the winter to protect the roots.

Uses: Lemon balm has many culinary uses. It can be added to fruit desserts, ice cream, custards, and pastries. It can be used to make tea, punch, flavored liqueur, or extra tangy lemonade. The leaves are best when fresh and can be used to season chicken, fish, and vegetables. You can be generous when cooking with lemon balm because the leaves have a delicate flavor.

The fresh foliage is terrific in flower arrangements and the dried leaves can be used to create lemon-scented potpourri.

Recommended:
Common lemon balm *(Melissa officinalis)*
Golden lemon balm *(M. officinalis* 'Aurea')
Variegated lemon balm *(M. officinalis* 'Variegata')

Lemon Grass

Cymbopogon citratus

TENDER PERENNIAL

Description: Lemon grass is a tropical plant and only grows well outside in the Southern or West Coast regions of the United States. It grows in large clumps with long, narrow, grass-like leaves and it rarely flowers. It can reach a height of 6 feet in some climates but generally stands 3–4 feet tall. The bright green, bulbous stems and leaves have a very strong lemon scent and flavor. It makes a very nice specimen plant in the garden. It grows in full sun to partial shade and should be propagated by division. It will survive in areas with mild winters, but should be heavily mulched in areas reaching 20 degrees. Areas with colder winters should grow lemon grass as a potted herb and bring it indoors in the winter. It does very well in greenhouses.

Uses: Lemon grass is commonly used in Thai and Vietnamese cuisine. It can be used whole or chopped, but in either case, the leaves should be bruised to release the flavorful oils. It can be used to flavor steamed vegetables, rice, curries, chicken, and fish. It has antiseptic properties and is used in some cosmetics. Commercially, the oil is used as an artificial flavoring for lemon candies. The fragrance holds up well when dried, which makes lemon grass an excellent addition to citrus potpourri.

Recommended:

Lemon grass *(Cymbopogon citratus)*

Lemon Verbena
Aloysia triphylla

TENDER PERENNIAL

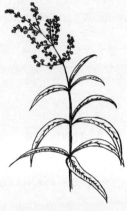

© Copyright Theresa Loe

Description: This strongly scented, woody shrub can reach a height of 10 feet, but generally stays about 4–5 feet in most areas. It has whorls of bright green leaves and spikes of pale, white flowers. It prefers full sun and is hardy only to about 20 degrees. In areas with cold winters, it must be potted up and brought indoors. It grows very well in containers, but should be fed regularly if grown year round as a potted plant. Keep in mind that lemon verbena is deciduous. Don't be alarmed if it loses all of its leaves in the winter. This extremely aromatic plant is best propagated from cuttings and is sometimes listed by its old name, *Lippia citriodora.*

Uses: Lemon verbena has always been a popular fragrance among women. Even today, the essential oil is used in some colognes. (In *Gone With the Wind,* lemon verbena was mentioned as the favorite cologne of Scarlet O'Hara's mother.) Fragrant infusions can be made from the leaves and used to scent bath waters. It can be used in many other cosmetic recipes as well.

The flavor of lemon verbena is very strong and lemony. It can be used in place of lemon juice in hot tea and iced drinks. It can be used as a flavoring in desserts, pastries, jellies, rice, and salad dressings. It is also a delicious seasoning in chicken and fish recipes. A tea brewed from its leaves is said to be mildly sedative.

Sprigs of this aromatic plant are exquisite in all types of fresh flower arrangements. They are so fragrant, they can be hung in a closet to freshen musty air. When dried, they can be added to potpourri recipes.

Recommended:
Lemon verbena *(Aloysia triphylla)*

Marjoram
Origanum majorana
TENDER PERENNIAL/HALF HARDY ANNUAL

Description: Sweet marjoram was believed to be a favorite herb of the goddess of love, Aphrodite. Wreaths of marjoram were worn by bridal couples in ancient Greece to sanctify marital bliss. Marjoram was also used as a strewing herb and was thought to impart disinfectant qualities when strewn in sickrooms. The leaves and oil have been used as a furniture polish for wooden floors, tables, and chairs.

There are many cultivated species of marjoram on the market. The best culinary marjoram is probably *Origanum majorana,* which is known as marjoram, sweet marjoram, or knotted marjoram. It is a Mediterranean herb that grows as a tender perennial in warm climates. In colder areas, it is grown as an annual. It prefers full sun and has small gray-green leaves. The white flowers are small and the seed clusters look like tiny knots. It reaches approximately 1–2 feet when flowering.

If you have difficulty growing sweet marjoram, you might want to try the hybrid *O.* x *majoricum.* It is a hybrid between *O. majorana* and *O. vulgare* var. *virens.* It is easier to cultivate and can be substituted for sweet marjoram in recipes.

For culinary purposes, do *not* try to use wild marjoram *(O. vul-*

gare subsp. *vulgare),* which is sometimes erroneously sold as oregano. It looks like oregano, but has pinkish-purple flowers. Although it is excellent for flower arrangements and crafts, it does not have a good culinary flavor. (I grow wild marjoram in my cut flower garden.)

Sweet marjoram can be grown from seed but the seeds you buy are not always true. You may have better luck buying the actual plant from a reputable nursery or taking divisions from someone's garden. Marjoram can also be propagated by layering.

Uses: Sweet marjoram is sweeter than oregano and can be used in many of the same recipes. Try adding it to red meat, chicken, and vegetables. It can also be used in vinegar, marinades, herb butter, cheese, soup, and stuffing.

Marjoram is mildly antiseptic and is found in some cosmetic recipes. It is also very good in wreaths and flower arrangements.

Recommended:
Sweet marjoram *(O. majorana)*
Golden marjoram *(O. majorana* 'Aureum')
Marjoram hybrid *(O.* x *majoricum)*

Mint

Mentha spp.

PERENNIAL

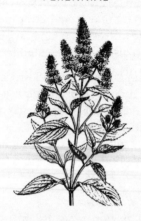

Description: Mint hybridizes very easily and there are literally hundreds of different varieties to choose from. Peppermint and spearmint are probably familiar to most people because they are used to flavor candy, gum, and toothpaste. But there are many other varieties worthy of a place in your herb garden. For example, you might want to grow apple mint *(Mentha suaveolens)* with its fuzzy, light green leaves and sweet apple fragrance. It can be used in fruit salads or as a garnish in ice tea. Another choice might be Corsican mint *(M. requienii)* with its tiny leaves and very potent fragrance. Unlike the other mints, Corsican mint prefers shade and grows in a mossy form just a few inches tall. If you want a plant with flea-repelling qualities, you should grow pennyroyal *(M. pulegium)*. It can be made into an infusion to rinse pets or strewn over bedding areas to deter fleas. It is also a moth repellant.

Almost all the mints prefer full sun (except Corsican mint) but can tolerate some shade. They generally grow 1–3 feet tall, depending upon the variety. You will read in gardening books that mint is a notorious spreader and can easily over take your entire garden. But don't let that deter you from growing it; it can be controlled. The plant spreads by root runners which travel either underground or across the topsoil. To prevent an invasion, you can sink barriers about 6 inches underground around the plants. You will still have to watch closely, though, because the runners can still travel over and around the barriers. Your second choice is to grow mint in containers. It does very well in pots, hanging baskets, and window boxes.

Mint is extremely easy to propagate by layering, divisions, or cuttings. Just about any little piece of mint that has a node can grow into a plant. (That is why it can get out of hand in the garden.)

Uses: Peppermint and spearmint have long histories as medicinal plants and they are still popular today. Peppermint tea helps relieve headaches, insomnia, and upset stomachs. Spearmint is often chewed to freshen the breath and is usually the more popular herb of choice in culinary dishes. Both herbs were used as strewing herbs. They were sprinkled on the floor of sickrooms and living areas to sweeten the air when stepped upon.

Mint can be used in both savory and sweet dishes. It is especially flavorful in tea, desserts, candy, cordials, jellies, and fruit recipes. It can also be used with lamb, duck, fish, and vegetables. (It is especially good with peas and carrots.) Mint is a classic flavoring with anything chocolate. Try using peppermint, spearmint, apple mint, and orange mint in your culinary adventures.

Mint is used in both homemade and commercial cosmetics and soaps. It is said to cool the skin in hot weather and soothe irritated, dry skin. It can also be used in sweet-smelling flower arrangements and potpourri.

Recommended:
Peppermint *(Mentha* x *piperita)*
Spearmint *(M. spicata)*
Apple mint *(M. suaveolens)*
Variegated apple mint *(M. s.* 'Variegata'): Also known as variegated pineapple mint.
Corsican mint *(M. requienii)*
Orange mint *(M.* x *piperita* var. *citrata)*
English pennyroyal *(M. pulegium* var. *erecta)*

Nasturtium

Tropaeolum majus

ANNUAL

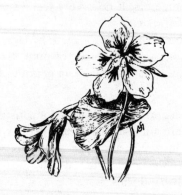

Description: Nasturtiums (lovingly referred to as "nasties" by some) are native to South America and first came to Europe from Peru via Spanish explorers in the 1500s. Within a few years they reached England. They soon became popular in the garden and kitchen. Nasturtiums are lovely trailing plants with flat, round leaves and colorful, trumpet-shaped flowers. The flowers come in all shades of yellow, red, and orange. They are sometimes referred to as "lark's heel" in old herbals because "unto the backe-part (of the flowers) doth hang a taile or spurre, such as hath the Larkes heel" (Gerard).

You can find both climbing and dwarf forms of this plant as well as variegated varieties. You can grow nasties in hanging baskets, tubs, pots, window boxes, or directly in the garden. Unless you have a slope or large area you wish to cover with flowers, you should grow climbing forms on a trellis or fence. A south facing wall or slope is usually best. This plant is propagated by seed in early spring. It prefers full sun to partial shade and will bloom from summer until fall in most areas. Don't overfertilize the soil before planting nasturtiums. They do best in very poor soil. (Fertile soil produces lush growth and few flowers.)

Uses: All parts of the nasturtium are edible. The leaves were once used as a remedy for scurvy and are now known to be high in vitamin C and iron. They have a strong, peppery flavor. The flowers have a more subdued flavor. Use both to give a bite to savory foods. Add fresh leaves or flowers to salad, sandwiches, cheese, and dip. All parts can be used to make a peppery vinegar. For a pretty appetizer, the flowers can be stuffed with cheese.

Recommended:
Nasturtium *(Tropaeolum majus)*
Variegated *(T. majus* 'Alaska')
Dwarf hybrid *(T. majus nanum* 'Tom Thumb')

Oregano
Origanum vulgare subsp. *hirtum*
TENDER PERENNIAL

Description: There is much confusion as to which plants are true culinary oreganos and which are not. There are many different *Origanum* species with very similar physical attributes. But when it comes to flavor, there are only a few worthy of culinary uses. Greek oregano *(Origanum vulgare* subsp. *hirtum)* is considered by many to be "True" oregano. It is sometimes listed in plant catalogs as *O. hirtum* or *O. heracleoticum* and has white blossoms. Wild marjoram *(O. vulgare* subsp. *vulgare)* is sometimes sold as oregano but it has pink flowers and no flavor. It can become very confusing! You may even find seed and plant catalogs which list a certain plant as "oregano" but give the botanical name for "wild marjoram." If you are looking for an oregano for cooking, you should avoid wild marjoram or you will be very disappointed. Wild marjoram is better suited to flower arrangements.

Your best bet for getting Greek oregano is to order from a seed catalog that lists the correct botanical name or take a cutting from someone who has a flavorful white blooming variety. (Oregano can also be propagated by root division.) If you decide to try seeds, do not cover them with soil because they need light to germinate. Greek oregano has a peppery flavor and grows in full sun to a height of approximately 2 feet. It has round, green leaves with a pungent scent.

Keep in mind that there is more to life than just cooking and there are several beautiful varieties of oregano to try besides Greek oregano. You might want to grow dittany of Crete *(O. dictamnus)* with its small hop-like bracts and a cascading growth habit. It is gorgeous in a hanging basket! There is also a pretty variety called Golden Creeping Oregano (*O. vulgare* subsp. *vulgare* 'Aureum').

Most varieties do not do well in humid weather. They can usually survive mild winters with a heavy mulching, but in extremely cold winters, the plants should be potted up and brought indoors. Bees and butterflies love all the oreganos.

Uses: Oregano is most associated with Italian cooking and makes an excellent addition to anything with tomato sauce (spaghetti, pizza, etc.). It did not catch on as a culinary herb in America until about 1940. Now it is extremely popular in all kinds of meat and vegetable dishes. It can be used with beef, game, pork, eggs, and breads.

Oregano tea has been used to relieve coughs, headaches, and indigestion. Fresh leaves can be added to bath water to help relieve achy muscles. The flowers can be used in wreaths, flower arranging, and other crafts.

Recommended:
Greek oregano *(O. vulgare* subsp. *hirtum)*
Dittany of Crete *(O. dictamnus)*

Parsley

Petroselinum crispum

HARDY BIENNIAL

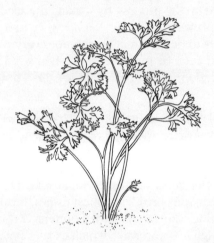

Description: Parsley is a very recognizable herb. Who hasn't seen a sprig of parsley lying on a plate in a restaurant? But parsley is much more than a garnish. It is indispensable in the kitchen and is quite beautiful in the garden.

There are two main varieties which are popular in America today: curly leaf parsley *(Petroselinum crispum)* and Italian flat-leaf parsley *(P. crispum* var. *neapolitanum)*. Both can be grown in full sun to partial shade and reach a height of 6–10 inches. When flowering, the clusters of greenish-yellow flowers can reach 2 1/2 feet. The leaves of parsley are triangular and deeply divided. Many people grow parsley as an annual, because when it flowers in the second year, the leaves are no longer useful in cooking. After flowering, the plant sets seed and dies.

Parsley is best propagated by seeds which are sown directly into the garden. It used to be believed that if parsley was trans-planted, misfortune would befall the household. I guess if you could call the death of your parsley plant "misfortune," then that statement is true. Parsley seedlings do not like to be transplanted and can go into shock or die if moved.

You have to be patient when growing parsley from seed. They can take up to 6 weeks to germinate. (There is an old saying that parsley seeds go to the Devil seven times before sprouting.) You can help speed up the process, by soaking the seeds overnight in water before planting.

Parsley likes to be grown in pots. It does very well in window boxes and can even be grown on a kitchen windowsill. Just be sure that the indoor plants receive at least 4–5 hours of sunlight per day.

Uses: Parsley is very high in vitamin C. It can be used generously in almost all savory recipes and tends to blend or enhance the other flavors. The Italian flat-leaf parsley has a slightly better flavor than curly leaf parsley and is usually the parsley of choice among chefs. The stems and leaves can be added to salads, soups, eggs, vegetables, rice, bread, and meat dishes. It can also be used to create delicious sauces and herbal butters.

Parsley is high in chlorophyl, which can act as a natural breath freshener. That's why it is a good ingredient to add to foods with a lot of seasoning or garlic. Parsley leaves can also be chewed to freshen the breath and cleanse the palate. The leaves have a nice bright green color, which makes them especially pretty in flower arrangements and wreaths.

Recommended:
Curly leaf parsley *(Petroselinum crispum)*
Italian flat-leaf parsley *(P. crispum* var *neapolitanum)*

Rose

Rosa spp.

PERENNIAL

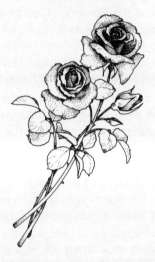

Description: The rose is a beloved flower which is as much adored today as it was hundreds of years ago. But is it an herb? You bet! It is used in cooking, crafting, and potpourri making. It also has numerous medicinal and cosmetic uses which date back thousands of years. It definitely deserves a place in the herb garden.

There are numerous mythological stories associated with roses, as well as many romantic associations. Roses have inspired art, literature, and folklore for thousands of years. The ancient Romans grew tons of roses and the ancient Greeks proclaimed the rose to be "the Queen of all flowers." Even Cleopatra is believed to have had an affinity for this flower. She had the palace floors covered, knee deep, with rose petals when she summoned Mark Anthony.

There are many different species of roses to choose from. Almost all have thorned stems, dark green leaves, and single or double petaled flowers. The roses mentioned in old herbals and stillroom recipes are "old roses" or antique roses, which means they were grown prior to 1867 when hybrids hit the market. To be absolutely authentic, you would want antique roses in your herb garden. But if you already have hybrid teas, you can still use their flowers in recipes. For cooking and crafting, you will generally want to choose the flowers which have the most fragrant petals. Be sure to taste the petals first and choose the ones with the best flavor.

Many old herbals mention the apothecary's rose *(Rosa gallica officinalis)* or the damask rose *(R. damascena)*. The petals of these roses were not only used in perfumes, but were also used medicinally. A rose syrup was made with honey for sore throats and a rose vinegar was applied to the forehead to reduce fever.

All roses need full sun and well-draining soil. They are generally heavy feeders and require a lot of water. They are susceptible to blackspot, rust, mildew, and aphids. Many people complain that roses are too much work. But in general, antique roses are more disease-resistant and require less care than the modern hybrid tea roses. If you choose to grow antiques, you will find that they do not take too much care and are well worth the effort. *(See* the "Source Guide" for mail-order sources of antique roses.)

Uses: Rose hips (the seed heads that form after flowering) are packed full of vitamin C. They are used to make tea, jelly, conserves, and wine. The flower petals are used to make syrups and gargles for sore throats. They are very astringent and cleansing, which is why they have a long history as cosmetic ingredients. The petals and essential oils of roses are used in sweet baths, bath oils, perfumes, and soaps. Pure rose essential oil is very expensive because it can take up to 60,000 roses to produce just one ounce of essential oil!

In the kitchen, rose petals can be added to salad, sandwiches, butter, jelly, desserts, and pastries. The petals are sometimes candied and used as a garnish.

Rose flowers and hips are traditionally used fresh in flower arrangements and posies. When dried, they can be used in a number of craft projects including potpourri.

Recommended:
Apothecary's rose *(Rosa gallica officinalis)*
Damask rose *(R. damascena)*
Cabbage or Provence rose *(R. centifolia)*

Rosemary

Rosmarinus officinalis

TENDER PERENNIAL

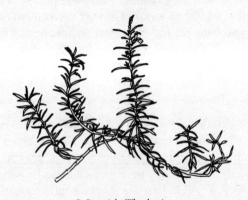

© Copyright Wheeler Arts

*"... I let it run all over my garden walls, not onlie
because bees love it, but because 'tis the herb sacred to
remembrance and therefore to friendship."*

—Sir Thomas More, Utopia

Description: Ancient Greeks believed that rosemary improved
memory. They wore wreaths of the herb on their head while
studying. In the Middle Ages, sprigs of rosemary were placed
under pillows to ward off evil spirits and prevent nightmares.
Rosemary has long been considered the symbol for remembrance
and love. Brides wore sprigs in their hair and had rosemary in their
bouquets. Even today, rosemary is sometimes used in flower
arrangements and bridal decorations.

Rosemary is an evergreen herb with aromatic, pine needle-shaped leaves and whorls of blue flowers. There are also white and pink forms. The different cultivars of rosemary can be divided into two groups: upright and prostrate (creeping). Both prefer full sun but will tolerate some shade. The upright rosemaries can grow between 2 and 6 feet tall. They make excellent hedges or shrubs in the garden. The prostrate rosemaries usually stay low to the ground and are perfect for trailing over walls and window boxes. Both types can be grown in pots and shaped into topiaries or bonsai.

Rosemary is best propagated by cuttings or layering. It is a tender perennial, which means that in very cold climates, it must be potted up and brought indoors. Here in Southern California, we are blessed with the perfect climate for rosemary. It grows outdoors all year round and reaches great heights with very little care. In fact, we periodically must cut it back, which allows us to use the thick, fragrant branches as skewers for grilling.

Uses: Fresh and dried rosemary can be added to all meat dishes. It is especially good in beef, game, and lamb recipes. It is also a nice seasoning for breads, vegetables, butters, cheese, soups, and salad dressings. Surprisingly rosemary can also be added to sweet recipes as well. Try it in pastries, cookies, and sorbets.

Rosemary is said to be astringent, antibacterial, and antifungal. Cosmetic uses for rosemary include hair rinses, dandruff shampoo, soap, and herbal baths. In crafting, rosemary is a common ingredient in potpourri and flower decorations.

Recommended:
Creeping rosemary (*Rosmarinus officinalis* 'Prostratus')
Tuscan blue rosemary (*R. officinalis* 'Tuscan Blue')
Pine scented rosemary (*R. officinalis* 'Pine Scented')
White blooming rosemary (*R. officinalis* 'Alba')
Pink blooming rosemary (*R. officinalis* 'Majorica Pink')
Golden rain rosemary (*R. officinalis* 'Joyce DeBaggio')

Sage

Salvia officinalis

PERENNIAL

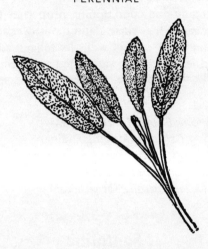

Description: The genus *Salvia* has literally hundreds of species to choose from. However, no herb garden would be complete without common sage *(Salvia officinalis)*, aka garden sage, with its velvety grayish-green leaves. Keep in mind, though, that there are many other varieties of *S. officinalis* worthy of a place in your herb garden. (*See* the "Recommended" list below.) There are also some ornamental *Salvia* species that are quite beautiful, such as Mexican sage *(S. leucantha)*. It has spikes of fuzzy lavender flowers that are beautiful in flower bouquets and hold their color when dried.

Most sage plants have colorful, long-throated flowers which are very attractive to hummingbirds. Although most are extremely easy to grow, there are a few, such as pineapple sage *(S. elegans)*, that are tender and will not survive harsh winters without being brought indoors. The rest will grow in full sun and can survive with just a heavy mulching for the winter. Most varieties grow to approximately 2–3 feet tall. Sage plants can be propagated by seeds, cuttings, or layering.

Uses: Sage is traditionally combined with thyme, rosemary, and marjoram in the kitchen. It can be used with poultry, pork, beef, venison, and game birds. It also works well in sausage, stuffing, soup, and bread. The flowers of the culinary varieties are edible and can be used in salad or as a garnish.

Sage's astringent and conditioning properties make it invaluable in facial steams, hair rinses, and mouthwashes. It has been used in perfume and soap as well. Its foliage adds fullness to flower arrangements, and the variegated varieties are perfect for handheld posies.

Recommended:
Common sage *(Salvia officinalis):* Culinary
Golden sage *(S. officinalis* 'Aurea'): Culinary
Tricolor sage *(S. officinalis* 'Tricolor'): Culinary
Pineapple sage *(S. elegans):* Culinary
Mexican sage *(S. leucantha):* Ornamental

Santolina

Santolina chamaecyparissus

PERENNIAL

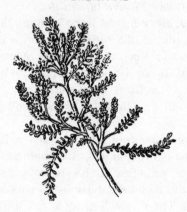

Description: Grey-leaf santolina is a woody shrub with silvery-white leaves that grows to about 2 feet. Although it is sometimes called lavender cotton, it is not a true lavender and is actually a member of the daisy family. It produces mustard yellow, button-shaped flowers in midsummer. The foliage is extremely aromatic and some find it offensive. It has a musky, medicinal scent, which makes it useful as a moth-repelling herb.

During the Elizabethan Era, santolina became a popular knot garden herb. It is extremely easy to shape into hedges and curves. When combined with other santolina species, such as green-leaf santolina *(Santolina virens)*, it can create many formal knot garden patterns.

The seeds of santolina are slow to germinate. It is probably best propagated by cuttings or layering. It prefers full sun and does not tolerate humidity very well. It is evergreen in temperate climates, but in cold areas, it will die back and should be mulched heavily to survive any snowy winters.

Uses: With its moth-repelling qualities, santolina sprigs can be placed among linens, woolens, and books. Dried santolina can be made into moth-repellant potpourris and sachets. The leaves hold their color well when dried and make excellent wreaths that are seldom bothered by bugs. The flowers can be dried for potpourri and other crafts. Although the foliage is excellent in flower arrangements, it should not be used in centerpiece arrangements. The strong fragrance may not be appreciated at the dinner table.

Recommended:
Grey santolina or lavender cotton *(Santolina chamaecyparissus)*
Green santolina *(S. virens)*

Savory

Satureja spp.

ANNUAL AND PERENNIAL

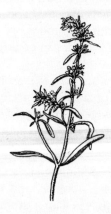

Description: There are about 30 species in the genus *Satureja*, but two are commonly grown as savory in American gardens. Summer savory *(Satureja hortenis)* is an annual, and winter savory *(S. montana)* is a perennial. Colonists brought both savories to America as medicinal herbs. They were used to relieve indigestion and soothe sore throats.

Summer savory grows 12–18 inches tall and has long narrow leaves with a delicate, peppery flavor. The flowers are a pinkish-white and are also edible. Winter savory is shorter (about 6–15 inches tall) with a spreading growth habit, which makes it valuable as a border and knot garden plant. It looks and tastes similar to summer savory but has thicker leaves and a stronger flavor. It is hardy to about 10 degrees.

Both savories grow in full sun and are much loved by bees. Summer savory can be propagated by seeds, layering, or cuttings. Winter savory is best propagated by cuttings or division.

Uses: Although both savories can be used in culinary dishes, most cooks prefer the more delicate flavor of summer savory. However, winter savory can be used just as well if young leaves are taken from the tips of the branches.

Savory can be used to season all meat dishes, especially beef and game meats. It is also delicious with beans, eggs, herb butters, and fish.

The leaves of the savory plant can be crushed and rubbed on bee stings to relieve the pain and the itch. Savory foliage is also very attractive in floral bouquets.

Recommended:
Summer savory *(Satureja hortensis)*
Winter savory *(S. montana)*

Scented Geranium

Pelargonium spp.

TENDER PERENNIAL

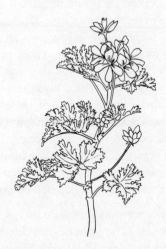

Description: Although scented geraniums belong to the same botanical family as true geraniums, they are not geraniums at all. They are pelargoniums. They look similar to true geraniums but have aromatic, strongly scented foliage. You can find varieties

with sweet fragrances such as rose, lemon, apple, nutmeg, co-
conut, peppermint, or chocolate! There are records of over 200
different scented geraniums, hybridized from about 75 different
varieties. You should definitely grow more than one of these very
versatile plants.

Most scented geraniums grow in full sun and are hardy only to
about 35 degrees. If you live in a colder area, you will have to dig
them up and bring them inside for the winter. What a treat that
will be! Scented geraniums do very well in pots and don't mind
being grown indoors provided they have a little fertilizer and
plenty of light.

Scented geraniums became popular in Europe as houseplants
in the 1600s. Their sweetly scented leaves were used for potpourri and tea. They were brought to America with the Colonists
and were very popular here as well. Thomas Jefferson grew
scented geraniums at the White House.

In the 1800s scented geraniums reached the peak of their popularity when the French began using their essential oil in perfumery. The rose-scented geranium became a cheaper alternative
to the extremely expensive attar of rose. During the Victorian Era,
scented geraniums were grown in low pots around the parlors so
that ladies' dresses would brush them as they passed by, filling the
room with fragrance. The Victorians also used them in pastries,
desserts, and jellies, as well as floral bouquets.

The flowers of the scented geranium are not spectacular, but
these plants are mostly grown for their fragrant foliage. The pretty
leaves are well veined and have deep lopes. They range in size
from 1/2 inch to several inches, depending upon the variety. They
fill the air with scent whenever they are even casually brushed.
Scented geraniums should be propagated by cuttings or layering.

Uses: In the kitchen, scented geranium leaves will add subtle flavor to any sweet recipe. They can be used in all kinds of cookies,
cakes, desserts, and pastries. Adding the leaves of rose or lemon
scented geranium to apple jelly creates a delicious treat.

Known for being slightly astringent, the leaves can be used in
cosmetics and facial steams. The leaves can also be dried for potpourri recipes. They hold their fragrance quite well over long pe-

riods of time. The essential oil from scented geraniums is used in potpourri making, perfumery, and aromatherapy.

Recommended:
Rose scented *(Pelargonium graveolens)*
Round leaf rose scented *(P. capitatum)*
Variegated rose scented *(P. graveolens* 'Lady Plymouth')
Lemon scented *(P. crispum)*
Lime scented *(P. nervosum)*
Apple scented *(P. ordoratissimum)*
Peppermint *(P. graveolens* 'Tomentosa')
Nutmeg *(P. fragrans)*

Sorrel, French

Rumex acetosa

PERENNIAL

Description: French sorrel is also known as broad-leaf sorrel, common sorrel, or garden sorrel. It has been used since ancient times as a medicinal and culinary herb. The Egyptians ate it to calm the stomach after indulging in rich foods. The Greeks made a tea from sorrel to reduce fevers and cool the body. It is rich in vitamin C and was used to prevent scurvy. It has been considered a popular salad herb since the Medieval days, and today the tangy leaves are popular in French cooking.

Sorrel grows in full sun to partial shade with clumps of bright green, oval-shaped leaves. It reaches 2–3 feet and has reddish-green flower stalks. It is best propagated by seed or division. For a healthy plant, you should dig up and divide sorrel every 2–3 years.

There is another sorrel which is sometimes referred to as French sorrel or buckler-leaved sorrel *(Rumex scutatus)*. Although it is not as common here in America as *R. acetosa,* it is preferred by some cooks because it has a less bitter flavor with a more lemony tang.

Uses: For culinary purposes, sorrel leaves should be picked young, before the plant goes into flower. They can be tossed into salads or sautéed with butter for a quick, delicious sauce. Sorrel goes well with egg and fish recipes. The fresh leaves can also be used to make classic French sorrel soup. Surprisingly, sorrel leaf juice can sometimes bleach out minor rust and mold stains in linen!

Recommended:
Common sorrel *(Rumex acetosa)*
Buckler-leaved sorrel *(R. scutatus)*

Tarragon, French
Artemisia dracunculus var. *sativa*

TENDER PERENNIAL

Description: "True" French tarragon *(Artemisia dracunculus* var. *sativa)* has slender, bright green leaves that have a peppery taste with anise overtones. It gets its name from the French word *esdragon* meaning "little dragon." It was so named because it has dragon- or serpent-type shaped roots. Tarragon grows to approximately 2–3 feet tall and cannot be propagated by seed because it very rarely flowers. Take cuttings or root divisions in early spring.

There is another plant which is sometimes erroneously sold as French tarragon. It is actually Russian tarragon *(A. dracunculoides)*, formerly known as *A. redowskii* and it has an inferior flavor. (If you ever see French tarragon seeds for sale, they are probably Russian tarragon.) Although Russian tarragon is pretty in flower arrangements, it has no value as a culinary herb.

Uses: French tarragon is popular in French cooking and is the primary flavoring in Bearnaise and remoulade sauces. It can be added to many savory foods including: eggs, chicken, fish, and salad dressings. When cooking with tarragon, use a light hand because it can easily dominate other flavors or overpower a dish. Only add it at the end of cooking times or it will taste bitter.

Tarragon is said to stimulate the digestive system. The leaves used to be chewed to numb the taste buds before taking medicine.

Recommended:
French tarragon *(Artemisia dracunculus* var. *sativa)*

Thyme
Thymus vulgaris
PERENNIAL

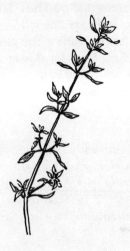

Description: There are hundreds of different species within the genus *Thymus*. Most can be classified as either upright (10–12 inches) or creeping (2–6 inches), and many are worthy of a space in your garden. The upright varieties are generally the best for culinary use, but the creeping thymes make excellent plants for rock gardens and pathways, releasing their fragrance when stepped upon. They all can be grown in hanging baskets, in window boxes, and along borders.

Indigenous to Mediterranean countries, common thyme *(Thymus vulgaris)* is one of the most popular in American gardens. It is a low-growing, evergreen herb with tiny, aromatic leaves and blossoms. Most thyme plants need full sun and well-drained soil. Continuous clipping promotes bushy growth. After several years, some plants may need to be replaced if they become too woody.

You can grow thyme from seed, but cultivars must be propagated asexually by cuttings, layering, or dividing.

Uses: It has been said, "When in doubt in the kitchen, use thyme." Thyme is extremely versatile as a culinary herb and can be used in just about any savory recipe. Try using it fresh or dried to season beef, fish, poultry, egg, and vegetable dishes. It makes a delicious herb butter and can be added to all kinds of sauces and marinades.

Thyme has many antiseptic qualities. The main oil, thymol, is a powerful antiseptic and explains why thyme has been a successful ingredient in lotions, salves, and mouthwashes.

Thyme is an excellent herb for flower arranging and wreath making because it can withstand long periods of time out of water without wilting. The delicate leaves can also be pressed to create all kinds of decorative crafts.

Recommended:
Common thyme *(Thymus vulgaris):* Upright
Lemon thyme *(T.* x *citriodorus):* Upright
Silver thyme *(T.* x *citriodorus* 'Argenteus'): Upright
Caraway scented thyme *(T. herba-barona):* Creeping
Woolly thyme *(T. pseudolanuginosus):* Creeping

Woodruff, Sweet

Galium odoratum

PERENNIAL

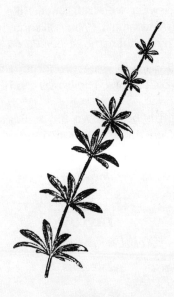

Description: The uses for this woodland plant date back to at least the 1300s, when it was used to scent linens, stuff mattresses, and freshen rooms as a strewing herb. In the medieval days, churches were decorated with sweet woodruff bundles. During the Elizabethan Era, it was extremely popular in wreaths, garlands, and sachets. It is traditionally used in the German celebration of May Day to create Maibowle, or May Wine. (May Wine is made by steeping sweet woodruff in a sweet white wine.)

Sweet woodruff is one of the few herbs which actually prefer shaded areas. It can be grown as an edging plant in a shady section of the herb garden or as a ground cover under trees or shrubs. It does well in pots and looks quite lovely in a hanging basket. It has a spreading habit and only reaches about 6–12 inches tall. Whorls of bright green, pointed leaves form like spokes of a wheel around the stem. The tiny, star-shaped white flowers appear in late spring or early summer. Sweet woodruff can be propagated by seed or root division. It will survive cold winters with just a heavy mulching.

Both the leaves and flowers of sweet woodruff are fragrant. But you will notice that the scent is very subdued while fresh. However, once dried, sweet woodruff smells like a combination of newly mowed hay and vanilla. (You will sometimes see woodruff listed in catalogs by its old name: *Asperula odorata.*)

Uses: The fresh flowers of sweet woodruff can be used in salad or as a garnish in cold drinks. The leaves can be used fresh to flavor May Wine.

Sweet woodruff is best grown for its fragrance and beauty. Dry the leaves and use them in potpourri and other fragrant crafts.

Recommended:
Sweet woodruff *(Galium odoratum)*

Yarrow
Achillea millefolium

PERENNIAL

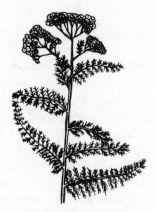

© Copyright Theresa Loe

Description: Some of the common names for yarrow include soldier's woundwort, carpenter's weed, and nosebleed. The name "soldier's woundwort" comes from its extensive use in treating wounds of all kinds. For centuries, it was a popular wound dressing and was used in this way up to the American Civil War. Native Americans used it to treat many ailments including bruises and sores.

There are many superstitions associated with this herb. One involves young girls placing a flannel sachet of yarrow under their pillows at night, so that they would dream of their future husbands. (Heck, it's worth a try.)

Yarrow is a great way to add color to the herb garden. The blossoms of common yarrow appear as tall, showy clusters of tiny white flowers, with a hint of pink. But you can find varieties with many other striking colors. Some seed companies sell seed mixtures, including pastel varieties which are quite lovely. The leaves of yarrow are long, narrow, and feathery.

Yarrow grows in full sun, to a height of 2–3 feet when flowering. It is a tough and adaptable plant and can become invasive. It can be propagated by seed or division. The seed should only be lightly covered with soil, as it needs some light for germination. As yarrow begins to creep into other areas, you will need to dig up sections and divide them to keep it under control.

Uses: Yarrow flowers work very well in fresh and dried flower arrangements. They hold their color extremely well when dried and can be added to potpourri and other dried craft projects.

Yarrow leaves are astringent and cleansing. They can be used in skin lotions and other cosmetics.

Recommended:
Flaming pink yarrow (*Achillea millefolium* 'Rubra')
Golden yarrow (*A.* x 'Coronation Gold')

Chapter 2

⟨≈⟩

Getting Started

Happy is the herb gardener through all the seasons and the years. That person enjoys a life enriched with rare fragrances at dawn and dusk and in the heat of noon.

—ADELMA GRENIER SIMMONS

PLANNING AN HERB GARDEN

We all know that a sprawling herb garden with winding paths and hundreds of plants would look spectacular in anyone's backyard, but it would also take a tremendous amount of time (or help) to maintain and use the herbs. If you don't have this kind of time or space, don't despair. Herb gardens come in all shapes and sizes and can be created almost anywhere! Herbs can be added to an existing landscape, planted in a small section of the yard, or even grown in containers on an apartment balcony or windowsill. No matter where you grow your herbs, you simply have to work within your boundaries and choose the herbs which give you the most pleasure.

There are unlimited ways to use herbs in the garden! Creeping rosemary can be placed on the edge of a small raised flowerbed, and in no time at all, it will be gracefully spilling over the edge. Corsican mint, chamomile, and creeping thyme can be planted between stepping stones to create a fragrant, living carpet. Sweet woodruff can be tucked beneath shrubs and shady corners of the yard. Santolina, upright rosemary, and lavender can be used to create fragrant hedges along existing perennial borders.

If you do want to design and plant a large or more complex herb garden, it can be a very rewarding experience as well. If you have the time to maintain them, knot gardens and formally structured herb gardens can be quite dramatic and impressive. If you start out small, you shouldn't have too much trouble with maintenance. You can always add on to the garden later. Just remember, no matter how many herbs you wish to grow, or how much space you have to grow them in, you'll find herb gardening well worth the effort.

No matter what size your finished garden will be, the best place to begin gathering garden ideas is from magazines and garden design books. Collect pictures, ideas, and clippings of what you like or think is appropriate for your garden space. After you have collected some ideas and you want to start formulating your garden design, you should ask yourself the following questions:

1. What do I expect from my garden? If you are interested in growing and using only a few specialized herbs, then you can probably find space for them in your existing landscape. They can be tucked into borders with very little effort. However, if you want to make an architectural impact with your garden, you will need to do some serious planning before you break ground. Think about what your expectations are and plan accordingly.

2. What type of herbs do you want to grow? This may have an influence on the type of design you choose, or you may discover that you want to plant a garden with a particular theme. (*See* "Theme Gardens," below.)

3. How much time do you want to spend gardening? The size and style of a garden directly influence the amount of time involved in maintaining it. For example, a large knot garden must be constantly pruned to keep its formal structure, but a small cottage garden can be neglected for small amounts of time and still look quaint. Before you decide on a design, think about how much time is involved in its upkeep and how much time you have available.

4. Where is the best location for your herb garden? Ideally, you will want a sunny, well-draining location, but do not be discouraged if you have less than ideal conditions. You can work within your limitations with some careful planning. If you do not have full sun, choose herbs which can tolerate partial sun and shade. If you do not have space, you may have to grow smaller herbs such as thyme, basil, and chives. Or you can plant in containers and hanging baskets. As you plan your garden, evaluate the potential site and choose the herbs which fit your conditions.

5. How much space do the plants need? All herbs have different growth habits, and these should be given consideration when laying out the garden plan. Some herbs, such as fennel, need a lot of space to grow, while others, such as thyme, take up very little space. As you choose your herbs for planting, be sure to look up how tall and wide they grow and give them ample space when you do your actual planting. Also, take note of invasive herbs such as mint. You must be careful where you place invasive herbs or they will take over a garden! They should be planted within sunken barriers, in planters, or in pots.

6. How should the garden be laid out? No matter how large or how small your herb garden is going to be, it is smart to draw it out on paper first, to save yourself digging time later. It is much easier to erase than to move an established plant! The general rule of thumb for borders and cottage-style gardens is to place taller herbs toward the back and shorter herbs toward the front. Be sure to include pathways or stepping stones in your design so that you have access to all the herbs for harvesting.

THEME GARDENS

If you find yourself drawn to a particular group of herbs with similar uses or colors, you may want to create a theme garden. It can be a fun way to organize the herbs you are planting. For example, if you enjoy fragrant herbs, you may want to create a "pot-pourri garden." If you like cooking with herbs, you might try planting a "culinary garden" or a "tea garden." If you are the whimsical type, a "fairy garden" or a "hummingbird garden" might be more your style. Look over the list below for theme garden ideas.

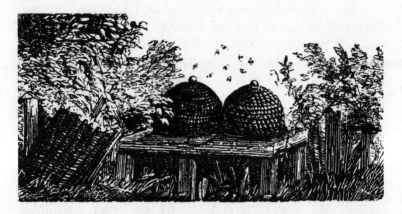

Beekeepers Garden: Bees are essential to the pollination of many plants and trees in the garden. Since they are attracted to the garden by color (see note) and scent, there are many aromatic herbs they can't resist. If you keep bees or have fruit trees, you may want to include the following bee-loving herbs in your garden: basil, borage, chamomile, dill, fennel, hyssop, lavender, lemon balm, marjoram, oregano, rosemary, sage, savory, and thyme.

Note: Bees are not attracted by the color red. This is because their eyes cannot perceive the long wave lengths in the red end of the spectrum. Many red flowers are pollinated by birds (such as hummingbirds) rather than bees.

Butterfly Garden: Butterflies add beauty and grace to the garden. They are attracted to the garden by color (see "Nectar Guides") and scent. (The female butterfly can sometimes smell a plant from up to a half-mile away.) They love many of the same herbs that bees enjoy (see list above). If you plant a butterfly garden, however, be prepared to give up some of the foliage to caterpillars.

NECTAR GUIDES

Butterflies and bees see a broader spectrum of light waves then we do, and some plants have developed a way to use this characteristic to their advantage. They attract these pollinating insects to their flowers by emitting what are called "nectar guides." These guides are bands of color (some of which are ultraviolet) that help the insect locate the plant. It is like a flashing neon sign to the butterfly!

Culinary Garden: A culinary or kitchen garden should be planted near the kitchen door so that a cook doesn't have to travel far to gather the fresh herbs. Plant basil, bay, borage, burnet, cilantro, chives, dill, hyssop, lavender, marjoram, mint, nasturtium, oregano, parsley, rose, rosemary, sage, savory, sorrel, tarragon, and thyme.

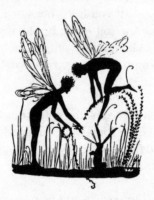

Fairy Garden: Children love to plant fairy gardens and set out little fairy treats at night. It is a great way to get them involved in horticulture. In case you don't already know, most garden fairies love to play among tiny leaved plants and colorful flowers (but they are very elusive). They are especially partial to Corsican mint, calendula, chamomile, dwarf sage, silver thyme, golden lemon thyme, and rosemary. Be sure to include flowers such as nasturtiums, pansies, primroses, and johnny-jump-ups. They also enjoy all kinds of ferns, moss, and lichens.

Fragrance Garden: Almost all herbs are fragrant, but some are more potent than others. This makes them appropriate for all kinds of crafts, cosmetics, and potpourri. A few of the most aromatic herbs are basil, chamomile, lavender, lemon balm, lemon verbena, mint, rose, rosemary, sage, scented geraniums, and sweet woodruff.

Hummingbird Garden: Hummingbirds absolutely love salvia (sage) plants, so plant as many as you can for these charming little creatures. They are also attracted to brightly colored flowers (especially red) so a mixture of flowers and herbs make a wonderful hummingbird haven. Try growing pineapple sage, Mexican sage, common sage, lamb's ears, mint, scented geraniums, and rosemary. You might also want to include some flowers such as delphinium, lily, red morning glory, or honeysuckle.

Shakespearean Garden: William Shakespeare wrote lovingly of many herbs and flowers. This type of garden is a fun way to celebrate his work. Decorate the garden with painted signs quoting herbal lines from Shakespeare such as, "Here's flowers for you; Hot lavender, mints, savory, marjoram; The marigold that goes to bed wi' the sun; And with him rises weeping . . ." (*The Winter's Tale,* Act IV, Scene III). The following herbs are mentioned in Shakespeare's writings: bay, burnet, calendula, chamomile, hyssop, lavender, lemon balm, marjoram, mint, parsley, rose, rosemary, savory, thyme.

Silver Garden/Moon Garden: A garden of silver-colored foliage can look quite magnificent, especially at night. Try combining the following herbs with white blooming flowers for a moon garden:

clary sage, common sage, grey santolina, lamb's ears, lavender, silver thyme, wormwood, and silver king artemisia.

Tea Garden: Many herbs can be used to create soothing and delicious teas. A tea garden should include chamomile, fennel, hyssop, lavender, lemon balm, mint, rose, rosemary, and scented geranium.

Growing in Containers

If you lack the room for a formal herb garden, container growing may be the solution for you. Herbs do very well in pots and can be moved around a balcony or patio to create a multitude of arrangements. Although they are perfect for apartment dwellers and small space gardeners, anyone can plant and enjoy container grown herbs. Even if you already have an herb garden, you may, at some time, want to plant herbs in pots, hanging baskets, or window boxes. It may be that your herb garden is planted too far from the kitchen and you need a few pots of culinary herbs sitting outside the backdoor. Or you may want to grow an invasive herb, like mint, and need to keep it contained and under control. No matter what the reason, potted herbs are fairly easy to maintain. Watering and occasional feeding will be your biggest chores.

POTTING

A container for herb growing should have drainage holes so that the plants do not become water-logged. (Nondraining containers should be used only if you are willing to monitor them more closely.) You may want to try clay pots, whiskey barrels, strawberry pots, or even unusual containers like wooden boxes or troughs. Choose a container which will accommodate a mature version of the herb you wish to plant. You want the roots to have plenty of room so that the plant will be happy and productive.

The soil used in the containers is important. You generally do not want to use regular soil out of the garden because its chemical and physical makeup is uncertain. It can become hard-packed and it may contain pests and disease spores. Your best bet is to purchase a commercial potting soil. If you feel that the commercial soil is too heavy or poorly draining, then you can add a small amount of perlite for aeration and vermiculite for moisture retention. (Small bags of perlite and vermiculite are available at garden centers.) To get the herbs off to a good start, add a small amount of slow-release fertilizer to the soil mixture. When you are ready to fill a container with soil, remember to place a rock or broken shard of pottery over the drainage holes to prevent the soil from falling out the bottom.

HANGING BASKETS

There are many herbs which lend themselves to hanging basket planting. Try planting mint, pennyroyal, creeping rosemary, sweet woodruff, or thyme.

MAINTENANCE

Once your herbs are potted, you will need to water them regularly. In hot areas, this can be a daily chore. In less arid climates, one to three times a week may be sufficient. You will have to determine your requirements and stick to a regular schedule. Watering is the most labor-intensive part of container growing, especially if you have many potted plants.

Frequent watering will quickly leach the nutrients from the potting soil. Since there is only a limited amount of soil in each pot, this is the one time that a frequent feeding routine should be maintained. A general, all-purpose plant food is fine. This can be a slow-release granule that is sprinkled into each pot, a foliar spray, or a liquid plant food.

Although I have a formal herb garden now, for years I grew my herbs strictly in pots. While renting a very small house a few years back, I grew more than 125 herbs in pots because I had no garden space. Through the years, I found that a monthly treatment

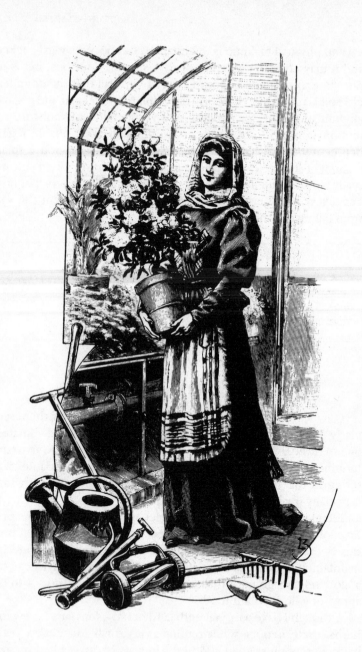

of fish emulsion or manure tea and an occasional feeding with an all-purpose liquid food kept the plants extremely lush and green. (When using a commercial plant food, it is usually best to dilute the mixture to half-strength. Too much nitrogen will result in too much foliage and not enough flavor.) For sources of organic fertilizers such as liquid sea kelp, check the "Source Guide" in the back of this book.

MANURE TEA

You can make your own fertilizer called manure tea. Place three cups of steer or chicken manure in some cheesecloth or a burlap bag and tie closed. (Manure is available at most nurseries and garden supply centers.) Place this bag in a 5-gallon bucket of water and steep for two days (The longer it steeps, the stronger it gets.) Then, remove the "tea bag." Add about 1 cup of this "tea" to 1 gallon of water and use this mixture to give your potted plants a light feeding about once a month.

HARVESTING AND DRYING HERBS

Herbs are so versatile that you will find yourself constantly picking sprigs for a variety of uses. This mild harvesting of your herbs will encourage plant growth and allow you to control the shape and size of the plant. But occasionally, you might want to harvest large quantities of your herb plants as they reach their peak. What can't be used fresh can be dried and stored in airtight containers for later use. During the winter months, when your herb choices and quantities are limited, your dried herbs will come in handy. Nothing should go to waste. The leaves, flowers, and seeds can be used in cooking or crafting. (The seeds can also be saved to plant next year.) The leftover herb stems can be used as fireplace starters (Chapter 9) or grilling herbs (Chapter 4). If your dried herbs become too old for culinary purposes, they can be used as grilling herbs also.

People usually associate harvesting with autumn. But herbs can be harvested throughout the growing season. In fact, for the best flavor and fragrance, an herb should be harvested just before it flowers, when its aromatic oils are at their peak. If you are harvesting for flowers only, harvest the plants just as the flowers begin to open. Seeds should be harvested when they are just ripened and about to drop to the ground.

Always harvest on a dry day, preferably in the morning before the heat of the sun has hit the foliage. Gather the harvested herbs into small bundles and tie using rubber bands. As the herb stems dry, they tend to shrink and the rubber band will shrink with them, thereby preventing the bundles from falling apart. Hang the herb bundles in a warm, dry area, out of direct sunlight. If it is humid, you may want to use a fan to increase circulation. If you are collecting the herbs for seeds, place the herb bundles inside paper bags with the stems sticking out and hang as usual. The bag will allow air to circulate but will also collect falling seeds as the herbs dry.

OVEN DRYING

Herbs can be successfully dried in the oven too. Place the herb leaves onto cookie sheets. Place them in an oven with the pilot light on or turn the oven on to its lowest setting. Leave the door ajar to let moisture escape. Be sure to watch the herbs closely. You don't want them to burn!

Depending upon the density of the leaves and the time of the year, your herbs should dry between seven and ten days. When completely dry, the leaves will be crisp and brittle. At this point, strip the leaves from the branches and place them in clean glass jars. Be sure to label and date the containers. Dried herbs are best used within one year for maximum flavor and fragrance. The jars should be stored out of direct sunlight such as in a dark cupboard.

Check the newly sealed jars after a few days. If moisture is visible, the herbs were not completely dry. They must be removed and redried to prevent mold from forming. (For more information on how to store herb flavors for later use, *see* Chapter 4, "Preserving and Using the Garden's Bounty.")

Chapter 3

⚜

The Basics

Most herbs are extremely easy to grow because they can tolerate a wide range of conditions and they generally have only three requirements:

1. Sunshine (though some herbs can grow in shade).
2. Some protection from harsh elements such as heavy wind and extreme cold.
3. Well-draining, moderately fertile soil.

SUNSHINE

Sun intensity varies in different regions, but for most areas, herbs need 6–8 hours of light per day to be at their best. This is considered "full sun." A full-sun location will produce lush plants with essential oil production at its peak. However, there are a few "full-sun" herbs which can tolerate partial shade (and some herbs which prefer shade). Just keep in mind that when "full-sun" herbs are grown in less than 6 hours of light per day, they might have a weaker flavor or fragrance and they might get leggy. The herbs which prefer shade, such as Corsican mint and sweet woodruff, do very well in partial shade with little change in growth habits. (Check the plant descriptions in Chapter 1 for the sun preferences of individual herbs.)

PROTECTION FROM THE ELEMENTS

Extremes in wind, temperature, and humidity can be difficult on all plants, and herbs are no exception. Although herbs will tolerate quite a bit before showing signs of stress, some of the following special circumstances can pose problems.

A windy area will tend to dry out the soil and damage plant foliage. If that wind is a cold one, it can do more damage than just extremely low temperatures alone. Windblown herbs will require extra water and staking. Hedges, fences, and walls are excellent solutions to this problem and add to the herb garden design.

If you live in an area with harsh, cold winters, be sure to note the climate considerations in the plant descriptions. Plants listed as "tender perennials" (such as rosemary) need to be brought indoors during cold winter months. Just pot them up and keep them by a very sunny window. (First let them sit outdoors in the pot for one week, to get over the shock of being uprooted.) While indoors, the dry, heated air can pose a problem for your herbs. Be sure to check the soil moisture often and water only if needed. Most other perennial herbs will do well in the winter with a heavy mulching for protection. Of course, annual herbs do not pose a problem because they are replanted each spring.

Note: Herbs such as bay, lemon verbena, pineapple sage, rosemary, and scented geranium do very well in pots. If you live in a Northern climate, you may want to grow these herbs in containers all year round so that a winter move indoors will be more convenient for you and the plants. Although they will not thrive indoors during the winter months, they should survive until spring. Watch closely for pests while indoors.

If high temperatures are your problem, you may want to plant your herbs in an area with afternoon shade to protect against the burning rays of the sun. Be sure not to water your herbs during the heat of the day or the leaves will steam. Early mornings and evenings are the best times to water. A drip system would be a good option for watering because there is less evaporation and the water would only go where needed.

Another problem with high temperatures is that some herbs such as cilantro and parsley will bolt in the heat and go to seed too quickly. To prevent this from happening, try to keep the flowers pinched off as much as possible. Planting these herbs in partial shade may help. Sometimes, certain perennial herbs will succumb to extreme heat. If this happens, you should treat them as annuals and replant them each spring.

If you live in a humid area, you have a difficult problem. Some herbs, especially gray-leaved herbs, are very affected by humidity. They tend to get powdery mildew and do not look very attractive when the temperature and humidity rise. If you want to grow silver-leaved herbs such as lamb's ears, lavender, or grey santolina, you will have to plant them in dry, sunny areas and hope for the best. This is another case where drip watering would be very beneficial. The less moisture you put on the leaves, the better.

Soil

Good soil is the key to any gardener's success. It provides nutrients and moisture to plants as well as giving them structural support. Soil is a combination of rock particles, organic matter, water, air, and microorganisms. It can vary from hard-packed clay to granular sand.

Clay soil tends to saturate with water easily. The soil is so hard packed, it causes the water to puddle up, thereby drowning the plants. Clay soil may have lots of nutrients but they are not readily available to the roots. On the other hand, sandy soil is the exact opposite. It is very drying to the roots because the water moves through too quickly. It usually lacks nutrients because they are washed out of the soil with the water.

The best soil is a combination of clay, sand, and humus called loam. It is light enough to allow air, water, and nutrients to move through the soil without drying out too quickly. For herbs, it is very important that the soil be well draining. With few exceptions, herbs do not like to have their feet wet all the time.

If you are planting a large area, you may want to invest in a soil analysis from your local community extension service or other soil lab. The test is relatively inexpensive and will provide you with a detailed report about what type of soil you have, what minerals are lacking, and what can be added to improve your soil.

MULCHING

No matter what type of soil you have, it will always benefit from the addition of compost and organic matter. Organic matter will loosen hard-packed clay soil and will help sandy soil retain moisture. It will also add natural nutrients to the soil, thereby feeding the plants. One way to add organic matter to your soil is through mulching.

Mulch is multifunctional. It helps to keep the soil cool in the summer and warm in the winter. It reduces weeds and helps retain moisture. As it breaks down, it adds nutrients to the soil and improves the soil for future generations of gardens.

The best mulch is the free kind you gather from your garden or neighborhood, i.e., homemade compost, grass clippings, chopped leaves, shredded brush, shredded bark, straw, or a mixture of any of the above. You can also buy bags of commercial mulches from your local garden center, but it can be expensive for large areas. For best results, place 2–3 inches of mulch over your herb garden twice a year: spring and fall. This is a natural way to slowly feed and improve your garden.

FERTILIZING

Herbs will thrive in only moderately fertile soil. In fact, if you overfertilize, you will have fast-growing foliage which lacks intense flavors and has very few flowers. Your best bet is to work on improving the soil each year, by adding organic matter as a mulch in the fall and spring rather than feeding with a commercial fertilizer. As the organic matter breaks down, it will energize the herbs naturally without overfeeding. If you still want to feed your plants occasionally, use an organic plant food which is diluted to half-strength.

The one time you will definitely want your herbs to be on a regular feeding schedule is when they are grown in containers. Frequent watering of container herbs will wash away the nutrients in the soil. Therefore, it is usually best to feed potted herbs frequently with a weak solution of liquid fertilizer. (*See* "Growing in Containers" in Chapter 2 for more information on feeding potted herbs.)

PROPAGATION

Propagation is a wonderful way to increase the number of plants in your garden, pass on your favorite plants to friends, and save money in the process!

SEEDS

Seed planting is probably the most versatile propagation method because there is such a wide assortment of herb seeds and they are fairly easy to obtain through mail-order or local garden centers. This makes herb plants accessible to almost anyone regardless of where they live. (*See* the "Source Guide" for mail-order companies.) You will find that there are seeds available for most herbs with the exception of some hybrids (which are either sterile or do not reproduce reliably from seed) and some herbs such as French tarragon, which very rarely produces seeds at all. (These types of herbs must be propagated from cuttings.)

Annual seeds are the easiest to grow because they germinate and mature faster than perennials. But with a little patience, many perennials can be sown from seed as well. Herbs can be sown directly into the garden or started indoors. (Borage, basil, chervil, dill, and parsley do not like to be transplanted and are best sown directly outside.)

For indoor planting, you will need clean, well-draining containers to sow your seeds. If you are doing a large number of seeds, you may wish to purchase a seedling flat from a nursery. Fill your containers three-quarters full with a sterile growing medium. This can be a soilless mix you buy at the garden center or it can be a mixture you prepare yourself. (There are probably as many growing medium recipes as there are gardeners, but one of the easiest combinations is equal parts commercial potting mix, peat moss, and perlite.)

Moisten your growing medium well and firm it down with your hands. If you are planting flats, sprinkle your seeds in rows about 2 inches apart. If you are planting individual containers, place a few medium-sized seeds into each pot or lightly sprinkle very small seeds over the surface of each pot. Cover with a thin layer of growing medium to a thickness approximately two to three times the diameter of the seed you are planting. Extremely fine seeds do not need to be covered; just press them down into the medium.

After planting, be sure to label your containers with the plant name and water lightly. Then, cover the containers with either a plastic bag or plastic wrap to hold in moisture until the seeds sprout. Except where noted below and in the plant profiles in Chapter 1, most seeds do not need light to germinate. Be sure to read the seed packet for any specific instructions.

Note: Chamomile, dill, feverfew, lemon balm, and yarrow must have light to germinate. Do not cover these seeds with dark plastic. The larger seeds can be very lightly covered with soil, but smaller seeds should just be pressed into the soil with no covering.

After the first two true leaves of the plant appear, your seedlings can be transplanted to individual pots until they are large enough to go outside. Harden off the seedlings before planting outside by gradually introducing them to the outdoors a few hours each day for several days. After about 1 1/2 weeks, they will be acclimated to the outdoors and will be ready for planting.

CUTTINGS

Most plants have the ability to regenerate themselves from small pieces of the stem called "cuttings." Soft-stemmed herbs are the easiest to propagate in this manner. Cuttings can be taken throughout the growing season, but fresh, new growth is the best candidate for a cutting.

Prepare pots or flats of a sterile growing medium for your cuttings. You can use the seedling mixture described above or you can use 100% perlite as your growing medium. Use a clean knife to cut a 3–5-inch, nonflowering sprig of the herb just below a leaf node (the place where the leaves join the stem). Remove the leaves from the lower half of the cutting. Dip the lower portion of this cutting into a powdered root hormone (available at your local garden center). Use a stick or pencil to make a small hole in your moistened growing medium and carefully place in the sprig and firm the medium around the stem. Water lightly. Create a mini-greenhouse by covering the pots with clear plastic which is held up with sticks above the actual cuttings. (You can also use an inverted glass jar in place of the plastic.) Keep the cuttings moist, out of direct sunlight, and covered until they show signs of growth, which means they have begun to root. Then, remove the clear plastic. Transplant to the garden after they show sufficient growth and the outdoor soil is warm.

DIVISION

Through the years, your herbs might become too big for their original location. Fortunately, some herbs such as chives, lemon grass, marjoram, mint, oregano, sorrel, tarragon, sweet woodruff, and yarrow grow in clumps which can be dug up when they become too large and divided into pieces for replanting. This process is called dividing and it should be done in the early spring or the fall, when the plants are fairly dormant. Although dividing temporarily sends the plants into shock, they will quickly bounce back if you divide gently and plant the divisions immediately.

To divide one of the herb plants listed above, simply dig up the entire clump. If you can't use your hands to divide the clump, use a clean knife or sharp shovel to separate the root ball into two or three smaller clumps. Immediately replant one of the clumps in the original location and plant the other clumps in another area (or pot them up for a friend). Water them well. Mix a weak solution of plant food (fish emulsion or liquid seaweed) and feed the transplanted divisions to encourage establishment.

LAYERING

Layering is the propagation method used to encourage plants to develop roots along their branches. These rooted branch sections can be severed from the mother plant to continue to grow on their own. There are several herbs which can be layered, including lavender, lemon balm, marjoram, mint, rosemary, sage, santolina, savory, scented geranium, southernwood, and thyme. Some herbs root in only a few weeks while others may take several months. But in either case it is a very simple way to propagate.

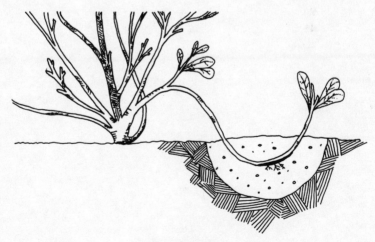

© Copyright Theresa Loe

Layering must be done during the growing season. Early spring is best. First, choose a low branch from the mother plant which can easily bend down to the ground. Hold the branch at about 8 inches from the end and press it down, taking note of where it comes in contact with the soil. At this point on the underside of the branch, wound the area by scratching off the outer layer of the plant stem. Sprinkle the wounded area with rooting hormone (available at the garden center). At the contact point in the soil work in a few handfuls of compost. Gently bend the branch down to the ground and bury it under a few inches of soil, being careful to leave at least 6 inches of branch tip above ground for photosynthesis. Use a rock or a U-shaped piece of wire to secure the branch in place and water well. Watch the layered piece carefully. When new growth begins, you can check under the soil for roots. If roots have formed, sever the plant from its mother but leave it in place for a few more weeks before transplanting.

Herbs in the Kitchen

Even if you have never cooked with herbs before, there is no reason to feel intimidated by these wonderful culinary plants. Just remember that, as with any cooking, herbal flavoring is truly a judgment call, with the cook deciding what suits her taste buds. Just follow the basic guidelines given below, and soon you will find that herbs have introduced you to a whole new world of culinary expression! If you are already an experienced herbal cook, the upcoming recipes should help further inspire your culinary adventures!

As you probably already know, a good cook always tastes the dish throughout the cooking process, not just at the end. This is especially important when using herbs in cooking. You will find that some herbs such as bay, oregano, rosemary, sage, and thyme need long cooking times in order to infuse their flavors into a dish. On the other hand, more fragile herbs, such as basil, cilantro, dill, parsley, salad burnet, and tarragon, must have short cooking times because they lose their flavorful oils rapidly when exposed to heat. For this reason, it is common for these fragile herbs to be used "raw" as a last-minute addition in some recipes.

The amount of chopping you do can also have an effect on the flavoring power of an herb. Whole leaves and coarsely chopped leaves do not fully release their volatile oils. However, when these leaves are finely chopped or minced, their oils are more fully released, thereby intensifying the flavors.

A mortar and pestle or a food processor can maximize this oil release.

When herbs are dried, these flavorful oils slowly lose their potency over time. The longer the herb sits on the pantry shelf, the less flavorful it will become. Therefore, fresh herbs and freshly dried herbs have a superior flavor in recipes. This is why it is important to use up dried herbs within a year if possible.

When cooking, keep in mind that a dried herb is a more concentrated form of a fresh herb. As herb leaves dry, they shrink and you actually have more herb leaves in the dried version than you may realize. When substituting dried herbs for fresh in recipes, only add half as much of the dried version. For example, if a recipe calls for 1 teaspoon fresh sage, use 1/2 teaspoon dried sage as a substitute. (When substituting a fresh herb for a dried, start out using twice as much of the fresh herb. If more is needed, you can add it later.)

As you work with herbs, you will learn that "season to taste" implies much more than just an increase in the salt and pepper. It suggests the addition of any number of aromatic herbs fresh from the garden! Be experimental and enjoy the flavors that these plants have to offer.

Chapter 4

కళ్ళ

Preserving and Using the Garden's Bounty

There is a huge array of methods for preserving the flavors of herbs for later use. Air drying herbs is probably the most common preservation method. (For information on herb drying techniques, *see* "Harvesting and Drying Herbs" in Chapter 2.) Although air drying is the most common and the easiest preservation method, it is important to know that it is not necessarily the best method for all herbs. Delicate herbs such as basil, chives, cilantro, dill, fennel, parsley, and tarragon tend to lose flavor when dried. Although they can be used in the dry state, they actually retain a more potent flavor when stored in a frozen state. They can be frozen quite successfully as "ice cubes" or as concentrated pastes. Although the freezing process causes herbs to lose texture, they will retain their wonderful flavors. Herb flavors can also be preserved by creating herb butters, sugars, syrups, jellies, and vinegars.

FREEZING HERBS

As you can see from the two methods listed below, preserving herbs by freezing is a very simple process. Herbs stored in this way can be used in liquid recipes such as soups, stews, marinades, or sauces.

METHOD 1

1. Wash and pat dry the herb leaves you wish to preserve.
2. These leaves can be chopped and stored directly inside small freezer bags or mixed with water and frozen in ice cube trays.
3. If you choose to make herbal ice cubes, place them inside freezer bags after they are frozen for easy storage.
4. Be sure to label and date the freezer bags because, once frozen, the herbs are indistinguishable.

METHOD 2

1. Gather a large handful of herb sprigs such as basil, tarragon, or dill.
2. Wash the herbs, but do not pat dry.
3. Stuff these sprigs very tightly into a small container with a lid. Stuff as many herbs into the container as possible.
4. Label and freeze.
5. When you want to use the herbs, just remove the whole frozen block and chop off the amount you need. The leaves chop nicely while frozen. Measure and use the herbs as if they were fresh.

Herb Paste

Herb pastes are similar to pestos except that there are only two ingredients: herb leaves and oil. You'll be surprised at how flavorful and versatile herb pastes can be! They can be used in sauces, marinades, stews, or soups. You can use them to create a quick herb butter or cream cheese dip. You can also use them as a "rub" on beef, chicken, or fish.

Pastes can be frozen as "ice cubes," or they can be stored in small containers. The oil coats the herb leaves and helps to retain the color. It also helps prevent the paste from becoming "rock hard" while frozen. This means that you can scrape a spoon across the top of the frozen paste and remove small amounts for cooking without defrosting the entire container. When cooking with the paste, just add 1/2 teaspoon at a time to get the desired amount of flavor. (Remember, it is concentrated.) With a small stash of pastes in the freezer, you'll have an ample supply of concentrated flavor at your fingertips throughout the year!

> **Note:** You should begin by making a paste from only one herb at a time. Later you can experiment with combinations such as poultry paste: basil, rosemary, and sage; or an Italian paste: oregano, thyme, and marjoram.

1. Place fresh herb leaves into a food processor or blender and process until finely chopped.
2. While the processor or blender is running, slowly add a vegetable oil, one tablespoon at a time. Only add enough oil to coat the herbs and form a paste. You do not want it to be too runny.
3. Remove the paste and either store it in an airtight container or place it into an ice cube tray to freeze before storing in a freezer bag.
4. Be sure to label the containers with the herb name and date. Freeze and use within six months for best flavor.

Herb Butters

Herb butters are a very simple way to add flavor to a meal. Typically they are used on breads and vegetables, but they can also be used to create delicious sauces, marinades, and basting mixtures. If you add a few spoonfuls of herb butter to hot pasta, you have a quick and easy meal.

Butters can be used fresh or they can be frozen in plastic wrap for later use. Be sure to label and date your frozen butters and use within four months for best flavor. Keep in mind that the basic recipe for herb butter can be changed to suit your needs. For example, a basting sauce may need a stronger flavor than a butter to be used on bread and would therefore have more herbs added. Try adding chopped shallots, scallions, dried red peppers, or grated citrus peel to your recipes for a more intense flavor. Be creative with your herb combinations!

Basic **H**erb **B**utter **R**ecipe

> *1 stick softened butter (1/2 cup)*
> *approximately 2 tbsp. chopped fresh herbs (1–3 different*
> * kinds)*
> *other flavoring such as spices, citrus peel or garlic*

Rosemary-Garlic Butter (for bread and vegetables)

1. Mix 2 tbsp. freshly chopped rosemary into the softened butter.
2. Add 1 clove of minced garlic and mix well.
3. Let mixture sit in the refrigerator for several hours before using.

Dill Butter (for bread and vegetables)

1. Mix 1 tbsp. dill weed, 1 tsp. dill seed, and 2 tsp. freshly chopped parsley into the softened butter.
2. Let the mixture sit in the refrigerator for several hours before using.

Lemon Herb Butter (for steamed green beans, asparagus, fish, or poultry)

1. Mix 1 tbsp. each of freshly chopped lemon thyme and lemon balm into the softened butter.

2. Add 2 tsp. grated lemon zest (the yellow portion of the peel).
3. Store in the refrigerator for several hours before using.

Tarragon Mustard Butter (for sandwiches, chicken, bread and vegetables)

1. Mix 1 tbsp. freshly chopped tarragon and 2 tsp. freshly chopped chive blossoms.
2. Add 1 tbsp. prepared mustard (regular, spicy, or Dijon) into the softened butter.
3. Store in the refrigerator for several hours before using.

HERBAL SPICE BLENDS

Herb blends can be used in place of salt in some recipes and are helpful in spicing up bland, fat-free diets. If you aren't counting calories, try adding herb seasonings to sour cream or cream cheese to create sinfully delicious dips and hors d'oeuvres.

There are numerous benefits from creating flavorful herb blends straight from your garden:

1. You can customize the seasonings to your own personal preferences.
2. You can be assured that the blends you create are completely free of preservatives, additives, and pesticides.
3. The ingredients are freshly dried and therefore have superior flavor and a longer shelf life than commercial blends.
4. The ingredients are free!
5. Herbal blends make inexpensive gifts for family and friends.

The following recipes yield small batches of seasonings so that you can experiment freely without feeling wasteful. However, they can easily be doubled or tripled for storage on your pantry shelf or for gift giving. Just be sure to use them up within one year for best flavor. Once you have tried a few of the following blends, don't be afraid to develop a few of your own!

To make the following herb seasonings, combine all ingredients and store in an airtight jar or container. Use 1 or 2 teaspoons at a time in recipes until you get the desired level of flavor.

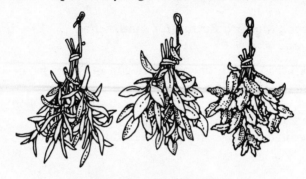

Beef Seasoning

This simple blend can be used in any red meat recipe.

1 tbsp. dried rosemary
1 tbsp. dried savory
1 tbsp. dried thyme
1 tbsp. dried parsley
1 tsp. garlic powder
1 tsp. ground black pepper

Poultry Seasoning

Sprinkle some of this seasoning on chicken or turkey. It can also be added to soups and casseroles.

1 tbsp. dried sage
1 tbsp. dried thyme
1 tbsp. dried marjoram
1 tsp. dried tarragon
1/4 tsp. ground white pepper

Seafood Seasoning

This recipe includes dill weed, which is the leafy portion of the dill plant, and dried lemon peel. You can use a commercially prepared dried lemon peel, which is available in the spice section of the supermarket, or you can dry your own. To dry the lemon peel, grate the zest (the yellow portion of the peel) of one lemon. Place it on a cookie sheet, in the oven, on its lowest setting. Watch closely and remove when completely dry (30 minutes–1 hour). Use some of this seasoning during cooking of any fish recipe or combine with butter for a fast seafood sauce.

2 tbsp. dried dill weed
1 tsp. dried dill seed
1 tbsp. dried lemon thyme (or common thyme)
1 tsp. dried lemon balm
1 tsp. dried lemon peel
1 tsp. fennel seeds

Vegetable Seasoning

This unusual blend can be combined with butter as a vegetable sauce, sprinkled over cooked vegetables, or added to the water of steaming vegetables.

2 tbsp. dried mint
1 tsp. dried lemon thyme (or common thyme)
1 tsp. celery seed

Popcorn Seasoning

Sprinkle approximately 1 tbsp. of this flavorful combination over freshly buttered popcorn for a new treat!

2 tbsp. dried oregano
1 tbsp. dried basil
2 tsp. salt (optional)
1 tsp. garlic powder
5 tbsp. Parmesan cheese

Italian Seasoning

Add this blend to spaghetti sauces, bread, lasagne, pasta, or anything requiring a taste of Italy.

2 tbsp. dried oregano
2 tbsp. dried thyme
1 tbsp. dried basil
2 tsp. dried rosemary
1/2 tsp. garlic powder

GRILLING HERBS

Dried herbs will lose much of their flavor after a year of sitting on the spice shelf. But don't throw them away! They can still be used as grilling herbs. Next time you are grilling meat or vegetables, sprinkle some of the dried herbs over the coals and close the lid. The burning herbs will give off a flavorful smoke which will help season the food! You can also accomplish the same thing with fresh herb sprigs. Toss a few bay leaves or sage sprigs over the coals the next time you are grilling beef or chicken!

Herbal Syrup

Herbal syrups are a very simple and "sweet" way to preserve herb flavors for later use. The finished syrups have a multitude of uses. Try them as sweeteners in hot tea or cold fruit drinks. They can be drizzled over cakes, ice cream, pastries, or fresh fruit. You can make syrup with almost any sweet herb such as lemon verbena, lemon balm, mint, rose petals, scented geraniums, or lavender. The herbs will color the liquid slightly, but if more color is desired, add a few drops of food coloring.

INGREDIENTS:

1–1 1/2 cups sugar
1/2 cup water
1 cup hard-packed fresh herbs

1. In a medium-sized sauce pan, combine all ingredients over medium-high heat. Bring to a boil, reduce heat, and simmer 3 minutes.
2. Remove from heat and set aside to cool completely. When cool, strain the mixture and pour into a decorative bottle with a tight-fitting lid.
3. Store in the refrigerator and use within 3 months.

Lemon Herb Syrup: Follow the recipe above using 1 1/2 cups sugar, 1/2 cup water, 1/2 cup lemon balm, 1/2 cup lemon verbena, and the yellow portion of one lemon peel. (You can use a potato peeler to easily remove peel.)

Mint Syrup: Follow the basic recipe using 1 cup sugar, 1/2 cup water, and 1 cup hard-packed spearmint or peppermint.

Rose Petal Syrup: Follow the basic recipe using 1 cup sugar, 1/2 cup water, and 1 1/2 cups fresh red or pink rose petals from fragrant roses. Stir in 1 tbsp. of rosewater after the mixture has cooled completely.

Herbal Sugar

Another "sweet" way to preserve the flavor of herbs is by making infused sugars. When the finished sugars are used in baking, pastry making, candy making, etc., they impart some of their delicate flavors into the baked goods. Herbal sugars can also be used to sweeten tea and fruit drinks. Any of the sweet herbs can be used: lemon verbena, lemon balm, mint, rose petals, scented geraniums, or lavender.

INGREDIENTS:

2 cups sugar
1 cup fresh herbs (choose one of the herbs listed above)

1. In a glass jar, place alternating layers of sugar and herbs, being sure that all the herb leaves are completely covered with sugar. Cover tightly with an airtight lid.
2. Set mixture aside for 2–3 weeks. Strain the sugar through a coarse sieve, removing all the herbs.
3. Store infused sugar in an airtight container and use within six months.

Herbal Jelly

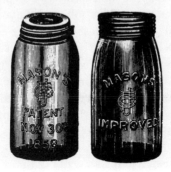

One of the easiest ways to make a flavorful herb jelly is to add herbs to a plain apple jelly. The apple flavor combines well with both sweet and savory herbs, creating a unique condiment. Jellies made with lavender, scented geranium, roses, or lemon verbena can be used on toast, scones, or desserts. Jellies made with mint, basil, rosemary, sage, or thyme are excellent condiments when served with various meat dishes.

INGREDIENTS:

5 cups sugar
extra herb leaves or sprigs for decoration in jar
4 cups apple juice
1 1/2 cups firmly packed fresh herbs
1 3/4 oz. package powdered pectin
6-7 canning jars with screw top lids—washed and
   sterilized in hot water

1. Measure sugar and set aside. Place an extra herb sprig in the bottom of each clean, sterilized canning jar.
2. Combine apple juice and fresh herbs in a large sauce pan over medium heat. Bring to a boil. Let the mixture boil 1

minute, then remove from heat and set aside to cool
completely (about 1 hour).

3. Strain out and discard the herbs.

4. Combine cooled apple juice and powdered pectin in a large
sauce pan. Bring to a rolling boil (one that cannot be stirred
down) and boil hard 1 minute.

5. Add the measured sugar and bring the mixture to a rolling
boil again. Allow mixture to boil hard for 1 minute. Then
remove from heat and skim off foam if necessary.

6. Ladle jelly into clean, sterilized canning jars. Wipe off the
tops of the jars and place on the lids and rings. Tighten
the jar rings until they are just snug; not too tight or too
loose.

7. Process the finished jelly in a water bath for 10 minutes.
Remove and let cool. Check the seal on each jar by pressing
down on the lid. If it pops up and down in the center, it is
not sealed. All unsealed jars should be stored in the
refrigerator and eaten within 2 weeks. Sealed jars can be
stored in the pantry and used within 1 year.

YIELD: SIX 8 OZ. JARS

LIQUID PECTIN

*Liquid pectin may be substituted for powdered in the
above recipe. However, the cooking sequence is a little different. To use liquid pectin, follow the above recipe substituting Steps 4 and 5 as follows:*

4. Combine cooled apple juice and measured sugar in a
large sauce pan. Bring to a rolling boil (one that cannot be stirred down) and boil hard 1 minute.

5. Add liquid pectin and bring mixture to a rolling boil
again. Allow mixture to boil hard for 1 minute. Then remove from heat and skim off foam if necessary. Continue with Step 6 above.

Rose Geranium Jelly: Follow the basic jelly recipe using 1 1/2–2 cups fresh rose geranium leaves as the herb. After the jelly is completely cooked, add 2 tbsp. rosewater and stir well. Before ladling the jelly into the jars, place one fresh rose geranium leaf in the bottom of each jar.

Rose Petal Jelly: Follow the basic jelly recipe using 2 cups of fresh red or pink rose petals from very fragrant roses. After the jelly is completely cooked, add 1 tbsp. rosewater and stir well. Don't bother adding a rose petal to each empty jar; they tend to turn brown and look unattractive when the hot jelly is ladled in.

Note: To prepare the rose petals for jelly making, you should rinse them under cool water. Pull the petals off and blot them dry between two tea towels. Rose petals have a very distinctive white or yellow portion at the base of the petal (where the petal joins the flower). Use scissors or your fingers to remove this portion from each petal. (It is bitter and should be removed when cooking with roses.) Then measure and use as directed in the jelly recipe.

HERBAL VINEGARS

Flavored vinegars have become quite popular in recent years and are considered a staple in the gourmet kitchen. They can be used to create delicious salad dressings, marinades, and sauces. You can create your own exotic and unique herbal vinegars with ingredients you grow yourself. They are inexpensive to create and they make wonderful gifts when accompanied by a recipe for their use. Virtually any culinary herb and spice can be used in the creation of flavored vinegars. You are only limited by your own imagination! Use the basic herb vinegar recipe below as a guide for your own creations or use one of the tried-and-true recipes that follow. To use your new creations, a recipe for basic vinaigrette and grilling marinade follow the vinegar section.

VINEGAR BASE

There are several different vinegars on the market that are appropriate for flavoring. The only one I do *not* recommend using is distilled white vinegar. Its flavor is really too harsh and it overpowers the delicate herbal flavors. However, you can use any of the following vinegars with good results.

White wine vinegar: has a light color and very good flavor. It is excellent for delicate herbs or sweet vinegars. It is also good for fruit vinegars.

Red wine vinegar: is ruby red and is best for strong or savory herb vinegars such as rosemary or sage.

Rice vinegar: has a clear color. This vinegar is sweet and is excellent for sweet herb or fruit vinegars.

Cider vinegar: has a caramel color. This vinegar is inexpensive and is fine for almost all herbal vinegars except fruit vinegars. (I prefer rice vinegar or champagne vinegar for sweetly flavored mixtures.)

Champagne vinegar: has a clear color. This is the best of all the vinegars, because it has a very delicate flavor. The down side is that it can be difficult to find in large quantities and it is usually the most expensive of all the vinegars.

GENERAL CONSIDERATIONS WHEN MAKING FLAVORED VINEGARS

1. Never use aluminum pans or utensils for heating or steeping your vinegars. Use enamel or glass containers and wooden spoons. The aluminum can react with the vinegar and produce an off flavor.

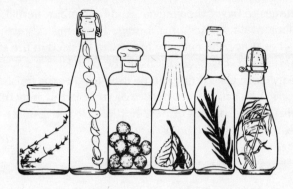

2. The longer you steep a vinegar mixture, the stronger the herb flavor will become.

3. Herb vinegar lasts indefinitely on the shelf because the acidity of the vinegar acts as a preservative. However, although it is perfectly safe to use, over time the flavor of herbal vinegar will deteriorate. For best flavor, it should be used within 6 months to a year.

4. You can use a double layer of cheesecloth to strain your vinegars, but the resulting product may not be crystal clear and a sediment might develop at the bottom of the finished bottle. This is not harmful, but is not aesthetically pleasing (especially for gift giving). For a clear vinegar, you should use coffee filters for a third or fourth straining after straining with cheesecloth first. The finished product will look as clear as the commercial brands!

5. Make sure that the fresh herbs you use are completely free from moisture before adding them to the vinegar. Any water on the leaves will result in a cloudy vinegar.

6. There are no hard-and-fast rules when it comes to measuring herbs for these vinegar recipes. The measurements given here are just approximations. You may add more or less of a particular herb as you feel necessary. You will soon discover that you can't go wrong with herb vinegar because they all taste wonderful!

7. Add fresh herb sprigs to the vinegar bottles before pouring in the finished product. It adds a nice decoration and con-

tinues to flavor the vinegar. And remember, herbal flowers
such as chive blossoms, borage blossoms, nasturtiums, or
other flowering culinary herbs can be used in the steeping
process and as decorations in the bottle.

8. Any clean glass bottle can be used to store the finished vinegars. You can use old bottles or you can buy new ones. For
mail-order sources of new bottles, *see* the "Source Guide"
at the back of the book.

Basic Herb Vinegar Recipe

INGREDIENTS:

4 cups vinegar
1 cup hard-packed fresh herbs
*other flavorings such as citrus peel, raspberries, garlic, or
    spices*

1. Heat the vinegar to very warm but not boiling. Add the herbs
   and spices. Pour the mixture into a clean glass container.
   Cover and allow to cool.
2. Let herbs steep for 1–2 weeks at room temperature. Strain
   the vinegar several times through cheesecloth and/or coffee
   filters to get a clear liquid.
3. Place a few fresh sprigs of the herb used inside clean glass
   bottles. Pour the strained vinegar into the bottles. Seal bottles
   with tight-fitting corks or lids.
4. Label and store your finished vinegars in a cool, dark
   cupboard. Use within 6 months to 1 year.

YIELD: **4 CUPS**

Classic Herb Vinegar Combinations

Rosemary/Garlic Vinegar: 4 cups red wine vinegar, 1 cup fresh rosemary, 5 cloves of garlic (cut in half). Use in salad dressings, beef marinades, and beef sauces.

Lemon Basil Vinegar: 4 cups white wine vinegar, 1 cup fresh lemon basil, the yellow portion of one lemon peel (use a potato peeler to remove peel). Use in salad dressings, poultry, or fish marinades and sauces. (You may substitute another basil for the lemon basil.)

Tarragon Vinegar: 4 cups white wine or champagne vinegar, 1 cup fresh tarragon. Use in poultry or fish marinades and sauces.

More Adventurous Herb Vinegars

Spicy Lemongrass Vinegar: 4 cups rice wine vinegar, 3/4 cup freshly chopped lemon grass, 2 tbsp. black peppercorns, 3 whole red chili peppers, yellow portion of one lemon peel (use a potato peeler to remove peel). After steeping, place a spiral of fresh lemon peel and 1 whole red chili pepper in the finished bottle for decoration. Use in salad dressings, poultry marinades, or Asian cooking.

Fresh Fennel Vinegar: 4 cups white wine or champagne vinegar, 1 cup fresh fennel leaves, 2 tbsp. fennel seed. After steeping, place a fresh sprig of fennel seed (if available) in the finished bottle for decoration. Excellent in salad dressings, vegetable dishes, chicken, pork, and fish marinades.

Salad Burnet Vinegar: 4 cups white wine or champagne vinegar, 1 cup fresh salad burnet, 1/4 cup fresh chives. This vinegar has a distinctive cucumber-like flavor and is delicious in salad dressings, cucumber salads, and vegetable dishes.

Basic Vinaigrette Salad Dressing

Vinaigrette is a great way to utilize a flavorful herbal vinegar and it requires only a few ingredients: oil, vinegar, mustard, salt, and pepper. The basic proportions are 3 parts oil to 1 part vinegar. The amount of mustard used can vary. You can change the flavor tremendously by changing the type of oil or vinegar used. Try olive oil, walnut oil, or vegetable oil in combination with any of the herbal vinegars you create. It is also nice to include some freshly chopped herbs if possible.

INGREDIENTS:

2 tbsp. herbal vinegar
6 tbsp. oil
1 tsp. prepared mustard
1 tsp. freshly chopped herbs
salt and pepper to taste

1. Combine all ingredients in a bowl and whisk until well combined. Pour into a glass jar with a tight-fitting lid. Set aside for at least 10 minutes.
2. Shake dressing again before pouring over fresh salad greens and serving.

Basic Grilling Marinade

This marinade is another way to utilize the vinegars you have made. It can be used on chicken and vegetables when grilling or as a basting sauce on any poultry recipe. Try using different vinegars to get different flavors. It is always nice to include some freshly chopped herbs in the recipe for added flavor. (For example, if you use a dill vinegar, include fresh dill weed in the marinade.)

INGREDIENTS:

1/4 cup herb vinegar
1/2 cup vegetable oil
3 tbsp. honey
1/4 tsp. garlic powder
1 tsp. freshly chopped herbs (optional)

1. Combine all ingredients in a bowl and whisk vigorously. Pour over chicken or vegetables to be marinaded.
2. Cover and refrigerate for 20–30 minutes before grilling.

Chapter 5

✺

Savory Herbs

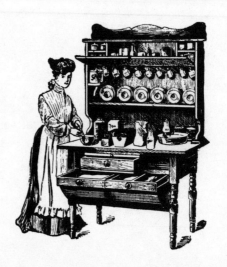

Hundreds of years ago, when there were no refrigerators or preservatives (other than salt), herbs were used to cover up the off flavors of different meats as they began to spoil. Fortunately, today we don't use herbs for this purpose! Instead, we use them to add extraordinary flavor to otherwise ordinary foods.

Savory herbs are generally used to flavor foods other than

desserts, such as appetizers, main dishes, and side dishes. They usually have a robust flavor and are delicious on their own or in combination with other herbs. Some herbs, such as basil, are useful in both savory and sweet recipes. So you may find a so-called savory herb used in a dessert. As you can see, there are no stringent rules in herbal cooking. Rather, there are just a lot of gray areas which leave the door open to experimentation. That's what makes herbal cooking so fun!

Some of the herbs which can be used in savory recipes are basil, bay, salad burnet, calendula, chives, cilantro, dill, fennel, hyssop, lemon grass, marjoram, nasturtium, oregano, parsley, rosemary, sage, savory, sorrel, tarragon, and thyme. This list is not complete, by any means. But it is a good start for creating delicious meals.

BOUQUET GARNI

One way to add savory flavors to food is with a bouquet garni. (*Bouquet garni* is a French term meaning "bundle of herbs.") It can be made with fresh or dried herbs that are tossed into soups, stocks, sauces, or stews for flavoring. The bouquet garni is always removed before serving. It is a nice way to flavor foods, especially clear soups or stocks, without cluttering up the broth with lots of little herb sprigs and branches.

The classic combination of herbs for a bouquet garni is parsley, thyme, and bay leaf. But you can add or subtract different herbs if you want to. That way, you can create your own bouquet garni combinations for your own specific needs and preferences. However, it is best to use only three or four different herbs at a time.

A fresh bouquet garni can be made by tying together a few sprigs of each herb with a cotton string (like a little posy). For added flavor, you can lay the fresh herb sprigs in a 4-inch piece of celery and tie it with cotton string. You can also wrap up some fresh sprigs of herbs in a blanched leek that is tied securely with cotton string. The leek will add flavor as well as hold the bouquet garni together.

For a dried bouquet garni, combine 1 teaspoon of each herb

inside a cotton tea bag and tie securely. Or tie the dried herbs up in a square of cheesecloth. Either way, the dried bouquet garni will keep the liquid you are cooking flavorful but clear.

Summertime Gazpacho with Fresh Basil and Chives

Basil is a very aromatic herb which has a flavor reminiscent of clove and pepper. This flavor combines well with any tomato dish, especially summertime gazpacho. Gazpacho is a delicious cold soup, which can be served as an appetizer or as a light luncheon meal. Cold soup may be new to some people, but once they taste the refreshing flavor, they will be hooked! Serve it with herbal bread or light sandwiches.

This recipe is a breeze to make if you have a food processor, because it only takes a few minutes and there is no cooking involved. If you don't have a food processor, you can use a blender. Just chop the vegetables into smaller pieces for processing. The finished soup should have some texture and crunch to it. If the soup seems too thick, you can add more tomato juice to thin it.

INGREDIENTS:

4 large, ripe tomatoes (or 5 medium tomatoes)
2 medium green bell peppers, coarsely chopped
1/2 onion, coarsely chopped
2 large cucumbers, peeled and coarsely chopped
1 clove garlic, cut in half
4 tbsp. freshly chopped basil
2 tbsp. freshly chopped chives
1 1/2 cups tomato juice
1 tbsp. lemon juice
1/4 tsp. Tabasco sauce (optional)
salt and pepper to taste
extra chopped chives for garnishing

1. Remove the core on the tomatoes and cut them in half, crosswise. Squeeze out the seeds. (You will lose some juice when you do this.) Then, coarsely chop the seeded tomatoes.
2. Place the tomatoes in the food processor and process until smooth. Pour the tomato puree into a large bowl.
3. Place the bell pepper and onion in the food processor and process until smooth. Pour the resulting puree into the bowl with the tomatoes.
4. Place the cucumber, garlic, basil, chives, and 1/2 cup of the tomato juice in the food processor bowl and process until very smooth and creamy. (Be sure the garlic gets processed well.)
5. Pour this mixture into the bowl holding the tomato and bell pepper puree. Add the remaining tomato juice, lemon juice, and Tabasco. Mix well. (If the soup is too thick, add more tomato juice.) Add salt and pepper to taste. (Use a light hand; the soup's flavor intensifies as it sits in the refrigerator.)
6. Let the soup sit in the refrigerator at least five hours to overnight. Then, taste it to be sure the seasoning is correct. Adjust seasonings if necessary. Serve chilled, with chopped chives sprinkled over the top.

YIELD: APPROXIMATELY 2 QUARTS

Stuffed Nasturtiums

These little gems are fun to make and a delight to eat. They can be served as appetizers or as a festive edible garnish on a luncheon plate. The flowers themselves have a delicate, peppery taste.

INGREDIENTS:

1 eight-ounce package cream cheese, softened
1 tbsp. prepared mustard
1 tbsp. finely minced red onion
2 tsp. freshly chopped parsley
2–3-dozen nasturtium flowers
pastry bag and star tip

1. In a small bowl, combine cream cheese, mustard, red onion, and parsley. Use a fork to combine all the ingredients well. Cover and let the mixture sit in the refrigerator for several hours to overnight.
2. Thoroughly wash the nasturtium flowers and allow them to dry on paper towels.
3. Meanwhile, take the cream cheese mixture out of the refrigerator and let it sit at room temperature for 30 minutes to soften.
4. Spoon the cream cheese mixture into a pastry bag fitted with a large star tip. Pipe the cheese into the individual flowers. Place the stuffed flowers on a plate and store in the refrigerator until ready to serve.

YIELD: **2–3** DOZEN

Herb Bread in Flowerpots

Herb bread just seems to be more delicious when it is served in small clay flowerpots! That's right, flowerpots! This bread is baked and served inside clean, unused flowerpots which have been seasoned with oil to prevent sticking. Once the flowerpots are seasoned, they can be used again and again for bread baking. Just keep them in the kitchen so that no one plants anything in them!

Clay flowerpots are safe for cooking as long as they are clean and American made (some foreign pots have too many impurities). For added safety, you can line the inside of the flowerpots with aluminum foil. (This will also prevent the dough and the herb butter from leaking out of the bottom.)

This recipe calls for using frozen bread dough, which is available from the freezer section of your supermarket. It comes in two forms: loaves or individual rolls. You can use either one for this recipe. If you would rather make your own homemade dough, you can use any standard white bread dough recipe.

This bread is made with fresh rosemary, but you can substitute many different herbs in its place. Try some of the substitution suggestions at the end of the recipe.

INGREDIENTS:

8 small clay flowerpots (clean and unused)
vegetable oil
1 loaf frozen bread dough (or 1 package frozen bread rolls)
1 tbsp. butter, melted
1 stick of butter or margarine
1 tbsp. finely chopped rosemary (see substitutions below)
aluminum foil
Parmesan cheese

1. Wash and dry the flowerpots. Brush the inside of each flowerpot with vegetable oil. Place the pots on a cookie sheet and bake them at 450 degrees for one hour. Remove the flowerpots and set them aside to cool.
2. Meanwhile, remove the frozen dough from the freezer and place it on a greased cookie sheet. Rub the outside of the dough with 1 tbsp. of melted butter to prevent it from drying out. Set the dough in a warm place for several hours or until it has risen to double its original size.
3. Line the flowerpots with aluminum foil. Trim the foil so that it is approximately 1/2 inch below the top of the pot and will not show when the bread is baked inside.
4. After the dough has risen to double the original size, melt 1 stick of butter in a small sauce pan. Add your herbs and stir well. Remove from heat.
5. Break off a piece of dough that is about the size of a golf ball (or take one frozen dough roll). Roll it into a ball and dip it into the herb butter mixture. Coat it well on all sides and place it inside the flowerpot which is lined with foil.
6. Continue until you have 3-4 balls inside each flowerpot. (The flowerpots should be filled about 1/2-2/3 full.) Sprinkle the tops with Parmesan cheese. Set the filled flowerpots in a warm place and let them rise again until they are double in size (approximately 30 minutes).
7. Preheat the oven to 350 degrees. Place the flowerpots on a cookie sheet and bake them for about 12 minutes or until the tops are golden brown.
8. You can serve the bread warm or cold. If you need to reheat the bread before serving, simply cover each flowerpot bread with aluminum foil and place in a 350-degree oven for 10-15 minutes. Keep in mind that if you serve this bread hot, the warm flowerpots will be sitting directly on your table. To prevent them from marking the table, you can set them in clay saucers or on coasters.

Herb Substitutions: You can dramatically change the flavor of your bread by substituting one of the following for the rosemary:

1. 1 tbsp. "Italian Herb Seasoning," from Chapter 4
2. 2 tbsp. freshly chopped chives and 1 clove garlic, minced
3. 1 tbsp. dried dill weed and 1 tsp. dill seed

YIELD: **6–8** FLOWERPOT BREADS

Grilled Focaccia with Savory Herb Toppings

Focaccia is an Italian flat bread. Here the focaccia is grilled on the barbeque. This adds a smoky flavor that you just can't get any other way. This recipe is not as complicated as it sounds. By using frozen bread dough, the preparation time is cut in half. The individual focaccia dough can be prepared up to 24 hours ahead of time and stored in the refrigerator. The toppings can be chopped ahead of time also. Then, when the grill is ready, the bread dough, oil, and toppings are taken out and grilled. Each frozen loaf of bread will yield three focaccias. They will be popular, so to be safe, count on one focaccia per guest.

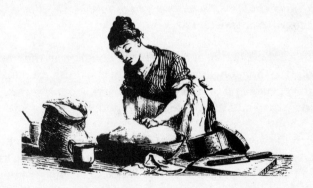

Once the frozen bread dough has risen, you must be very careful when you handle it. If you overwork it, it will not roll out properly. Instead, it will keep springing back on you. If this happens, set the dough aside for about 15–20 minutes to rest and then try rolling it out again.

You should prepare a few toppings from each topping group listed below. Then, make several different focaccias by using different combinations of those toppings. Have fun with it! You can't go wrong! This bread makes a great appetizer. Grill it right in front of your guests and serve it hot. Or, you can grill it ahead of time and serve it cold on a buffet table. If served cold, use a pizza cutter to slice it.

INGREDIENTS:

2 loaves of frozen bread dough
vegetable oil
cutting board and rolling pin
parchment paper or wax paper
herb and vegetable toppings:

Topping Group 1: *1/4 cup of any of the following herbs (finely chopped): rosemary, sage, marjoram, mint, dill, chives, basil*

Topping Group 2: *1/3 cup of any of the following (finely chopped): scallions, red onion, black olives, mozzarella cheese, Parmesan cheese*

1. Remove the 2 loaves of frozen bread dough from the freezer and place them on greased cookie sheets. Brush each loaf with vegetable oil to prevent it from drying out. Set them in a warm place until they have risen to double their original size (2–3 hours).

2. When the dough is ready, brush your cutting board and rolling pin with vegetable oil to prevent sticking. Use a knife to cut off 1/3 of one loaf. Carefully place this piece of dough on the cutting board without deflating it. Use the rolling pin to roll it out into a free-form circle. (If you have trouble keeping the bread from springing back as you roll it out,

follow the steps detailed in the introduction of this recipe.)

3. Place the rolled-out circle on a piece of parchment paper (or wax paper) and set it on a plate. Place another piece of parchment paper on top of it.
4. Cut another 1/3 piece off the dough loaf and follow the same procedure to roll it out. Place it on the parchment paper stack and place another piece of parchment paper (or wax paper) on top of it. Continue with the remaining bread dough.
5. After all the dough is rolled out, wrap the entire stack of uncooked focaccias with plastic wrap. Place them in the refrigerator until you are ready to grill.
6. Meanwhile prepare a few toppings and place them on a plate in individual piles. Cover with plastic wrap and set them in the refrigerator until you are ready to grill.

Hint: Try adding hickory or mesquite chips to the grill coals just before grilling the bread! This will give the bread a unique hickory flavor that can't be beat! You should be able to find barbeque wood chips wherever you buy charcoal. Soak them in water first so that they will smolder and smoke rather than burn.

To Grill the Bread:

1. When the grill is ready, remove the top piece of parchment paper from the top piece of focaccia dough. Brush the dough with oil to prevent sticking. Sprinkle the dough with your toppings of choice.
2. Carefully place your hand under the piece of parchment paper that the dough is resting on and flip the dough onto the grill (facedown), like a pancake. Immediately remove the back piece of parchment paper and brush that side

with oil while the bottom is grilling. Add your toppings
to the exposed side and cover the grill. Cook for 1–2
minutes.
3. Open the grill and use a large spatula to flip the bread. Cover
and cook for 1–2 minutes longer.
4. Remove the bread and continue with the next piece of
focaccia dough.
5. When all the bread is grilled, serve immediately or let cool
and serve cold.

YIELD: **6** FOCACCIAS (**3** PER LOAF OF BREAD)

Homemade Herbal Croutons

Croutons are very easy to make at home and they can turn an
ordinary salad into something gourmet. They can also be sprinkled over winter soups for an added crunch. Both the dill and
the garlic-herb versions of this recipe are simple and delicious.
Try using different breads such as whole wheat, rye, and sour-
dough.

INGREDIENTS:

1/3 cup butter (3/4 stick)
1 tsp. dill seed
1 tbsp. fresh dill weed (or 2 tsp. dried)
1 tbsp. freshly chopped chives (omit if you don't have fresh)
4–5 cups of French bread, cut into 1-inch cubes

1. Preheat oven to 350 degrees. In a small sauce pan, melt
butter. Remove from heat and add the herbs. Stir well and set
aside.
2. Place bread cubes in a large bowl. Drizzle one-half of the
butter mixture over the bread cubes and then stir gently.
Drizzle the remaining butter over the bread cubes and gently

stir again until they are well coated, but not soggy. (Different breads absorb differently, so you may not need all the butter in the recipe.)

3. Spread the buttered bread cubes, in a single layer, on an aluminum foil–lined cookie sheet. Place in the preheated oven and bake for approximately 16-20 minutes or until the cubes are crispy on both sides and slightly browned. Watch them closely so that they do not burn.

4. Remove and let cool. Store leftovers in an airtight container.

Garlic-Herb Croutons

Follow the recipe above, substituting the following for the dill and chives:

INGREDIENTS:

1 glove garlic, minced
1 tbsp. freshly chopped sage (or 2 tsp. dried)
1 tsp. freshly chopped thyme (or 1/2 tsp. dried)
1 tsp. freshly chopped parsley (or 1/2 tsp. dried)
1-2 tsp. grated Parmesan cheese (sprinkled over croutons
as they come out of the oven)

YIELD: APPROXIMATELY 4–5 CUPS

Chicken Fajitas

Fajitas are very popular throughout the Southwest and are a nice change from everyday chicken recipes. They are basically just warm tortillas filled with spicy chicken, onion, and bell peppers. They are simple to make and can be served with Spanish rice, re-fried beans or a salad. Sour cream, guacamole, and salsa should be served as condiments with the fajitas. (A recipe for quick gua-camole follows.)

INGREDIENTS:

4 skinless, boneless chicken breasts
1 tbsp. vegetable oil
1/4 tsp. chili powder
1/4 tsp. ground cumin
1 onion, roughly chopped
1 red bell pepper, cut into strips
1 green bell pepper, cut into strips
2 tbsp. water
1 tbsp. freshly chopped cilantro
flour tortillas
sour cream
guacamole
medium-hot salsa

1. Cut the boneless chicken into 1-inch cubes. Heat the oil in a nonstick skillet. Add the chicken, chili powder, and cumin and sauté over a medium-high heat until the meat is fully cooked and starting to brown (about 10–12 minutes).
2. Add the onion and bell peppers to the skillet. Continue to sauté until the onions begin to brown and caramelize.
3. Add 2 tbsp. of water to the skillet. Continue to stir the fajitas for 1–2 minutes as the water deglazes the pan and creates a sauce. Add the cilantro and heat through.
4. Fill warm tortillas with the fajita mixture. Add a generous spoonful of sour cream, guacamole, and salsa to each plate. Serve immediately.

YIELD: **4** SERVINGS

Quick Guacamole

Guacamole is an avocado dip. You can serve it as a condiment with the fajitas described above or as an appetizer with tortilla chips. This guacamole is quick because you use a commercial salsa instead of homemade. This eliminates the peeling and seeding of the tomatoes and jalapenos, which can take time. Try to make this within a few hours of serving. The lemon juice will help prevent the avocados from browning, but with time the avocados begin to oxidize.

INGREDIENTS:

2 ripe avocados, peeled and pit removed
2 tbsp. fresh lemon juice
1/2 onion, finely chopped
2-4 tbsp. chunky salsa
1 tbsp. freshly chopped cilantro
salt to taste

1. Chop the avocados and place in a medium-sized bowl with the lemon juice. Use a fork to mash the avocados.
2. Add the onion, salsa, and cilantro. Mix well. Add salt to taste. Store covered in the refrigerator until ready to serve.

Roasted Rosemary Chicken with Wild Rice Stuffing

❧❧❧

There is something very comforting about the aroma of roasted chicken on a cold winter day. This rosemary chicken can definitely be classified as a comfort food. It is tender, moist, and flavorful! The wild rice stuffing should be made ahead of time and allowed to cool before stuffing the bird. (This is to prevent bacteria from forming.) If you choose not to stuff the bird with wild rice, try filling the bird's cavity with a handful of rosemary branches and a few slices of lemon. The results will be equally delicious.

A 5–7-pound, stuffed bird will take about 2 1/2–3 1/2 hours to cook. The bird is done when the juices run clear and the leg joint moves very easily. To be safe, you may want to purchase an inexpensive instant-read thermometer. They are invaluable in the kitchen. The chicken is done when the thermometer reads 160 degrees in the thickest part of the breast.

INGREDIENTS:

5–7 lb. roasting chicken
wild rice stuffing (recipe to follow)
2 tbsp. vegetable oil
1 tbsp. freshly chopped rosemary (or 2 tsp. dried)

1. Preheat oven to 350 degrees. Remove giblets and rinse inside and outside of the bird. Pat dry with paper towels.
2. Fill the cavity of the chicken with cold, wild rice stuffing.
3. Place the bird in a shallow, medium-sized roasting pan. Brush the outside of the chicken with oil and sprinkle with the rosemary.
4. Loosely cover the chicken with aluminum foil. Roast in the preheated oven for 2 1/2–3 1/2 hours or until the juices run clear and the leg joint moves easily. (The thickest part of the

breast should register 160 degrees on a meat thermometer when done.)
5. When the chicken is done, remove it from the oven and let rest for 10–15 minutes before slicing.

YIELD: **4** PORTIONS

Herbal Wild Rice Stuffing

This recipe makes more than enough stuffing for a 7-pound chicken. The extra stuffing can be placed in a small casserole pan and cooked alongside the chicken during the last 30–45 minutes of cooking time. More than just a stuffing, this wild rice recipe can be made anytime as a side dish too!

This recipe calls for long-grain brown rice because it has a delicious, nutty flavor. Long-grain white rice may be substituted, but your cooking time in Step 1 may be shorter.

INGREDIENTS:

3/4 cup wild rice (rinsed)
1 1/2 cups long-grain brown rice
3 3/4 cups chicken broth
2 bay leaves (fresh or dried)
1 tbsp. olive oil
1 cup finely chopped celery
1 cup finely chopped onion
1/2 cup finely chopped leeks (white portion only)
2 cloves garlic, minced
1 tbsp. freshly chopped sage leaves (or 2 tsp. dried)
1 tbsp. freshly chopped marjoram leaves (or 1 tsp. dried)
1/4 tsp. salt
1/4 tsp. pepper

1. In a large sauce pan, combine wild rice, brown rice, chicken broth, and bay leaf. Bring to a boil, reduce heat, and cover. Simmer for 30–45 minutes or until all the liquid is absorbed by the rice.
2. Meanwhile, in a large skillet, combine oil, celery, onion, leeks, garlic, and herbs. Sauté on medium-high heat for 3–4 minutes. Stir constantly to prevent the onions and garlic from browning. (You only want to sweat the vegetables, not brown them.) Remove from heat and set aside.
3. When the rice is done cooking, remove from heat and add the sautéed vegetables. Add the salt and pepper and stir well. Set rice aside to cool completely before stuffing the chicken (or serve immediately as a side dish).

YIELD: 6–7 CUPS

*P*an-*F*ried *R*ed *S*napper *with* *F*ennel *S*eed *and* *L*emon *G*rass

This recipe is fast! If you mix up the herb bread crumbs ahead of time, you can bread the fish, fry it, and serve it in less than 10 minutes! And by using a nonstick frying pan, you greatly reduce the amount of oil needed. The three-step breading procedure described below is the best way to get an even crust that won't flake off while cooking. You can use the same procedure to bread other types of fish too.

You'll find that the lemon grass and fennel in this recipe create a sensational flavor combination and they do not overpower the delicate flavor of the fish. If the lemon grass is too difficult to cut with a kitchen knife, use scissors.

Since this recipe uses a nonstick skillet, only 1 tbsp. of oil is needed. If you use any other type of skillet, you may need more oil to prevent sticking.

INGREDIENTS:

4 red snapper fillets
1 cup unseasoned bread crumbs
4 tsp. finely chopped lemon grass leaves
2 tsp. fennel seed
4 tsp. dried marjoram
1/2 tsp. ground black pepper
1/2 tsp. garlic powder
1 tbsp. freshly grated lemon zest
1 cup flour
2 eggs, beaten
1 tbsp. vegetable oil
2 lemons, cut into wedges (to serve with the fish)

1. Rinse the red snapper fillets and pat dry with paper towels. Set aside.
2. In a small bowl, combine the bread crumbs, lemon grass, fennel seed, marjoram, pepper, garlic powder, and lemon zest. Mix well.
3. Place 3 plates in a row on the counter. (This is going to be your breading assembly line.) On the first plate, pour out the flour. On the second plate, pour out the beaten eggs. On the third plate, place the herbed bread crumbs.
4. Pour 1 tbsp. of vegetable oil into a nonstick frying pan and place over medium-high heat. Take one fillet and dredge it in the flour then dip it into the egg. Next, dredge it in the herb bread crumbs. (Be sure to get a thick coating of bread crumbs on the fillet.)
5. Place the breaded fillet in the hot pan and repeat the breading procedure with the remaining fillets. Pan-fry all the fish fillets over medium-high heat for approximately 3–4 minutes per side or until the outside is golden brown and center is flaky. (Depending upon the size of the skillet and the fillets, you may only be able to cook two or three at a time.)
6. Serve immediately with lemon wedges.

YIELD: **4** PORTIONS

Beef Stew with Bay and Savory

This is a rather traditional beef stew that I have made for years. For a different flavor, substitute fresh rosemary for the fresh savory. Serve this hardy meal with a crusty bread.

INGREDIENTS:

2 tbsp. vegetable oil
1 1/2 lbs. beef stew meat, cut into 1-inch cubes
1 cup flour
2 cups beef broth
1 cup tomato juice
1 15 oz. can stewed tomatoes (about 2 cups)
1 onion, roughly chopped
2 bay leaves (fresh or dried)
1 tbsp. freshly chopped savory
2 gloves garlic, pressed
1/4 tsp. ground black pepper
4 large carrots, cut into 3-inch pieces
3 stalks of celery, cut into 3-inch pieces
4 small white potatoes, cut in half
salt to taste

1. Heat the oil in a Dutch oven. Rinse the stew meat, pat it dry with paper towels, and dredge it in the flour.
2. Cook the floured meat in the oil until browned. Add beef broth, tomato juice, stewed tomatoes, onion, bay leaves, savory, pressed garlic, and black pepper. Stir and cover. Simmer over low heat for 1 hour, stirring occasionally.
3. Add carrots, celery, and white potatoes to the stew. Stir well. Cover and simmer an additional 30–45 minutes or until potatoes are fork tender.
4. Add salt to taste. Serve immediately.

YIELD: **4** SERVINGS

Roasted Potatoes with Rosemary and Oregano

These hardy potatoes are a great accompaniment to any meal. The aroma coming from the kitchen as they roast will be enough to make everyone's mouth water! This recipe serves six, but if you want to serve only four, reduce the amount of potatoes to 2 pounds. Leftovers are easily reheated the next day, either in the microwave or a low oven. When using red or white potatoes, you should leave the skin on. However, if substituting russet potatoes, peel them before roasting.

INGREDIENTS:

1/4 cup vegetable oil
2 tbsp. freshly chopped rosemary
1 tbsp. freshly chopped oregano
1/4 cup chopped scallions
1 glove garlic, minced
1/4 tsp. salt
1/4 tsp. pepper
2 1/2–3 lbs. red or white potatoes, quartered (halved if small)

1. Preheat oven to 350 degrees. In a large bowl, combine oil, herbs, scallions, garlic, salt, and pepper. Mix well.
2. Add the quartered potatoes to the oil and herb mixture. Stir well until all the potatoes are well coated.
3. Place the potatoes in a medium-sized roasting pan. Roast, uncovered, in a 350-degree oven for 45–60 minutes or until they are browned on the outside and fork tender in the center. Stir them occasionally while roasting. Serve them hot out of the oven.

YIELD: **6** SERVINGS

Garden Salad

❧

This garden salad is a colorful mixture of fresh flowers and greens. It is as beautiful as it is delicious. Be sure that the flowers are pesticide-free and washed thoroughly—especially nasturtiums and calendulas. (Sometimes, little insects wedge themselves down inside the petals.) Some flowers, such as borage and pansies, should be served whole. Large flowers, such as calendulas, should be separated into individual petals. (Nasturtiums can be served either way.) Blossoms from chives, hyssop, and mint should be roughly chopped.

INGREDIENTS:

*4 cups mixed greens: butter lettuce, endive, and spinach
    leaves
1/2 cup fresh sorrel leaves
1/2 cup peeled and sliced cucumber
1/2 cup shredded carrots
2 tbsp. roughly chopped salad burnet leaves
1 tsp. finely chopped basil leaves or flowers
1 cup of edible flowers such as borage, calendula, chives,
    hyssop, mint, nasturtium, and pansies*

1. In a large bowl, toss together the mixed greens, sorrel, cucumber, carrots, salad burnet, and basil.
2. Add the edible flowers and toss gently. Add "Honey-Dill Dressing" (*see* below) and serve immediately. You can use any salad dressing with this recipe. However, heavy, creamy dressings will coat and cover many of the pretty flowers and leaves. A light dressing would be a better choice.

Honey-Dill Dressing

INGREDIENTS:

6 tbsp. olive oil
2 tbsp. herbal vinegar (or apple cider vinegar)
1 small shallot, finely chopped
1/2 tsp. prepared mustard
1/2 tsp. honey
2 tsp. finely chopped fresh dill leaves
pinch of salt and black pepper

1. In a small bowl, combine all ingredients. Whisk until thoroughly mixed. Pour over salad and serve.

Salad Tip: You will find that you can add a variety of herbs and flowers to any plain green salad. Next time your salad needs a little sprucing up, try adding fresh basil, mint, lemon balm, chives, dill, fennel, or salad burnet leaves for flavor. Add any of the flowers listed in the garden salad recipe for color.

Vegetable Medley
with Fennel and Thyme

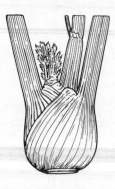

To make this recipe, you will need small fennel bulbs (the bottom portion of the fennel plant, minus the stalk). Unfortunately, this means that you must harvest out the entire plant. You may want to grow several crops of fennel strictly for this purpose and pick the bulbs when the plant is still fairly young. The best fennel for this recipe is Florence fennel *(Foeniculum vulgare* var. *azoricum). (See* the description of fennel in Chapter 1.) If you don't want to use up your fennel crop, you can buy fennel bulbs in the vegetable section of some supermarkets. Either way, the fennel imparts a delicate anise flavor which deliciously combines with the garlic and thyme.

INGREDIENTS:

2 small fennel bulbs (or 1 large)
2 tbsp. vegetable oil
1 cup sliced carrots
1/2 onion, sliced
1 cup sliced zucchini
1 glove garlic, minced
1 tsp. fresh thyme (1/2 tsp. dried)
salt and pepper to taste

1. Julienne the fennel bulbs. (Slice into small strips.)
2. Place the oil in a large skillet, over high heat. Add the fennel, carrots, and onions. Sauté over high heat until the onion becomes translucent.
3. Add the zucchini, garlic, and thyme. Sauté for approximately 3 minutes or until the zucchini is heated through. Add salt and pepper to taste and serve.

YIELD: APPROXIMATELY 4–5 CUPS (4 SERVINGS)

Chapter 6

Sweet Herbs

Although it may sound unusual to use herbs in sweet recipes, it was actually a very ordinary practice throughout history until just recently. Many old herbals and history books make mention of herbal candies, drinks and desserts. This is probaby due to the fact that up until Medieval times, sugar was extremely scarce and herbs were used as sweeteners in many recipes. Then, during the Victorian Era, when there was a renewed interest in gardening, herbs and flowers were once again popular additions to cakes, candies and pastries. A whole new set of herbal sweets were developed

There are many herbs which lend themselves to sweet recipes. Some of them, such as rosemary and basil, have the unique quality of being useful in both sweet and savory dishes. Below is a list of herbs to try in your own pastry, cookie or dessert recipes. Keep in mind that this list is only offered as a starting point for some sweet experimentation. It is in no way complete. As you expand your herbal knowledge, you will find more herbs to add to the list. Hopefully, the recipes in this chapter will provide a little inspiration for your sweet herbal journey.

Herbs to try in sweet recipes: basil, borage flowers, lavender, lemon balm, lemon verbena, mint, pineapple sage, rose, rosemary, scented geranium, sweet woodruff.

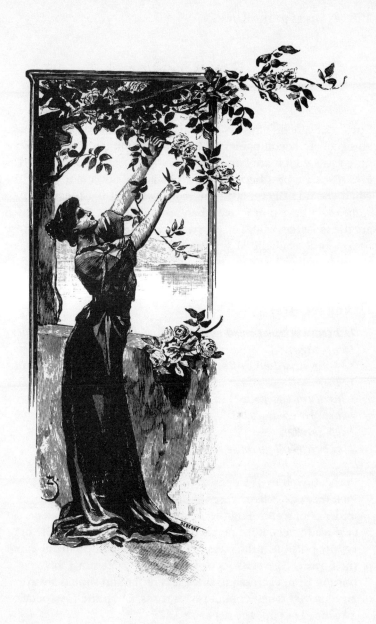

Rose Cookies

These delicate cookies taste just like shortbread and would make an excellent accompaniment to an afternoon tea! Be sure to use only roses which are completely pesticide-free. Pink, red, or yellow roses are best because their petals will add color to the finished cookie. Always taste the roses before using them because some roses have more flavor than others. Choose the roses which are the most flavorful. The rosewater is added to enhance the rose flavor. It is available at gourmet shops, health food stores, or through mail-order.

INGREDIENTS:

1/4 cup chopped fresh rose petals
1 cup sugar
3/4 cup unsalted butter, softened
1/4 tsp. salt
1 medium egg yolk
1 tbsp. rosewater
1 tsp. vanilla
1 1/2 cups all-purpose flour

1. Preheat oven to 375 degrees.
2. Pick roses (2–3 large roses should be enough) and rinse under cool water. Pull the petals off and blot dry between two tea towels. Rose petals have a very distinctive white or yellow portion at the base of the petal (where the petal joins the flower). Use scissors or your fingers to remove this portion from each petal, since it is bitter and should always be removed when cooking with roses. Chop the rose petals, measure 1/4 cup, and set aside.
3. In a medium mixing bowl, combine sugar, butter, salt, and egg yolk. Beat until creamy.
4. Add rosewater and vanilla. Mix well.

5. In a small bowl, combine rose petals and flour. Stir gently. Add this flour mixture to the sugar mixture and beat until well combined. It should resemble sticky cookie dough.
6. Line a cookie sheet with parchment paper (or use a nonstick cookie sheet). Drop rounded teaspoonfuls of dough, about 2 inches apart, onto the cookie sheets.
7. Bake for 16–20 minutes or until golden brown around the edges and firm in the center.
8. Immediately remove the cookies and let them cool on wire racks.

YIELD: APPROXIMATELY **25** COOKIES

Lavender Scones

In this recipe, dried lavender is used to infuse the liquid with its delicate flavor. Then more lavender is added to create speckles of color. This scone recipe is very versatile because you can substitute lemon verbena for the lavender to create a completely different treat! Serve these scones hot or cold with either tea or coffee. No matter how you serve them, don't forget to include generous helpings of butter and jam!

INGREDIENTS:

3/4 cup half and half
2 tbsp. dried lavender blossoms
1 3/4 cup all-purpose flour
1/4 cup sugar
1 tsp. baking soda
1/4 cup vegetable shortening
2 tsp. dried lavender
1 tbsp. sugar
1/2 tsp. ground cinnamon

1. In a small sauce pan, heat half and half until very warm (not boiling). Remove from heat and stir in the 2 tbsp. lavender. Set aside to steep for 20–30 minutes. Strain mixture and discard herbs.
2. Preheat oven to 425 degrees.
3. In a medium mixing bowl, combine flour, sugar, and baking soda. Stir to mix well.
4. Add shortening and use a pastry blender, two knives, or your fingers to cut in the shortening until the mixture resembles coarse meal.
5. Add the strained half and half and 2 tsp. dried lavender to the flour mixture. Use a fork and then your fingers to combine into a soft dough.
6. Turn the dough out onto a lightly floured surface. Form a ball and then gently roll the dough out into a 1/2-inch thick circle (about 9 inches in diameter).
7. Combine the 1 tbsp. sugar with the 1/2 tsp. cinnamon and sprinkle a light coating of this mixture over the top of the dough.
8. Place on a parchment-lined cookie sheet (or nonstick) and bake at 425 degrees for 12–15 minutes or until golden brown.
9. Remove the cookie sheet from the oven and let cool for 5 minutes. Cut the circle into eight wedges like a pizza. The scones may be eaten now or placed on a rack to cool completely. (They can also be reheated later in the microwave.)

Lemon Verbena Variation: Omit the lavender and substitute 1/4 cup whole, fresh lemon verbena leaves for the 2 tbsp. dried lavender. Add 2 tsp. grated lemon zest (the yellow portion of the peel) to the flour. Follow the remaining instructions as written.

YIELD: 8 SCONES

Lemon Verbena Strawberry Shortcake

୬ଌୢୠଈୖ

This is a new version of an old American classic. The lemon verbena adds a nice, tart accent to the sweet strawberries. The biscuits used to create this dessert are actually quite delicious on their own. If you don't use them all for the strawberry shortcake, you can serve the leftovers with tea. They are also delicious when sprinkled with powdered sugar. Yum!

INGREDIENTS:

3/4 cup half and half
1/4 cup whole lemon verbena leaves
1 3/4 cup all-purpose flour
3 tbsp. sugar
2 tsp. baking powder
1/2 tsp. baking soda
1/4 tsp. salt
1 tbsp. lemon zest
2 tbsp. vegetable shortening
2 tbsp. butter
5 cups sliced strawberries
1/4 cup sugar
whipped cream
extra lemon verbena leaves for garnishing

1. In a small pan, heat the half and half until hot, but not boiling. Remove from heat, add lemon verbena, and let steep for 20–30 minutes. Strain mixture and discard herbs.
2. Preheat oven to 425 degrees.
3. In a medium-sized bowl, combine flour, 3 tbsp. of sugar, baking powder, baking soda, salt, and lemon zest. Mix well.
4. Add shortening and butter to the flour mixture. Use a pastry blender, two knives, or your fingers to cut the shortening

and butter into the flour until the mixture resembles coarse meal.

5. Add the half and half to the flour mixture. Use a fork and then your fingers to combine into a soft dough. Roll dough out on a floured board to 1/2 inch thick. Use a 3-inch biscuit cutter to cut out six circles. (You may have to reroll scraps to get six.)

6. Place circles on a parchment-lined (or nonstick) cookie sheet and bake at 425 degrees for 10–12 minutes or until golden brown. Place on a rack to cool.

7. When you are ready to assemble the shortcakes, mix the strawberries and the 1/4 cup sugar together in a small bowl.

8. Cut each biscuit in half horizontally. Place the bottom half on a plate, and top with a generous helping of strawberries. Place a scoop of whipped cream over the strawberries and place the biscuit top over the whipped cream.

9. Add a small dollop of whipped cream to the top of each shortcake stack and place a few lemon verbena leaves on for garnish. Serve immediately.

YIELD: 6 SHORTCAKES

Lemon Balm Tart

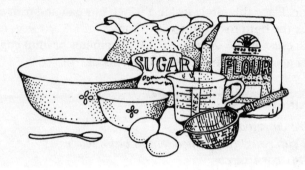

Colorful flakes of lemon balm create a beautiful mosaic in this pastry crust, which can be used to make all kinds of pies and tarts. The filling for this 9-inch tart is tangy and creamy. It is sure to be a hit at your next party. Serve with a sprig of lemon balm as a garnish.

CRUST:

> 1 1/4 cups flour
> 1/4 tsp. salt
> 2 tbsp. sugar
> 2 tsp. grated lemon zest (yellow portion of peel)
> 2 tbsp. finely chopped lemon balm leaves
> 1/3 cup vegetable shortening
> 3-4 tbsp. cold water

1. Preheat oven to 425 degrees. In a large bowl, combine flour, salt, sugar, lemon zest, and lemon balm. Stir well.
2. Add shortening and use two knives, a pastry blender, or your fingers to cut in the shortening until the mixture resembles coarse meal.
3. Add 2 tbsp. of cold water and mix with a fork until it begins to form a dough. Knead the dough with your hands. If the

dough feels too dry, add some of the remaining water, a little at a time, until a soft dough forms that holds together. (You may not need all the water.)

4. On a lightly floured board, roll out dough to a 1/8-inch thick circle. Place this circle inside a 9-inch tart pan and trim edges. Prick the bottom of crust with a fork.

5. Bake crust at 425 degrees for 13–16 minutes or until edges are a golden brown. Remove and let cool.

FILLING:

1 1/2 cups water
1/2 cup roughly chopped lemon balm leaves
4 tbsp. cornstarch
1/2 cup sugar
pinch of salt
1/3 cup freshly squeezed lemon juice
3 medium egg yolks, slightly beaten
2 tsp. lemon zest (yellow portion of peel)
2 tbsp. unsalted butter

1. In a small sauce pan, combine water and lemon balm leaves. Bring water to a boil, remove from heat, and cover. Let herbs steep 20–30 minutes. Strain mixture and discard herbs.

2. In a medium, heavy-bottomed sauce pan, whisk together strained water, cornstarch, sugar, and salt. Bring mixture to a boil, stirring constantly. Boil for 1 minute.

3. Remove pan from heat and stir in lemon juice. Pour a small amount of this hot cornstarch mixture into the beaten egg yolks. Stir well. Then, pour the egg yolks back into the cornstarch mixture and stir well. Return the pan to the stove.

4. Bring mixture to a simmer and cook for 4 minutes over medium-low heat or until an instant-read thermometer reads at least 165 degrees for 1 minute. Stir constantly so mixture does not burn.

5. Remove the pan from the heat and stir in lemon zest and butter. Stir until butter is melted and completely incorporated. Pour the finished lemon filling into the baked tart shell. Let cool completely before serving. Store any leftovers in the refrigerator.

YIELD: ONE 9-INCH LEMON TART

Open-Faced Rosemary-Apple Pie

This pie recipe makes a very unusual presentation and your guests will have trouble distinguishing the secret ingredient—rosemary. It adds a wonderfully subtle flavor which, when combined with the marmalade, makes a very delicious accent. If you don't want to take the time to make your own pie crust, a ready-made or a boxed crust will work almost as well. Just hide the box so your guests won't know!

CRUST:

1 1/4 cups all-purpose flour
1/4 tsp. salt
2 tbsp. sugar
1/3 cup vegetable shortening
3-4 tbsp. cold water

1. In a medium-sized bowl, combine flour, salt, and sugar. Mix well.
2. Add shortening and use two knives, a pastry blender, or your fingers to cut in the shortening until the mixture resembles coarse meal.
3. Add 2 tbsp. of cold water and mix with a fork until it begins to form a dough. Knead the dough with your hands. If dough

feels too dry, add some of the remaining water, a little at a time, until a soft dough forms that holds together. (You may not need all the water.)

4. On a lightly floured board, roll out dough into a 1/8-inch-thick circle. Place on a parchment-lined (or nonstick) cookie sheet and cover with a piece of plastic wrap. Set in the refrigerator until filling is ready.

FILLING:

5–6 Granny Smith apples
juice of 1 lemon
1 tsp. vanilla
2 tsp. chopped rosemary leaves
3 tbsp. sugar
1 tsp. cinnamon
1/2 tsp. allspice
1 tsp. cornstarch
4 tbsp. orange or lemon marmalade
1–2 tbsp. butter
aluminum foil

1. Preheat oven to 400 degrees.
2. Peel, core, and slice apples and place in a mixing bowl with the lemon juice. Add vanilla and stir apples well to coat.
3. In a small bowl, combine sugar, cinnamon, allspice, and cornstarch. Sprinkle over apples and mix well.
4. Remove the rolled-out crust from the refrigerator and remove plastic wrap. Place the marmalade in the center of the crust and spread evenly to within 2 inches of the edge. Carefully place a layer of apple slices in a spiral pattern, starting at the center of the crust and stopping 2 inches from the edge. Continue placing spiral layers until all apples have been used.
5. Fold the crust edges over twice and roll up over the edge of the apples. If necessary, place rolled strips of aluminum foil around the edges to hold crust in place.

6. Pour any remaining juice from the apple mixture into the center of the pie and dot the apples with pieces of the remaining tablespoon of butter. Bake at 400 degrees for 40–45 minutes. (Remove foil during last 5 minutes.) Serve warm or cold with whipped cream.

YIELD: **1** PIE

Chocolate Mint Pudding

Don't let the thought of making chocolate pudding from scratch intimidate you. It is incredibly easy and sinfully delicious! You'll be amazed at how creamy, minty, and rich the final product is! Tremendously better than any store-bought pudding, this dessert is sure to satisfy any chocoholic! If you don't have spearmint, fresh peppermint leaves may be substituted.

INGREDIENTS:

2 cups milk
1 cup roughly chopped, fresh spearmint leaves
3 oz. semisweet chocolate
1 oz. unsweetened chocolate
1/2 cup sugar
pinch of salt
2 tbsp. cornstarch
2 medium egg yolks, slightly beaten
1 tsp. vanilla
1 tbsp. butter, cut into pieces
extra mint sprig for garnishing

1. In a small sauce pan, combine milk and spearmint. Heat over a medium flame until milk is very hot, but not boiling. Remove from heat, cover, and set aside for 20 minutes. Strain

mixture and discard mint. Remove approx. 1/2 cup of the milk and set aside.

2. Melt the chocolate in the top half of a double boiler, stirring occasionally.

3. In a large sauce pan with a heavy bottom, combine melted chocolate with only 1 1/2 cups of the mint-flavored milk. Whisk or stir vigorously to combine. (Do not be concerned if the chocolate creates small flakes; they will melt later.)

4. Place the pan over medium heat and add sugar and salt. Bring to a boil.

5. In a separate bowl, combine the cornstarch with the reserved 1/2 cup mint-milk mixture. Mix well. Pour this into the chocolate mixture and return to a boil, stirring constantly. (Be careful not to burn the bottom; lower heat if necessary.) The chocolate mixture will thicken considerably after boiling for about 30–60 seconds. When this happens, remove from heat.

6. Pour a small amount of the chocolate mixture into the slightly beaten egg yolks. Mix well and then pour the yolks back into the chocolate. Return the pan to the stove and cook over a medium-low flame for 3 minutes, stirring constantly.

7. Remove from heat and stir in vanilla and butter. Stir well until the butter melts and is well incorporated. (The pudding will continue to thicken as it cools.) Pour pudding into 4–5 half-cup serving dishes and let cool. Serve with fresh mint sprigs as garnishes.

YIELD: **4–5** HALF-CUP SERVINGS

Basil-Lemon Sorbet

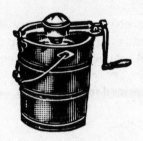

This light dessert is the perfect finish to a spicy meal! The coolness of this icy white sorbet with its lemonade flavor is very refreshing, and the hint of basil makes it very exotic. The lemon zest is included for extra flavor.

INGREDIENTS:

2 cups water
1 cup sugar
1/2 cup roughly chopped fresh basil leaves
1/3 cup freshly squeezed lemon juice
1/2 tsp. lemon zest (yellow portion of the peel)

1. In a small sauce pan, bring the water and sugar to a hard boil. Stir for 1 minute and then add the basil. Remove from heat, cover, and let mixture sit for 20 minutes.
2. Strain the basil water into a bowl and set aside to cool completely. (Placing it in the refrigerator will speed up the cooling process.)
3. Add lemon juice and zest. Stir well.
4. Pour into your ice cream maker and freeze according to the manufacturer's instructions.
5. Store in the freezer, but place sorbet in the refrigerator 15 minutes before serving to soften. Eat within 1 week.

YIELD: APPROXIMATELY 2 CUPS

Rosemary-Orange Sorbet

This sorbet recipe is very unusual and very delicious. The combination of rosemary and orange complement each other very well and create a flavorful summertime treat. Use freshly squeezed orange juice if possible. Try serving small scoops of this sorbet in wineglasses with a sprig of fresh rosemary as a garnish. Very elegant!

INGREDIENTS:

2 cups water
1/2 cup sugar
1 tbsp. roughly chopped, fresh rosemary leaves
1 cup orange juice
1 tsp. orange zest (the orange portion of the peel)

1. In a small sauce pan, bring the water and sugar to a hard boil. Stir for 1 minute and then add the rosemary. Remove from heat, cover, and let sit for 15 minutes.
2. Strain the rosemary water into a bowl and set aside to cool completely. (Placing it in the refrigerator will speed up the cooling process.)
3. Add the orange juice and zest. Stir well.
4. Pour into your ice cream maker and freeze according to the manufacturer's instructions.
5. Store in the freezer but place sorbet in the refrigerator 15 minutes before serving to soften. Eat within 1 week.

YIELD: APPROXIMATELY 2 CUPS

Minty Fruit Salad

For a quick and easy lunchtime treat, try this refreshing mint and fruit salad. You can use peppermint, spearmint, or apple mint to get a variety of flavors. If your mint is blooming, try adding chopped mint blossoms to the salad for extra flavor and color. The advantage of using the concentrated apple juice is that it eliminates the need for sugar. Any combination of fruit is delicious in this salad. Add the fruits you prefer or have in season.

INGREDIENTS:

1/2 cup frozen apple juice concentrate
1/4 cup chopped fresh mint leaves
1/2 cantaloupe, cut into 1-inch cubes (about 5-6 cups)
1/2 honeydew melon, cut into 1-inch cubes (about 5-6 cups)
1 cup seedless grapes
1 tsp. freshly chopped mint leaves

1. In a small sauce pan, combine apple juice and 1/4 cup mint leaves. Bring to a boil, remove from heat, and set aside to cool. Strain.
2. In a large bowl, combine fruit and 1 tsp. freshly chopped mint. Pour half the apple juice mixture over the fruit and stir well. Taste and add more juice to sweeten if necessary. Serve immediately.

Pineapple Sage Variation: For a different twist on this simple salad, try substituting fresh pineapple sage for the mint. Be sure to include some fresh pineapple in the mixed fruit!

YIELD: APPROXIMATELY 2 1/2-3 QUARTS (DEPENDING UPON FRUIT USED)

Herbs in the Home

❧❧❧

Beginning in sixteenth-century Europe, many homes had a "stillroom," where the housewife or maid concocted herbal medicines, soaps, cordials, tinctures, and aromatics for the home. It was usually next to the kitchen, and had its own fire and still for distilling important potions such as lavender oil or rosewater. It was from here that all the preparations were developed to keep the household clean, fragrant, and healthy. Many of these women kept stringent notes on how to create these recipes in stillroom books, which were passed down through generations.

Luckily for us, it is no longer necessary to have a special room to distill essential oils and create fragrant potions. But that doesn't make the thought of recreating some of those old recipes any less romantic. Many of the concoctions of the past can be adapted for modern purposes. For example, in Medieval times, herbs were strewn all over the floor so that their scent would be released when stepped upon. Although herb strewing is impractical today, herb powders can be sprinkled over carpeting and vacuumed up to achieve the same effect. Some of the old stillroom recipes for cosmetics can be easily recreated today by using just a few fresh ingredients right out of the garden and kitchen.

Historically, herbs have also been used in the home as decorations. It was an ancient practice to bring the fragrances of the garden indoors through freshly cut flowers and herbs. But herbs have other decorative qualities as well. They can be pressed flat and dried to be used in a variety of whimsical designs and decorations. They can even be used to decorate gift wrap!

Many people are familiar with the culinary aspects of herbs. But it is fascinating to explore the soothing, fragrant, and decorative history of herbs and how these attributes can be adapted to our modern way of living. This section focuses on some of these herbal characteristics and how we can use them in our own homes.

Chapter 7

❦

Beauty from the Garden: Herbal Cosmetics

Throughout recorded history, there is evidence that people all over the world created botanical cosmetics for both beauty and fragrance. The early Egyptians used ointments and perfumes for personal adornment and ancient rituals. The Romans used herbs in skin preparations and fragrant baths. During the sixteenth and seventeenth centuries, most well-to-do Europeans had a stillroom in their household, where essential oils were distilled from plants and used to create colognes, bath waters, and pomades (a perfumed ointment for the hair or scalp). In Colonial America, women grew herbs outside their kitchen doors for many purposes including beauty products. They made soaps, perfumes, lotions, and room deodorizers. But the romance of homemade cosmetics is probably best captured by the Victorian women, who would whisper beauty secrets to each other over afternoon tea or write of fragrant concoctions in their private journals.

Many of these old-time botanical toiletries and fragrances have been handed down through generations by mothers, daughters, alchemists, midwives, and house servants. Today, we can combine the best of this historical knowledge with today's technology to create our own personalized, all-natural beauty potions.

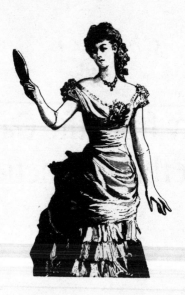

It can be very nostalgic to gather fragrant ingredients from the garden to make old-fashioned toiletries. But there are also some great advantages to creating your own homemade cosmetics:

1. You are guaranteed that everything is fresh and preservative-free.
2. You can choose ingredients specifically geared for your own skin and hair type.
3. You can personalize them by using your favorite essential oils for fragrance.
4. You can present them as gifts in creative packaging with the recipe attached.

Ingredients and Where to Find Them

Some of the ingredients listed in the following recipes may sound a bit exotic, but most can be found in your local supermarket, pharmacy, health food store, or your own herb garden. What you can't find locally can be ordered from some of the mail-order companies listed in the "Source Guide" at the back of this book. (Dried herbs such as chamomile and calendula can sometimes be found in the "bulk tea" section at the health food store.)

Almond Oil, Sweet: This makes an excellent all-purpose body oil because it is very emollient. Look for it in health food stores, in some grocery stores, or from one of the mail-order sources listed in this book.

Aloe Vera Gel: This is the sap from the aloe vera plant, which has antifungal and moisturizing properties. Aloe has a long history of medicinal uses including soothing dry, irritated, or burned skin. It can be found at some pharmacies, in health food stores, or through mail-order sources.

Apricot Kernel Oil: This oil can be found in health food stores, in some supermarkets, and through mail-order. It is a light oil which soaks into the skin well.

Beeswax: When used in conjunction with borax, beeswax acts as an emulsifying agent in cosmetics. It also gives a protective layer to the skin and holds in moisture. It can be found in many health food stores, candle supply houses, beekeeping stores, or one of the sources listed in the "Source Guide." I prefer to use pure, unbleached beeswax, which has a brown color and a sweet, honey scent. Some people like the bleached beeswax "pearls" or "beads" because they are easier to measure. If you wish to use them, be sure they do not have other additives. Beeswax has a very long shelf life and will not turn rancid.

Borax Powder (Sodium borate): This naturally occurring mineral is a water softener and can be found in the detergent section of the supermarket. In cosmetics it is used as an emulsifier, stabilizer, and preservative. It is only mildly alkaline so it can be help-ful in cleaning the skin without drying it out.

Castor Oil: Castor oil is a heavy, emollient oil which can be used in a variety of cosmetic recipes. It can act as a fixative in colognes because it dissolves readily in alcohol and then helps slow evap-oration of the volatile oils after it is applied to the skin. It can be found in the health food section of supermarkets, in health food stores, in pharmacies, and through mail-order.

Cream of Tartar: This is a by-product left after the fermentation of grapes into wine. It is an acid which is used in baking to stabi-lize beaten egg whites, among other things. It is used in some foot bath recipes in combination with baking soda to create an effer-vescence. Cream of tartar can be found in the spice section of the supermarket. If you can't find it, tartaric acid, which is at your local pharmacy, may be used in foot baths.

Essential Oils: The term "essential oil" is used throughout this book. It is important to understand that there is a big difference between an "essential" oil and a "fragrance" or "craft" oil. An essential oil is the volatile oil of a plant. It holds the fragrance and other properties of that plant which are valuable for culi-nary and therapeutic uses. The essential oil is stored in differ-ent areas of the plant, depending upon the plant variety. The extraction can be very labor-intensive and, therefore, a very ex-pensive process.

A "fragrance" or "craft" oil is a cheaper, synthetic version of an essential oil. It may have a similar fragrance, but it does not pos-sess the same therapeutic properties. It is *not* recommended that you use *any* synthetic oils or synthetic ingredients in homemade cosmetics. Not only will they lack the deep aromas and charac-teristics of pure essential oils, they may also cause allergic reac-tions to the skin. (Some pure essential oils can cause skin irritations as well. *See* "Allergic Reactions," below.) Sources for reputable pure essential oils are given in the "Source Guide" at the back of this book. They can also be found at some health food stores.

Glycerine: This thick, clear liquid occurs in the fat of most animals and vegetables in combination with fatty acids. It is a very common ingredient in commercial cosmetics because it is able to hold moisture against the surface of the skin and helps prevent drying. It mixes well with water and dissolves in alcohol. It can be found at pharmacies and through mail-order.

Grapeseed Oil: This oil is a bit more expensive but is far less greasy than other oils. It is very good for delicate, sensitive skin. It can be found in some health food stores or through mail-order.

Jojoba Bean Oil: This oil is terrific in body products because it is very similar to the skin's naturally secreted oils. It can be found at most health food stores or through mail-order.

Oatmeal: This morning cereal actually makes a wonderful cosmetic ingredient! It has mild cleansing properties and is beneficial to dry, sensitive skin. Be sure to buy the old-fashioned oats in the cereal section of the supermarket, not "quick-cooking" oats.

Sunflower Oil: This is a light and inexpensive oil which can be found in most health food stores and supermarkets and through mail-order.

Tincture of Benzoin: Tincture of benzoin is an alcohol-based product made from a gum resin secreted from the *Styrax benzoin* tree. It can usually be found in the antibacterial section of the pharmacy. You can also create your own by ordering Gum Benzoin *(Styrax benzoin)* through the mail and making a tincture using grain alcohol or vodka. (*See* "tinctures" in the terminology section of this chapter.) It is used in cosmetics as a preservative.

EQUIPMENT

There is really no special equipment required other than standard kitchen items such as pots, pans, and measuring tools. It is best to use stainless steel, enamel, or glass when making cosmetics to prevent a chemical reaction. Wash all equipment and storage containers in hot soapy water before using to make sure that everything is immaculately clean. (Any bacteria on your equipment will cause your cosmetics to prematurely spoil.)

Allergic Reactions

Most of the commercial cosmetics on the market today are made with synthetics and preservatives which can be very irritating to people with sensitive skin. Although homemade cosmetics are free from synthetics and preservatives, there is still the possibility of an allergic reaction to a particular herb or other ingredient. If you have sensitive skin or are worried about allergies, it is wise to do a patch test on each new cosmetic before spreading it all over your face or body. Once a particular sensitivity is known, that ingredient can be avoided, allowing your homemade creations to be problem-free.

PATCH TEST

Patch Test for Homemade Cosmetics: Place a small amount of the cosmetic mixture onto the inside crease of your arm and cover it with a Band-Aid. Wait 24 hours. If you have no reaction, then the cosmetic is safe to use. However, if you have any redness, hives, or swelling, then you are allergic and should avoid that mixture!

Patch Test for Just Herbs: Chop approximately 1 teaspoon of the herb in question and mix it with a small amount of plain water. Place this mixture onto the inside crease of your arm. Cover with a 100% cotton ball and a Band-Aid to hold in place. Leave the patch on for 24 hours. Remove the patch and check for a reaction. If you see no reaction, then the herb is safe to use.

PRESERVATIVES

Some of the ingredients in homemade cosmetics such as tincture of benzoin or alcohol have preservative properties and can help prolong the life of your mixtures. However, none of the recipes will last as long as commercial cosmetics. Try to use up your mixtures within a few months unless otherwise advised in the recipe. Lotions and creams have a longer shelf life if stored in the refrigerator. Colognes, bath bags, and bath oils can be stored on a shelf or in a dark cupboard away from direct sunlight. If you ever notice a bad smell coming from one of your mixtures, it has probably spoiled and should be discarded.

FIXATIVES

Fixatives are used in perfumery and potpourri making. They "fix" or hold the fragrance and make it long-lasting. Castor oil, tincture of benzoin, and glycerine can be used in cosmetics as fixatives. Some essential oils such as sandalwood and patchouli also have this property.

TERMINOLOGY

TINCTURES

A *tincture* is the result of steeping plant material in a solvent (usually alcohol or vinegar) to extract the essential elements of that particular plant. The mixture is a concentrated form of the plant's key elements, which can then be easily added to cosmetics. To make a tincture, the solvent is usually heated and the plant material is added and allowed to steep. Then the mixture is strained and bottled for later use. Although this method is similar to making a tea, the tincture is more concentrated because the alcohol is able to dissolve and hold more of the plant's compounds than just water alone.

INFUSION

An *infusion* is the result of steeping plant material in plain hot water (like tea). An infusion is not as concentrated as a tincture but does contain some of the essential elements of the plant material. It can be used in hair rinses, colognes, and toilet waters.

BAIN-MARIE

Bain-marie is a fancy term for a hot water bath which is a cooking method used to heat ingredients slowly. In cosmetics, a bain-marie refers to a pan of water on a stove which has a bowl sitting on top of it. The water in the pan is brought to a simmer and the cosmetic ingredients are placed in the bowl. The steam from the pan gently heats the bowl and prevents the ingredients from overheating. A double boiler is a type of bain-marie.

PERFUMES, COLOGNES, AND TOILET WATERS

Many of the old herbals use the terms *perfume, cologne,* and *toilet water* interchangeably. However, by today's standards, there are differences. A perfume has a strong fragrance and usually contains up to 30% aromatic oil. It is very concentrated and is only dabbed on the skin in small quantities. A homemade perfume can be very costly to make, so this chapter will cover less-expensive body fragrances: i.e., colognes and toilet waters.

A cologne has a softer fragrance than perfume and only contains 1–5% aromatic oil. It usually contains alcohol but may also contain water or oil. Cologne can be used like a perfume, added to bath water, or used as a body splash after a shower.

A toilet water is even lighter in fragrance than a cologne and usually consists of an herbal infusion (herbs brewed in hot water, like tea). It is almost always used as a body splash and is expected to impart softening qualities to the skin.

Most homemade colognes and toilet waters contain some

amount of alcohol to help preserve the mixture. Alcohol also increases evaporation when it is applied to the skin. It is through this evaporation that the fragrance molecules enter the air and allow the essences to be detected by the nose. Unfortunately, recipes with large amounts of alcohol can be very drying to the skin. To counter this dryness, a small amount of glycerine or oil is usually included in the recipes.

Gardener's Hand Salve

Our hands are exposed to more harsh elements than any other part of our body, and yet, most of us neglect them completely. Gardeners should be especially careful with their hands because garden activities can expose them to cuts, scrapes, bacteria, and infection. Many of the ingredients in this salve (calendula, aloe vera, and tea tree oil) can be very helpful in healing and preventing these problems.

Calendula *(Calendula officinalis)* is very healing and is known for its anti-inflammatory and antibacterial properties. Aloe vera has anti-inflammatory and moisturizing properties and tea tree essential oil *(Melaleuca alternifolia)* is extremely antiseptic. These components combine to form this very healing salve. Just smooth it on your hands at night after a long day in the garden.

INGREDIENTS:

1/4 cup sweet almond oil
1 tbsp. dried calendula flowers
4 tsp. grated or finely chopped beeswax
6 drops tea tree essential oil
1 tsp. aloe vera gel
1/8 tsp. tincture of benzoin

1. Heat oil in a pan over a low flame until just warm. Remove from heat and add calendula flowers. Stir well, cover pan, and sit aside for 2 hours.

2. Strain out flowers and pour oil into a double boiler or bain-marie. Add beeswax. Heat the oil mixture while stirring constantly until the wax is completely melted. Immediately remove from heat and stir in tea tree essential oil.
3. Pour warm oil mixture into a mixing bowl. Add the aloe vera and tincture of benzoin. Use a whisk or electric mixer to beat the mixture vigorously until well blended (about 3 minutes).
4. Pour into a clean container with a tight-fitting lid. Set aside to cool. Store in the refrigerator and use within 3 months.

YIELD: APPROXIMATELY 2 OZ.

Chamomile Moisturizing Lotion

Chamomile has wonderful soothing and anti-inflammatory properties. To reap the benefits of this healing herb, this recipe combines a chamomile infusion with moisturizing oils to create a lotion that is very beneficial to sensitive or dry skin.

Of the three possible oils you can use in this lotion, grapeseed oil is the least greasy. It just vanishes into the skin!

INGREDIENTS:

1/3 cup distilled water
2 chamomile tea bags or 2 tsp. dried chamomile flowers
1/4 tsp. borax powder
1/2 cup sweet almond oil, grapeseed oil, or sunflower oil
1 tbsp. grated or finely chopped beeswax
8 drops roman chamomile essential oil, lemon essential oil, or other favorite essential oil

1. In a small pan, heat the distilled water to almost boiling. Add the chamomile and set aside for about 10 minutes.
2. Strain out the chamomile and add the borax powder. Reheat the water over a low flame until the borax is completely dissolved (about 1 minute). Remove from heat and set aside.

3. In a double boiler or bain-marie, combine oil and beeswax. Heat the oil mixture while stirring constantly until the wax is completely melted. Immediately remove from heat and stir in essential oil.
4. Pour warm oil into a mixing bowl. Use a whisk or an electric mixer to beat oil while slowly adding the warm water mixture. Beat the entire mixture for about 2 minutes.
5. Pour into a clean container, label, and store in a cool, dark place. Use within 5 months.

YIELD: APPROXIMATELY 6 OZ.

HOW IT WORKS . . .

A lotion or a cream is actually an emulsion: a mixture of oil and water which is stabilized so that it will not separate. As the oil and water mixture is beaten, tiny droplets of one liquid are dispersed throughout the other liquid. Under normal circumstances, oil and water repel each other and will eventually separate with the oil on top, water on the bottom. However, if an emulsifying agent such as borax or wax is added, the tiny droplets are coated and no longer repel the other liquid. The emulsion is formed and retains its mixed state for long periods of time.

Moisturizing Hand and Body Cream

This moisturizing cream is nongreasy and very versatile. You can use sweet almond oil, apricot kernel oil, or jojoba oil to create a very luxurious mixture. The aloe vera gel in this recipe makes the cream extremely soothing to the skin. Unfortunately, the addition of fresh aloe also requires this cream to be kept in the refrigerator. You will find that the chilled cream is actually quite refreshing! However, if you wish, you may substitute 2 tablespoons of water for the 2 tablespoons of aloe gel. The resulting cream is almost as nice and does not need to be refrigerated.

INGREDIENTS:

1/4 tsp. borax powder
2 tbsp. aloe vera gel
2 tbsp. distilled water
5 tbsp. sweet almond oil, apricot kernel oil, or jojoba oil
2 tsp. grated or finely chopped beeswax
10 drops lavender essential oil

1. In a small pan, combine the borax, aloe, and water. Heat gently until the borax is dissolved. Set aside.
2. In a double boiler or bain-marie, combine the oil and beeswax. Heat the oil mixture while stirring constantly until the wax is melted. Immediately remove from heat and stir in the lavender oil.
3. Pour the warm oil into a mixing bowl. Use a whisk or an electric mixer to beat the oil while slowly adding the warm water mixture. Beat the entire mixture for about 2 minutes.
4. Pour into a clean container with a tight-fitting lid. Label and store in the refrigerator. Use within 30 days. (If the aloe vera gel was omitted, the cream may be stored in a cool, dark place and used within 3–4 months.)

YIELD: APPROXIMATELY 4 OZ.

Lavender Cologne

Lavender, with its sweet and refreshing fragrance, has always been considered a valuable herb throughout history. Among the many royals who fancied lavender, Queen Elizabeth I of England was one of the most enthusiastic. She drank large amounts of lavender tea and spent exorbitant amounts of money on lavender perfume. She even commanded that her royal gardeners provide freshly cut lavender flowers, at a moment's notice, every day of the year! Not an easy task!

Although it may not be practical to expect fresh lavender blossoms every day, this cologne captures the essence of those lavender blossoms in a tincture which can be enjoyed anytime. Be sure to make more than one batch and give it as a gift to a special friend!

INGREDIENTS:

1/2 cup vodka
2 tbsp. dried lavender blossoms
12 drops lavender essential oil
1/4 tsp. castor oil

1. Place vodka in a glass jar and add dried lavender. Cover and let sit for 1 week.
2. After 1 week, strain out the lavender and add the essential oil and caster oil to the vodka. Cover the jar and shake vigorously.
3. Pour the cologne into a decorative jar. The cologne does not need to be refrigerated, but be sure to store it out of direct sunlight. Always shake mixture before using and use within 6 months.

YIELD: 4 OZ. COLOGNE

Victorian Toilet Water

For this old-time recipe, an herbal infusion is created using either the robust pine scent of rosemary, the cooling fragrance of lemon verbena, or the delicate perfume of rose-scented geraniums. Any one of these herbs helps create this lightly scented toilet water which can be used as a refreshing body splash after bathing.

INGREDIENTS:

1/2 cup fresh herb leaves (or 1/4 cup dried)
1 cup distilled water
1/4 cup vodka
1 tbsp. glycerine

1. Gather 1/2 cup fresh leaves of either rosemary, lemon verbena, or scented geranium from the garden (or substitute 1/4 cup dried).
2. In a small pan, heat the water to a boil.
3. Remove from heat and add the herb leaves. Stir, cover, and set aside for 1 hour.
4. Strain the herb infusion and add vodka and glycerine. Stir well.
5. Pour into a decorative bottle. Store in the refrigerator and use within 1 month.

YIELD: **12 oz.**

> *Sweet perfumes work immediately upon the spirits for their refreshing, sweet and healthful ayres are special preservatives to health and therefore much to be praised.*
>
> —Treatise of Fruite-Trees, 1653

Herbal Body Spritz

An herbal body spritz is a very easy way to revive your neglected skin throughout the day. Simply combine distilled water and essential herbal oil in a plastic spray bottle. Spritz your face, arms, and legs whenever you need a refreshing "wake-up call." The water will help moisturize your skin while the essential oil will impart some of its therapeutic components.

On hot summer days, keep a bottle of peppermint-scented

spritz in the refrigerator. Whenever the heat of the day gets to you, cool down with an aromatic misting. Keep a small 2 oz. bottle of lavender-scented spritz in your purse to soothe and refresh your skin throughout the work day.

Choose an essential oil from the list below and enjoy!

Essential Oils to Try:

Lavender *(Lavandula officinalis):* Very soothing.
Peppermint *(Mentha* x *piperita):* Has a cooling effect on the body.
Rose *(Rosa* spp.): Extremely expensive but very good for dry, sensitive skin.
Spearmint *(Mentha spicata):* Nice for irritated skin.

INGREDIENTS:

1 cup distilled water
10–12 drops of your favorite essential oil

Combine ingredients in a plastic spray bottle. Shake vigorously before each use. Spray the body spritz on your face, arms, and legs anytime you need a refreshing pick-me-up. The spritz does not need to be refrigerated. Use within 6 months.

YIELD: 1 CUP BODY SPRITZ.

Effervescent Foot Bath

In water, baking soda acts as a water softener and skin soother. When combined with an acid (in this case, cream of tartar), it creates carbon dioxide, which will fizzle away the stresses of the day. The carbon dioxide also helps release the peppermint oil into the air, which acts as another stress reliever. The herbs in this recipe will create an infusion in the bath water, thereby releasing their therapeutic properties. Use dried sage for aching muscles or lemon balm to cool your tired feet.

INGREDIENTS:

1/2 cup baking soda
1/2 cup cream of tartar (or tartaric acid)
6 drops peppermint essential oil
4 tbsp. dried sage or lemon balm

1. In a small bowl combine all ingredients and mix well. This mixture can be stored in an airtight jar for later use (or gift) or it can be used immediately.
2. To make a foot bath: Pour the dry bath mixture into a large owl. Add approximately 8–10 cups warm (not hot) water. Stir vigorously and immediately submerge your feet in the warm bath water. The foot bath will fizz for several minutes as the mixture dissolves. Soak feet for 10 minutes and then rinse.
3. Apply a moisturizing lotion to your feet and put on a pair of cotton socks. Your feet will love you for it!

YIELD: 1 FOOT BATH

Sweet Bath Bags

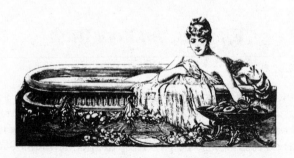

It may sound romantic to sprinkle herbs and flowers into your bath water, but it is not recommended. What doesn't stick to your body will probably clog up your drain! A sweet bath bag is an old-fashioned solution to this dilemma. An herb-filled bag is tied onto the bathtub spout so that as the tub is filled, the bath water flows through the bag, releasing the skin softening properties. While in the bath, you can use the bag as a washcloth, which will further release the soothing components.

You can personalize the mixture by choosing your favorite herb from the list below. The oatmeal and borax are included to soothe dry skin and soften the water. This recipe is so easy to make that you may want to prepare several batches at once. Keep the filled bags inside airtight jars until ready to use. (They make thoughtful gifts too.)

There are several things you can use to "bag" up this mixture:

1. You can sew sachet bags from 6-inch by 8-inch pieces of 100% cotton fabric. Just fold the fabric lengthwise with right sides together. (It will then be 8 × 3.) Stitch one of the 3 inch sides and the open 8 inch side. Leave the other 3 inch side open. It will be the top of the bag. Turn inside out and fill with your potpourri mixture. Tie the filled bath bags with ribbon or cotton string.

2. You can purchase large muslin "tea bags" from a health food store or one of the mail-order sources listed in this book. The "tea bags" should be 100% cotton and have draw-string ties.

3. You can use antique handkerchiefs! Just place the mixture in the center and tie closed with ribbon to form sachets.

4. Cut 10 inch circles from cotton fabric. Place 1/4 cup of mixture in the center and tie with ribbon.

INGREDIENTS:

1/2 cup borax
1/2 cup dried herbs (see Step 1 below*)*
2 cups oatmeal

1. Choose the herb you wish to use in the bath bag. Use rosemary or sage for a stimulating and invigorating bath. Use

chamomile or lavender blossoms for a calming and relaxing bath.
2. Combine all ingredients in a small bowl and stir well.
3. Place 1/4–1/2 cup of the mixture into each bag or handkerchief and tie securely.

YIELD: 6–12 BATH BAGS

"Garden-Fresh" Scented Bath Oil

This bath oil is one of the most luxurious gifts you can make for yourself or a friend! The dried flowers add color and elegance, the base oil nourishes and pampers the skin, and the fragrant essential oils soothe the spirit. It is important that the flowers and spices used are completely dry. Any moisture will make the final bath oil cloudy. If you choose to use rose buds or rose petals, choose light-colored flowers. Deep colors such as red tend to turn black when dried.

The spices listed are more for show than for fragrance. Choose the ones you have available. The sweet almond oil makes an excellent base oil. The jojoba oil can add more nourishing properties to the bath oil, but is not necessary. If it is difficult to find, simply substitute more almond oil in its place.

INGREDIENTS:

dried flowers and herbs such as: lavender, larkspur, love-in-a-mist, globe amaranth, lemon verbena, miniature rose buds, rose petals, calendula petals, etc.
1 cinnamon stick
4 whole allspice (optional)
2 whole star anise (optional)
6 oz. glass bottle
4 oz. sweet almond oil

2 oz. jojoba oil (optional)
10 drops lavender essential oil
5 drops lemon or orange essential oil
raffia or ribbon for decoration

1. Place sprigs of the dried herbs and flowers inside the clean 6 oz. bottle. They will add color as well as some fragrance to the final product. Break the cinnamon stick in half and add it to the bottle. Add the other spices to the bottle if you choose to use them.
2. In a clean bowl, combine the almond oil, jojoba, and essential oils. Stir well. Using a funnel, pour the oil mixture into the bottle until full. Tie the top with raffia or ribbon.
3. Let the mixture sit for 1 week to allow the scents to blend. To use: add 1–2 tbsp. of the bath oil to your bath water for soft and supple skin.

YIELD: **6 OZ.**

FOR TIRED, PUFFY EYES . . .

Chamomile has wonderful anti-inflammatory properties! Take two chamomile tea bags, dip them in cool water, and squeeze out the excess. Lie down and place one tea bag over each eye. Relax for 10 minutes.

Rose-Scented Facial Steam

Victorian women had a real love affair with roses. They were valued not only for their unequaled beauty, but for their fragrance, flavor, and medicinal uses as well. During the Victorian Era, the nighttime ritual of steaming the face with rose-scented water was very popular. This old-fashioned method is actually very efficient at cleansing the pores and softening the skin. Be sure to deeply inhale the rose fragrance as it can be very soothing and relaxing at the end of the day.

For variety, you can substitute one of the herbs listed below for the rose petals and scented geranium leaves.

Note: If you have very sensitive skin or tiny spider veins on your skin, it is *not* recommended that you ever use a facial steam.

INGREDIENTS:

> 1 1/2 cups fresh rose petals
> 1/2 cup fresh rose-scented geranium leaves
> 8 cups distilled water

1. Wash your face with a mild cleanser and pat dry.
2. In a large pan, bring the water almost to a boil and then remove from heat. Add rose petals and scented geranium leaves and stir well.
3. Set the pan on top of a towel on a sturdy surface. Hold your face over the steaming pan and use a towel to make a tent over your head to catch the steam. Keep your eyes closed and your face at least 10 inches away from the water's surface to prevent burning.
4. Inhale deeply and sit quietly for 6–8 minutes.
5. Rinse your face several times with cool water. Pat dry and apply a moisturizer.

Other herbs can be used in a facial steam. Try one of these or a combination! You will need approximately 1–2 cups of loosely packed fresh herbs to 8 cups of distilled water.

Chamomile: *Healing and soothing.*
Fennel leaves: *Astringent.*

Peppermint: *Cooling and refreshing.*
Rosemary: *Healing and stimulating.*

YIELD: **1** FACIAL STEAM

Herbal Hair Rinse

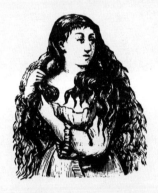

An herbal hair rinse is one of the easiest beauty products to make!
Basically, it is just a cold herbal tea (an infusion) which is used as
the final rinse after you shampoo. It does not remove tangles, but
can add shine and luster to your hair.

Choose the appropriate herb from the following:

Chamomile blossoms—*for light brown or blond hair.*
Sage or rosemary—*for dark hair.*
Lavender or basil—*for any hair type.*

INGREDIENTS:

8 cups water
1 cup fresh herbs (1/2 cup if dried)

1. Bring the water almost to a boil. Remove from heat and stir
   in herbs. Cover and let steep for 2 hours.

2. Strain mixture.
3. To use, simply pour the herbal rinse over your hair as the final step after shampooing. Do not rinse out.
4. Store any leftover rinse in the refrigerator and use within 1 week.

YIELD: 1 QUART

Chapter 8

⚜

Herbal Flower Arranging

> The joy of being able to cut flowers freely, lavishly, to decorate the house and to give to friends is an end that justifies a lot of gardening effort.
>
> —T. H. EVERETT

Flower arranging is a fun way to express creativity and bring a bit of the garden indoors for others to enjoy. By adding freshly cut herbs to floral arrangements, you can create unusual designs which make memorable impressions on family and friends. Herbs are terrific as floral bouquets because they hold up well and they add their own unique texture, fragrance, and charm.

There is no reason to feel intimidated about flower arranging. You can easily create charming arrangements on your own with just some basic knowledge and a little practice. The more you practice, the better you will get. You don't have to be a professional floral designer in order to create impressive arrangements. However, if you feel you need extra help, enroll in a floral design class at your local community college or park/recreation center. You will soon discover that flower arranging is an extremely rewarding craft because it is a celebration of the garden and gives pleasure to everyone who sees your work.

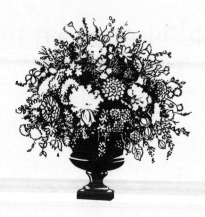

Suggested Materials and Tools

Plant Material: Almost all herbs work well in flower arrangements. Add cut flowers and other greenery to your herbs for added interest and color.

Floral Foam: This material is sometimes referred to by the brand name "Oasis." This is a green, spongy material which is used to hold the cut flowers and provide water. It usually comes in foam "bricks," which can be purchased at craft stores and floral supply stores. It can easily be cut with a knife to the desired size. Floral foam should be soaked for one hour in fresh water before being used in arrangements.

Scissors/Floral Knife/Clippers: A pair of sharp, clean scissors or a floral knife is needed for cutting plant material. Garden clippers may be necessary for woody items.

Containers: Just about any container can be used for flower arranging, as long as it is sturdy enough to hold the arrangement without tipping over. Try using watering cans, teapots, and flowerpots. Be sure to clean containers thoroughly to help reduce bacteria. If baskets or flowerpots are used, line them with papier-mâché liners from floral supply stores or plastic trash bags which are cut to size.

Florist Wire: Florist wire is a metal wire which comes on a paddle or spool. It is available in different gauges (thicknesses) from craft stores and floral supply stores. For flower arranging, a 24 or 26 gauge wire is usually sufficient. The wire is used in wreath and garland making and is used to wrap groups of plant material together securely.

Floral Stem Tape: This paper-based tape comes on a roll in either green, brown, or white. It has a sticky surface which is exposed as it is gently stretched. If you wrap it around a small grouping of stems, it sticks to itself and holds the stems together securely without pins. It can also be used to cover a wired stem, thereby hiding the "mechanics."

Green Floral Tape: This is different from floral stem tape. It is more like green masking tape and is found in craft stores and floral supply stores. It is used to tape floral foam into containers. Usually two pieces are taped in a crisscross fashion across the top of the floral foam and onto the container. The tape holds well, even when wet. It is not an essential tool, but can be very helpful with top-heavy arrangements.

Floral Frogs: Sometimes called pinholders or hairpin holders, these small metal objects are set in the bottom of the floral container and help hold the plant stems in place. Some of them look like mini "beds of nails" and the stems are embedded on the spiked ends. Others are just made of metal meshing that allows the stems to poke through. They come in all shapes, sizes, and colors. You can sometimes find used ones at garage sales for a few cents. You can purchase new ones at floral supply stores. They are usually only a few dollars, depending upon the size.

Preparing Your Plant Material

Herbs are very long-lasting in water and floral foam. However, it is important to note that in order for any plant material to hold up well, it must be picked and conditioned properly before being arranged.

Pick your materials in the morning, after the morning dew has dried but before the heat of the day hits them. Cut the stems at a 45-degree angle to obtain a maximum surface for water absorption. Use very sharp scissors or a sharp florist knife to cut stems. For woody stems such as rosemary, use pruning shears. Remove the foliage on the bottom half of the stems. After cutting, immediately place the plants in a bucket of room temperature water (not ice cold).

Conditioning

Conditioning means to process the plant material so that it will last longer in the arrangement. Usually this means soaking the plant material in water for several hours to rehydrate and prevent shock. But for really long-lasting arrangements, a chemical floral preservative may be added to the water to feed the plants and prevent bacteria from forming. Using a commercial chemical preservative is an optional step. (*Do not use a chemical preservative on any herb or flower to be eaten!* Use it only on plant material to be arranged.)

Commercial preservatives can be purchased from floral supply stores, nurseries, or even your local florist. Each brand comes with instructions on how much preservative to add to your water. Let your herbs and flowers soak in this preservative solution for several hours or overnight and use the mixture to water your finished arrangement.

WHAT IS IN A COMMERCIAL FLORAL PRESERVATIVE?

1. Antibacterial agents (bacteria will clog pores of the stems and cause arrangements to wilt faster).
2. Dextrose (to feed the plants).
3. Acidifiers (acidity inhibits bacteria growth).

You can make your own floral preservative by adding 1 teaspoon household bleach to each gallon of water! Although this will not feed the plants, it will keep the bacteria levels down.

CARE OF FLORAL ARRANGEMENTS

1. Keep fresh flowers out of direct sunlight.
2. Change the water frequently to prevent bacteria buildup.
3. Recut the stems in vase arrangements once per week.

BASIC FLORAL DESIGN STEPS

1. Prepare your container for the arrangement; i.e., clean it and add floral foam.
2. Place in your greenery and/or your tallest plant material to give an outline of the arrangement. This will determine the size and shape of your finished design. Work within this outline.
3. Begin adding flowers and herbs to fill in the outline. Don't crowd your flowers. (This is a tough one, because the tendency is to put *all* the flowers you have in one arrangement.) Of course, you don't want to waste the beautiful plant material, but try to use restraint. Place the leftover flowers in a small vase.
4. Pay attention to the textures of the plant material. By varying the textures you get a more interesting design.

5. Use odd (rather than even) numbers of flowers. They are easier to work with and they form a more pleasing pattern.
6. Place larger, heavier flowers at the heart or center of your design.
7. Place smaller, brighter flowers at the outer edges.

Design Shapes

Flower arrangements can be made in many different shapes, but there are four designs which lend themselves to herbal arranging: round, triangular, S-curved, and vegetative.

1. ***The Round or Oval Arrangement:*** This is the type of arrangement you see used as a centerpiece or coffee table display because it looks good from all angles. The trick to making a nice round arrangement is to make all the stems appear as though they are radiating from one central point.

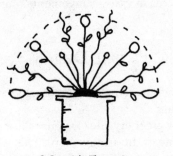

© Copyright Theresa Loe

2. ***The Triangular and L-shaped Arrangement:*** Triangular arrangements are great against walls and in corners. When you step back and look at this arrangement, it has a very clear triangle outline. It should be equally balanced on both sides and the stems should appear to radiate from one central point. An L-shaped arrangement is basically 1/2 of a triangular arrangement. It is asymmetrical with the heavy, dark-colored flowers placed toward the center.

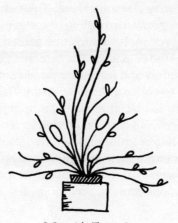

© Copyright Theresa Loe

3. *The S-Shaped Arrangement:* Sometimes called a *Hogarth Curve,* this type of design resembles a very curvy *S*. It must be designed on a pedestal or stemmed container like a candlestick. The heavy, darker flowers should be at the center with wispy greenery forming the *S*.

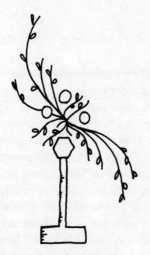

© Copyright Theresa Loe

4. *The Vegetative Arrangement:* This casual design style is also known as a *garden grouping* or *cottage garden* design. The arrangement resembles a miniature garden and appears to be growing out of the container. They are best displayed against a wall. Short greenery and leaves are placed around the edges of the container to conceal the floral foam. Then each variety of flower or herb is placed in small groupings as if they are growing in clusters. Tall, vertical groupings are placed toward the back, first. Shorter groupings are then placed toward the front. The plants intermingle to form a "cottage garden" look. Avoid exotic flowers. Use cottage plants in soft pastel colors such as feverfew, delphinium, oregano, roses, and carnations.

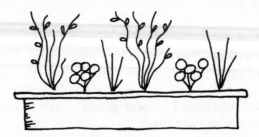

© Copyright Theresa Loe

Basic Round Arrangement for Beginners

This arrangement is very simple to make and looks quite lovely on a coffee table or as a centerpiece. The container should be a very pretty bowl with high sides, such as a crystal candy bowl, round flower vase, or rose bowl. You will need five medium- to large-sized flowers such as lilies, carnations, roses, and gardenias. They will be the main focus of the arrangement. Your greenery (or background material) will be herbal. Sage, marjoram, artemisia, or oregano are perfect choices for the greenery. Variegated varieties such as golden sage are even better! The accent material will also be herbal (accent material is anything that is light and airy such as baby's breath). Try using the seed heads of fennel, dill, salad burnet, or parsley as your accent material.

This arrangement calls for a floral frog (*see* "Suggested Materials and Tools" above). If you do not have one, you can still make the arrangement. A frog just makes it a little easier to keep the greenery in place. But it is not necessary.

MATERIALS:

1 crystal or glass bowl
5 flowers (see above)
greenery material (see above)
few sprigs of accent material (see above)
1 small flower-arranging frog
clippers

1. Cut and condition all of your plant material. Make sure that your container and floral frog are clean.
2. Cut your greenery to about 4–6 inches long and place it in your container. Continue until the entire container is loosely filled (not packed) with the greenery material. (Be sure to keep the arrangement in a round shape.)
3. Cut each flower to about 4–6 inches long. Place it in the container so that each flower is evenly space throughout the greenery.
4. Add a few sprigs of your accent material and you are done!

FRESH HERBAL WREATHS

Decorating with wreaths has origins in ancient cultures all over the world. Wreaths symbolized everything from "good luck" to "victory." Today, they are usually hung on front doors or walls as a symbol of hospitality and welcome. If they are laid flat on a table, wreaths can become centerpieces and punch bowl decorations. By using fresh herbs and flowers from the garden, you can create inexpensive, colorful, and aromatic versions of this old-time decoration. The other advantage to using fresh herbs is that they can be allowed to dry right on the wreath base, which then creates a fragrant, long-lasting dried flower decoration. By adding a few dried flowers or a ribbon, you have a decoration that will last a year or more.

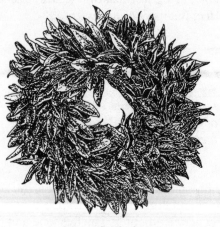

© Copyright Wheeler Arts

A wreath is not just a Christmas decoration. It can be made anytime of the year and is actually most delightful in the spring and summer. It is during this time that the garden is at its peak and the choices of plant material are endless. Easter wreaths, May Day wreaths, and Mother's Day wreaths are fun to create and they add a new twist to each holiday.

Plant Material: Most herbs do very well in wreaths, with the exception of some delicate herbs such as basil, borage blossoms, dill, and fennel. If you use these delicate herbs, their foliage will wilt quickly. More durable herbs would be bay, borage leaves, feverfew, hyssop, lamb's ears, lemon verbena, marjoram, mint, oregano, rosemary, sage, santolina, savory, southernwood, sweet woodruff, tarragon, thyme, wormwood, and yarrow. Any type of woody plant usually does well also. Feverfew is excellent in all types of flower-arranging projects. The flowers hold up very well both in and out of the water.

Wreath Base: The wreath base is the framework of the wreath. It can be a heavy wire circle, a floral foam wreath, a grapevine wreath, a moss or straw wreath, etc. You can purchase the wreath base at a floral supply or craft store. (Mail-order sources are given in the "Source Guide.") You can also fashion your own out of heavy twigs and wire. Many people prefer the grapevine or straw wreath bases because they are sturdy and natural looking.

MATERIALS:

several small buckets of fresh plant material
one 10–12-inch wreath base
1 paddle or spool of 24 gauge florist wire
garden clippers
ribbon

1. Pick your plant material and place it in small buckets of water until you are ready to design your wreath. Cut the plant material so that each sprig is about 6 inches long. For an interesting design, you may want to choose several different textures and shades of green herbs. If herbs such as feverfew, hyssop, mint, marjoram, and thyme are flowering, be sure to include them for extra color.
2. Wrap a length of wire around your wreath base and twist it securely. Do not cut the wire. You are going to use this wire to wrap each bundle of herbs onto the base in one continuous piece.
3. Take a handful of one herb variety (about 5–8 stems, depending upon its size) and lay it on the wreath base. Wrap the spool of wire around the bundle's stems once or twice to secure it. Pull tightly.
4. Take another small handful of a different herb and lay it in the same direction on the wreath base so that its leaves cover the stems of the first bundle. Wrap the wire around to secure it. Sometimes you will need to lay bundles next to each other in order to cover the sides of the wreath base. Continue in this manner until you have covered the entire base with herbs. To attach the last bundle, lift the leaves of the first bundle and tuck the stems underneath. Wrap as usual.

5. Tie off the wire by wrapping it several times and twisting it around itself to secure. Make a loop of wire and attach it to the back so that the wreath can be hung easily.

> The technique described here can be used to create a dried wreath too! Instead of attaching fresh bundles of herbs, use dried bundles of herbs. Incorporate a few pods, dried flowers, and ribbon to give a festive look.

GARLAND

Oh Brignal banks are wild and fair,
And Greta woods are green,
And you may gather garlands there
Would grace a summer queen.

—Sir Walter Scott, 1813

Garlands have been used as decorations since ancient times but they became popular in America during the Colonial era. Frugal housewives made garlands of fruits and vegetables and hung them to dry—this was one way to preserve food for the harsh winters. Later, garlands became popular Christmas decorations as well. Today, garlands can be used to decorate windows, fireplaces, mirrors, tables, and even hats all year round! They are popular at weddings and garden parties too.

There are several different ways to make a garland. One of the easiest is to attach bundles of fresh herbs to a rope or string. A long rope can be used to make a swag and a short string can be wrapped around a hat base. Use the same plant material that is described in "Fresh Herbal Wreaths," above. For this technique of garland making, you need foliage that can hold up fairly well out of water.

MATERIALS:

1/4-inch-thick rope or cording cut to desired length
fresh herb sprigs cut 3–5 inches long
other decorations such as straw flowers, fresh flowers,
  baby's breath, etc.
Spool or paddle of florist wire, 24 or 26 gauge
ribbon for the ends

1. Tie a knot onto each end of the rope and then tie one end of the rope to a stationary object, such as a doorknob or post.
2. Beginning at the end that is tied to the stationary object, gather a small bundle of cut herbs and lay them on the rope with the cut ends pointing toward to you. Wrap the wire around the ends of the herbs several times to secure them onto the rope. Do not cut the wire; just leave it on the spool as you work. Take another small handful of herbs and lay them in the same direction so that their leaves cover the wired stems of the first bundle. Wrap the wire around their stems several times to secure them to the rope. Continue in this fashion, working down from the tied end of the garland. As you work, you can add baby's breath, straw flowers, or fresh cut flowers throughout the garland.
3. When you reach the end of the garland, tie off the wire. Add a large, festive bow to each end of the rope. Once hung, the garland will look fresh for about three days to one week (or longer), depending upon the plant material used and the climate. (Obviously, high temperatures will dry out the garland faster.)

TOPIARY

Creating a topiary or standard from a live plant has been a popular gardening technique for hundreds of years. It involves meticulous pruning and care. However, you can create a freshly cut topiary in just a few minutes with plant material from the garden.

The results may last for only a week or two, but you don't have to put in months of pruning to achieve it.

A topiary like this one can be used as a centerpiece or hallway decoration. If you make a fragrant pair of topiaries, you can set them on either side of a doorway or mirror. Craft cement, called plaster of Paris, is used in this project because it cures quickly. It is available at craft supply stores. It not only holds the doweling "stem" in place, but adds weight to the bottom of the pot, which prevents toppling over. Once you make the topiary structure, it can be used again and again throughout the year. Just add fresh floral foam and plant material when you need it for a special occasion.

If you can't find plaster of Paris, you can use dry floral foam or sierra foam (for dried flower arranging) in the bottom of the pot to hold the doweling. The only problem with this is that it will not be as sturdy and will not have the added weight to keep it from toppling over. But in a pinch, it will work.

MATERIALS:

2 plastic flowerpot saucers, 4-inch diameter
1 nail
a hammer
one 2–3-foot piece of 1-inch doweling
6–8-inch clay flowerpot
plaster of Paris
1 block floral foam
floral tape to hold down floral foam
hot glue gun
gray Spanish moss
raffia and/or ribbon
several small buckets of plant material, cut into 6–8-inch
  lengths

1. Nail one of the plastic saucers onto one end of the doweling. Set the second saucer inside the first as a liner. This will form the top of the topiary and hold the floral foam without leaking.

2. Place some plastic or paper in the bottom of the clay flowerpot to plug up the hole. Add water to the plaster of Paris (according to the instructions on the bag) and pour it into the flowerpot, leaving 1 inch of space from the top of the pot. Immediately place the doweling into the cement to form the stem of the topiary. Set it aside to dry completely.
3. Cut a piece of the floral foam to fit inside the 4-inch plastic saucer. Soak it in water for at least an hour and then set it in the plastic saucer. Place two pieces of floral tape across the top and onto the saucer in a criss-cross fashion to hold the foam securely.
4. Use the hot glue gun to cover the doweling and bottom of the plastic saucer with moss. You want the doweling to look like a mossy stem and you don't want any of the plastic to show. Place some moss over the cement in the flowerpot to conceal it. (A piece of raffia or ribbon can be glued to the bottom of the saucer and wrapped down the stem to the top of the flowerpot for added interest if you wish.)
5. Begin placing plant material into the floral foam, forming a round ball shape. Be sure to place some greenery over the edge of the saucer to hide the mechanics of the arrangement.
6. Add flowering herbs, flowers, and pods to the arrangement until the topiary is completely filled in. Add a bow if you wish.
7. Water the topiary lightly every day and keep it out of direct light. It should last for a week or more (just like a regular flower arrangement).

Chapter 9

Scenting the Home

There are many old-fashioned ways to bring fragrance into the home with herbs. One of the oldest is through the use of potpourri. Potpourri is an aromatic mixture of flowers, herbs, spices, and essential oils which can be used to scent and freshen a musty room, closet, or drawer. Although the term *potpourri* was not specifically used for this preparation until the about eighteenth century, the practice of making aromatic mixtures, like potpourri, dates back to ancient Egypt. Since the Victorian Era, potpourri recipes have become an increasingly popular way to add fragrance to the home. However, there are many other ways to scent the home, and the recipes in this chapter go beyond typical potpourri recipes. They offer new ways to use potpourri, freshly cut herbs, and fragrant essential oils.

Using herbs to scent the home is not only a great way to bring in the outdoors, it's practical too! It's nice to use these aromatic recipes rather than relying on commercial products which use synthetic fragrances and chemicals. The all-natural preparations are far superior in scent, and they are inexpensive to make. For example, some herbs such as lavender and pennyroyal have insect-repelling qualities and can be used by themselves or in potpourri mixtures to repel certain bugs. They can be hung fresh in cupboards, sprinkled over a pet's bedding, or tucked in with woolen articles. Their fragrance will beat out commercially made moth balls any day of the week!

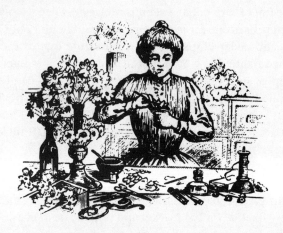

TERMINOLOGY

Fixatives: In perfumery and potpourri making there is one important ingredient which helps the product retain its scent for longer periods of time. This ingredient is called a *fixative.* It is especially important to use a fixative when you are making potpourri as sachets or moth repellants because they must last for longer than a few weeks. The fixative will "fix" or "hold" the scent of the mixture.

There are several natural materials which have fixative characteristics. For many years, the most common fixative was orris root *(Iris germanica),* which is the tuber of the Florentine iris. It is an excellent fixative and is readily available from craft and fragrance supply companies. However, many people are allergic to orris root (especially in powdered form). It can cause red, irritated eyes and an itchy nose. If you are not allergic to orris root, you will find that it is a superior product. But if you are making fragrant products to sell or give as gifts, you may want to use an alternate fixative.

There are several other plants, resins, and barks which can be used as fixatives in recipes, such as oakmoss *(Evernia prunastri)*, cellulose fiber (corn cobs), calamus root/sweet flag *(Acorus calamus)*, gum benzoin *(Styrax benzoin)*, patchouli *(Pogostemon cablin)*, and cedar chips. You can substitute one of the abovementioned fixatives for orris root in any recipe. For quick, primitive recipes, such as vacuum cleaner sachets, you can even use vermiculite (from your local garden center) as an inexpensive fixative. But vermiculite is limited in its fixative qualities and is not appropriate for potpourris which are to be seen. (It looks tacky and strange.)

Oakmoss has a woodsy scent and is one of the most popular alternatives to orris root. As with all the fixatives listed in this chapter, it can be purchased through mail-order. Cellulose fiber is a fairly new fixative on the market and is made from cut or ground corn cobs. It is very absorbent and you may need to increase the amount of essential oil you use in order to get a strong fragrance. You will find most of the abovementioned fixatives in two forms: cut/sifted or powdered. The cut form is usually best because the powdered form tends to leak from sachets and create a dusty film. The cut form also seems to hold the fragrance longer.

You will notice that some of the potpourri recipes in this chapter include a fixative. Others are either not potpourri or are for immediate use (such as "simmering herbs") and therefore do not need a fixative.

Sachets: Sachets are small bags or bundles filled with potpourri, perfumed powder, or just fragrant herbs. The Victorians called them "sweet bags." There are several things you can use to package sachets. For a simple sachet, you can place several spoonfuls of the mixture in the middle of a cheesecloth square or a fabric square, which is then tied with string. Or you can purchase cotton tea bags to fill with your herb mixture (*see* the "Source Guide" for mail-order sources). For a more romantic look, you can place some of the sachet mixture inside an antique handkerchief and tie it closed with a festive ribbon. If you have the time to sew, rectangular fabric bags are quite charming when filled with potpourri and tied with ribbon. No matter how the sachet is packaged, it will smell wonderful and add a bit of the garden to your home.

S*weet* B*ags*

These sweet bags are just general, all-purpose sachets, filled with the sweet fragrances of the garden. They can be used to perfume drawers, closets, and cupboards that are filled with linens, clothes, or stationery. Sweet bags can also be hung on bedposts, doorknobs, or the backs of chairs to add fragrance to the room.

A sweet bag is definitely worth making for yourself or a dear friend. It also makes an excellent present for someone who is ill or bedridden. When tucked inside bed pillows, it cheers them up with the wonderful perfumes of the outdoors. Since a sweet bag is more likely to be seen, you should make it out of old hankies or pretty pieces of fabric. Keep your eye out for such items at flea markets and garage sales.

Recipe 1: Lemon Sweet Bag

MATERIALS:

1/2 cup oakmoss, cut and sifted
8 drops essential oil of lemon
4 drops essential oil of lavender
1 cup dried lemon verbena leaves
1/2 cup dried lemon grass leaves
1/2 cup dried rosemary leaves
4 handkerchiefs or 6 eight-inch squares of fabric
matching ribbon

Recipe 2: Sweet Woodruff Bag

MATERIALS:

1/2 cup oakmoss, cut and sifted
6 drops rose oil or rose geranium oil
4 drops carnation or cinnamon oil
1 1/2 cups dried sweet woodruff
1 cup dried rose-scented geranium leaves
1 vanilla bean, chopped into pieces
1 tbsp. whole allspice
1 tbsp. whole cloves
5 handkerchiefs or 6–8 eight-inch squares of fabric
matching ribbon

1. Choose one of the recipes above and gather the ingredients.
   In a medium-sized glass jar with a tight-fitting lid, combine
   oakmoss with the essential oils. Shake well. Set aside for 3
   days to infuse the oakmoss with essential oil fragrance.
2. Add the remaining ingredients to the jar and shake well.
   Set aside for at least 2 weeks to allow the fragrances to
   blend. Fill the handkerchiefs or fabric squares with a few
   heaping spoonfuls of the sachet mixture. Tie securely with
   ribbon.

YIELD: **4–8 SWEET BAGS**

Moth-Repelling Sachets

Long before we had insecticides and moth balls, herbs were used
to help deter insects from the household. Recipes using insect-
repelling herbs were passed down from mother to daughter for
centuries. Moth-repelling herbs were probably considered the

most valuable because many families had articles of woolen clothing that they could not afford to lose to hungry moths.

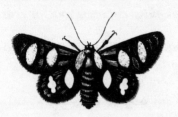

Today, moths can still be a problem and there are many aromatic materials which can be combined to successfully keep these little critters at bay. I like to make these sachets in the spring when I am packing up my sweaters for the summer. Moth-repelling materials include cedar chips, eucalyptus leaves, lavender, patchouli leaves, pennyroyal, santolina, and southernwood. Small, inexpensive bags of cedar chips can be purchased at a pet store, where they are sold as pet bedding. Patchouli leaves have an earthy scent and have fixative qualities as well as moth-repelling characteristics. Santolina has a very strong fragrance and should be used in moderation or it can be overpowering in a moth sachet. All the plants mentioned can be collected and dried at home or purchased through mail-order. (Cotton tea bags are also available through mail-order.)

Recipe 1: Lavender Moth Repellant

*1/2 cup cut oakmoss, cut orris root, or crushed patchouli
   leaves*
15 drops essential oil of eucalyptus or lavender
1 cup dried lavender blossoms
1 cup dried eucalyptus or pennyroyal leaves
1 cup cedar shavings
*10–12 cotton tea bags or 10–12 eight-inch squares of fabric
string (if using fabric)*

Recipe 2: Woodsy Moth Chaser

1/2 cup cut oakmoss, cut orris root, or crushed patchouli leaves
15 drops essential oil of cedar, pine, or eucalyptus
1 cup dried southernwood
1/2 cup dried santolina
1 cup cedar shavings
1 tbsp. whole cloves
2 whole cinnamon sticks, crushed
8–10 cotton tea bags or 8–10 eight-inch squares of fabric
string (if using fabric)

1. Choose one of the recipes above and gather the ingredients. In a large glass jar with a tight-fitting lid, combine oakmoss, orris root, or patchouli with the essential oil. Shake well and set aside for 1 week.
2. Add the remaining ingredients to the jar. Stir well. Set the mixture aside for another 2 weeks so that the fragrances can blend.
3. After 2 weeks, stuff the tea bags or fabric squares with the moth-repelling mixture and tie closed. For maximum protection, place at least 2 bags in each of your drawers. Use 3–4 bags in closets. Occasionally squeeze the bags to release the fragrance. Replace the sachets each year with fresh ones. The old moth sachets can be replenished with a fragrant essential oil and used as general drawer sachets.

YIELD: **8–12** SACHETS

Carpet Freshener

❧❦❧

There are many commercial carpet fresheners on the market which are sprinkled over the carpeting and vacuumed up. The problem with these fresheners is that their scent is very artificial and overpowering. They are also expensive to use all the time. One solution is to create a homemade freshener using baking soda and pure essential oils. This recipe uses lavender or rosemary, but you can substitute your favorite essential oil, if you wish. If you have pets, add a few drops of pennyroyal oil to help deter fleas.

MATERIALS:

4 cups baking soda
2 tsp. ground cloves
20 drops pure essential oil of lavender or rosemary

1. Combine all ingredients in a glass jar with a tight-fitting lid. Shake well. Let mixture set for 24 hours before using.
2. To use: Pour a small amount of the freshener into a fine sieve. Gently shake the sieve over your carpeting, dispersing a light layer of the freshener. Wait 10–15 minutes and then vacuum as usual. Keep any unused freshener in an airtight container.

YIELD: **4** CUPS

FLEA POWDER FOR PET'S BEDDING

Pennyroyal is known for its flea-repelling qualities. Combine 1 cup of baking soda with 10 drops of pennyroyal oil. Follow the instructions above for sprinkling the powder over the pet's bedding areas. Vacuum or shake out their bedding area after about 15–20 minutes. Pennyroyal oil can be very irritating to the skin if not diluted. Do *not* use the pure oil directly on your pet!

Vacuum Bag Sachet

೧⊷૭

As you vacuum, the bag fills with animal hair and debris and can give off an unpleasant odor. One way to eliminate this problem (and freshen the air as you vacuum) is to place a vacuum sachet inside the vacuum bag. Keep a small jar of sachets next to your vacuum bags and toss one inside every time you replace the bag. Use a combination of several dried, aromatic herbs such as lavender, lemon balm, lemon grass, lemon verbena, mint, rose, rosemary, scented geranium, or sweet woodruff.

This recipe calls for vermiculite, which is an ingredient in soil mixtures for potted plants. It is a mica-type mineral which was heated until it expanded into accordion-shaped particles. These particles are very absorbent. In soil, they help retain water. But when used in this unconventional way, they help retain the scent of the sachet. You can purchase small bags of vermiculite at your local garden center.

MATERIALS:

1 cup vermiculite
1 cup baking soda
15 drops of essential oil of mint, lavender, or
    eucalyptus
1 cup dried herbs, crushed (see list above)
3 cinnamon sticks, crushed
10–12 cotton tea bags or 10–12 eight-inch squares of
    heavy cheesecloth
thin string or twine (if using cheesecloth)

1. Combine vermiculite, baking soda, and essential oil in a glass jar with a tight-fitting lid. Cover and shake well. Set aside for 3 days.
2. In a large bowl, combine the ingredients in the jar with the dried herbs and cinnamon. Stir well. If using tea bags, fill

them with the mixture and tie the drawstring closed. If using cheesecloth, place a few spoonfuls of the herb mixture in the center of each cheesecloth square. Draw up the sides and tie with a piece of string.
3. Place one sachet inside the vacuum bag each time you replace it. Store all unused sachets in an airtight container.

YIELD: **10–12** SACHETS

Simmering Herbs

༶᠅༶

One of the easiest and quickest ways to scent the home is with simmering herbs. By boiling water which is infused with herbs and spices, you release the fragrance quickly into the air with the steam. In just a few minutes, the entire house will smell wonderful. This is a nice way to freshen your home before a party. Just be sure to set a timer so that you do not forget about the herbs and allow the pan to boil dry!

The measurements given here are approximations. You can add or subtract different herbs and spices to get various fragrances. Try using basil, lavender, lemon balm, lemon grass, lemon verbena, mint, rose, rosemary, scented geranium, or sweet woodruff to create your own recipes.

Recipe 1: Lemon

3 cups water
1 cup mixed fresh herb leaves of lemon verbena, lemon
    balm, and lemon-scented geranium
1 strip of fresh lemon or orange peel
2 sticks of cinnamon (or 1 tsp. ground)
1 tsp. whole cloves (or 1/2 tsp. ground)
10 drops of lemon or orange essential oil

Recipe 2: Vanilla Rose

3 cups water
1 cup fresh rose petals
1/2 cup fresh rose geranium leaves
1/2 vanilla bean, chopped
1 tsp. whole allspice (or 1/2 tsp. ground)
1/4 tsp. vanilla extract

Recipe 3: Lavender

3 cups water
1/2 cup dried lavender blossoms
10 drops lavender essential oil

Recipe 4: Holiday

3 cups water
1 cup fresh rosemary leaves
1/2 cup mixed pine needles
1/2 cup fresh-cut juniper pieces (tips of branches)
2 whole cinnamon sticks, crushed (or 1 tsp. ground)
1 tsp. whole cloves (or 1/2 tsp. ground)
5 drops rosemary or pine essential oil

1. Combine all the ingredients from one of the recipes above in a small sauce pan and bring to a boil.
2. Reduce the heat and let the mixture simmer for 15–20 minutes. Set a timer so that you don't forget to turn it off! You can reuse the mixture several times, but you may have to add more water.

And still she slept an azure-lidded sleep,
In blanched linen, smooth, and lavender'd.

—JOHN KEATS

Clothes Dryer Sachet

Nice alternatives to commercial dryer sheets, with their artificial fragrance, are clothes dryer sachets. Although they will not prevent static like the store-bought brands, they do make the clothes sweet-smelling. They can be made out of fabric squares or old cotton socks. (Children's socks are best because they are the perfect size for about 1/4 cup of the sachet mixture.) Cotton tea bags can also be filled with the sachet mixture. One dryer sachet will last for several loads. The heat from the dryer will release the fragrance of the herbs, giving your clothes a springtime scent.

   If you choose to make fabric sachets, be sure to use white fabric. Colors might bleed on the wet clothes.

MATERIALS:

   1 cup dried lavender blossoms
   1/2 cup dried rosemary blossoms
   1/2 cup dried lemon verbena
   10 drops lavender essential oil
   8 eight-inch squares of white cotton fabric or 8 small
      cotton socks
   cotton string or white ribbon

1. Combine the dried herbs and the essential oil in a medium-sized bowl. Mix well.
2. If using fabric squares, place approximately 1/4 cup of the herb mixture in the center of each fabric square. Pull up the sides of the square and tie closed with the string or ribbon. If using socks, fill each sock with 1/4 cup of the mixture and tie closed with string or ribbon.
3. Store the sachets in an airtight container. Use one sachet at a time in the clothes dryer with each load. The sachet may be used many times before it loses its scent. Be sure to crush it

in your hand a few times before each use to release the aromatic oils of the herbs.

YIELD: APPROXIMATELY 8 SACHETS

SCENTED DRAWER LINERS

Can't afford those expensive scented drawer liners that are so popular now? Make your own! Choose a cute, inexpensive roll of wallpaper or pick up some old samples from a wallpaper store (they throw out old designs periodically). Open the wallpaper, facedown, onto a long table and sprinkle some dried herbs all over it. (Try dried lavender, lemon verbena, mint, or rosemary.) Then, place 5–6 cotton balls which have been dipped in your favorite essential oil on the paper. (Lavender oil is excellent for this project.) Roll the wallpaper up (with the herbs and cotton balls enclosed) and place it inside a plastic trash bag. Seal the bag shut. Set it aside for 2–3 weeks. Then, unroll the paper and discard the herbs and cotton balls. Cut the paper to fit inside your clothing drawers or linen closet. (You may need to use tacks in the corners to get the paper to lie flat.)

Closet Bouquets

Closet bouquets are nice to use when you are having house guests. They are small bouquets of mixed, fresh-cut herbs which are tucked inside closets or set on top of linens to freshen them. Place them all around a guest room to give your guest a fragrant and pretty welcome present. These small bouquets can also be tucked into luggage for traveling. The traveler will arrive at his or her destination with a suitcase full of fragrance. Just be sure to wrap the bouquets in a thin towel or tissue paper before packing, to prevent them from soiling clothes.

Use the most aromatic herbs you can and be sure to include a few flowers for color. Try using basil, chamomile blossoms, lavender, lemon balm, lemon verbena, mint, rose, rosemary, sage, scented geranium, thyme, sweet woodruff, and yarrow. For added moth-repelling qualities, include pennyroyal, southernwood, or wormwood.

MATERIALS:

several small bunches of fresh herbs (see list above)
rubber bands
ribbon

1. Assemble several small bouquets of the fresh herbs. (Be sure to use several different kinds of aromatic herbs.) Wrap the ends of the bouquets with rubber bands and tie with a ribbon bow.
2. Set the bouquets in drawers, on closet shelves, and on top of bathroom towels.

CAR BOUQUETS

Try making one of the closet bouquets described above and setting it inside your car to make it sweet smelling! Just set it on the dashboard. In the summer, the heat of the sun will completely dry the bouquet in about 24 hours and give the car a wonderful springtime fragrance. After a week, you can remove the bouquet and use it as a fireplace herb or add it to a potpourri recipe!

Fireplace Herbs

Fireplace herbs are small bundles of dried herbs which are tossed into a burning fire to release their fragrance while they burn. These bundles can be made out of leftover herb twigs after the leaves are removed for other purposes, or they can be 4-6-inch branches which are cut and dried specifically for this purpose. Many of the aromatic herbs make good fireplace bundles. Try using basil, lavender, lemon grass, lemon verbena, mint, rosemary, or sage.

MATERIALS:

4-6-inch dried branches of aromatic herbs
cotton string

Tie the dried herb branches into small bundles using the cotton string. Toss one or two bundles into a fire whenever you want to release a smoky herbal fragrance into the room.

Chapter 10
Herbal Treasures

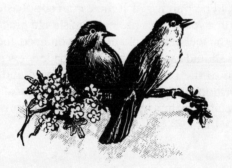

The pleasure one gets from an herb garden is increased many times over when that garden is somehow shared with others. Herbal treasures are crafts, gifts, and wrapping techniques which allow the colors and textures of the garden to be shared with friends and family. As you grow your own herbs, you will want to use them in every decorative way possible. This chapter explores some of the decorative uses of herbs.

Leaf **P** *rint* **S** *tationery*

༺৽৽৽༻

Herbal stationery is a breeze to make with this technique. Fresh leaves are coated with paint and pressed onto paper, leaving their herbal impression behind. Different shades of green can be blended to create one-of-a-kind note cards and stationery sheets. The best herbs for this project are those with flat leaves and heavy veins such as basil, bay, borage, salad burnet, cilantro, feverfew, lamb's ears, lemon balm, mint, nasturtium, parsley, sage, and scented geranium. All you need to print with these leaves is an all-purpose paint brush. However, if you want to use lacy or unusually shaped foliage (like dill or fennel) in this project, you will probably need to purchase a soft rubber roller called a brayer, to coat the leaves. A brayer is basically a rubber rolling pin with a handle and can be purchased at most craft supply stores.

The first time you try this project, you should practice on scrap paper to get the feel of how much paint you need and how much pressure you should use. Once you have made a few samples, you can move on to the real printing with colored and/or textured paper. Try printing on envelopes too! If you are really brave, you can try using fabric paints to decorate shirts and aprons. This project is so easy that kids can do it too!

MATERIALS:

fresh leaves from one of the herbs mentioned above
newspaper
several paper plates
acrylic or watercolor paints in various greens and grays
a flat, 1/4–1/2-inch-wide paint brush
paper towels
plain stationery and note cards for printing

1. Make sure your leaves are clean, dry, and free from bug bites. Lay the newspapers on your work surface to protect it from

paint. Keep a small stack of newspapers to paint on. If you are using acrylic paint, place several dots of different colored paint (about the size of a dime) onto one of your paper plates. If the paint seems too thick, thin it out with a few drops of water. If you are using watercolors, you can dip the brush directly into the paint and blend the colors on the paper plate.

2. Choose a leaf for your first print. Lay it on a piece of newspaper, facedown, so that the underside (the side with the veins) is facing upward. Use the paint brush to paint a thin layer over the entire underside of the leaf. You can paint part of the stem if you wish or you can leave it unpainted for easy handling.

3. Gently pick up the painted leaf and place it, painted side down, onto a piece of paper. While holding the leaf down with one finger, carefully cover it with a piece of paper towel. Gently press it with your fingers (do not rub). Be careful not to move the leaf or it will smear.

4. Remove the paper towel, and then carefully remove the leaf. You should have a nice impression of the herb. You might be able to make a second impression with the same leaf without repainting.

5. Repeat the printing procedures with various leaves and various colors. Be sure to use a fresh area of the newspaper to paint on. Let the finished stationery dry completely (about 24 hours) before using.

TIPS

- Try blending two or three colors together on one leaf. For a natural look, you can use different shades of green or gray. For an autumn look, you can use various shades of orange and rust.
- For stationery, you can place your prints in several areas: across the top of the page, in the upper left corner and lower right corner, or around the entire perimeter of the page.
- Use heavy paper, folded in half, to make note cards.

- To use a brayer with acrylic paint: Place a small amount of paint on a paper plate. Roll the brayer through the paint several times to get an even coating on its surface. Lay the leaf to be printed, facedown, on a piece of newspaper. Roll the brayer over the leaf several times to coat it. Carefully pick up the leaf and continue with Step 3 above. You can use the brayer on lacy foliage or on flowers such as lavender blossoms.

Planted Herb Basket

A planted basket, filled with fragrant herbs, is a terrific hostess gift or housewarming gift. It can also be a nice alternative to flowers for a sick friend. Long after flowers would have wilted, a planted basket is still lush and green. The leaves can be harvested directly from the basket and used in cooking or brewed for tea.

When choosing the herbs for your basket, keep in mind that the container is shallow. Low-growing herbs that do not have long tap roots are best. Choose very young, immature plants so that they can survive for several months in the confined quarters. Many of the herbs will not be able to reach full maturity in the basket, so be sure to tell the receiver of the gift that the herbs should be transplanted into the garden within 6 months. Pick three or four herbs with various types of foliage for an interesting look. You might want to try basil, chamomile, chives, Corsican mint, feverfew, hyssop, lemon balm, marjoram, mint, oregano, parsley, creeping rosemary, sage, savory, French tarragon, thyme, and sweet woodruff.

MATERIALS:

1 medium to large basket
2 heavy-duty plastic trash bags
potting soil
slow-release fertilizer

several small herb plants (see list above)
ribbon

1. Line the basket with two layers of plastic trash bags. This will make the container watertight. (Don't worry about trimming the plastic to the edge of the basket until after it is filled with soil.)
2. Fill the lined basket with potting soil. Add a small amount of slow-release fertilizer and mix it in well. Carefully trim the plastic to the top of the basket edge.
3. Lightly moisten the soil, being careful not to make it water-logged. (Remember, there are no drainage holes.) Plant your herbs in the basket, placing the tallest herb either in the center or the back of the basket. Tie a large bow and attach it to the basket.
4. The planted basket should be watered only when it is beginning to dry out and should be set in front of a very sunny window where it will get at least 4 hours of sunlight per day.

Dried Herbal Picture Frame

These picture frames are completely covered with natural ingredients from the garden. Gray Spanish moss (available at craft stores or through mail-order) covers the entire frame and acts as a foundation for building small clusters of dried botanicals in the corners. Air-dried or pressed flowers can be added for color. Miniature rose buds which have been allowed to air-dry are especially pretty. Dried bay leaves, chamomile blossoms, lavender blossoms, sage leaves, and thyme are good choices for this project.

You can use an inexpensive frame from a garage sale, thrift store, or discount store. Then, just add a special photo and you have a very inexpensive, yet personal gift for a treasured friend.

MATERIALS:

1 picture frame
Spanish moss
hot glue gun and glue
dried herb leaves and flowers
cinnamon sticks, whole allspice, and star anise

1. Use the hot glue gun to attach the Spanish moss over the entire picture frame. Be sure to cover the outside edges.
2. Glue very small pieces of dried sprigs, leaves, flowers, and spices on the corners of the frame in a pleasing design. Start with the leaves and end with the single flowers and spices.
3. Carefully remove any residual "spider webs" of glue. Keep the frame out of direct sunlight to reduce fading.

Pressed Herbs

Herb leaves and flowers can be pressed flat until they are completely dry. These pressed plants are little preserved pieces of the garden, which can be used to create very romantic projects and whimsical designs. You don't need an expensive flower press to dry herbs in this way. An old telephone book and a few bricks can do the job just fine. The pressed herbs won't last forever, but they should hold their color for at least a year if they are kept out of direct sunlight.

PRESSING THE PLANT MATERIAL

When you collect your plant material from the garden, choose leaves and flowers that have interesting shapes. Almost all the herbs mentioned in this book work well as pressed leaves and flowers with the exception of rose blossoms, which are too large. (Roses must be separated into individual petals to press.) You may also want to include ferns, pansies, lobelia, and ivy in your plant material.

Lay some of the plant material onto pieces of paper towel. Starting at the back of a telephone book, open a page and lay one of these paper towels inside. Then, carefully fold over some pages and lay down another paper towel of herbs. Continue until all the leaves and flowers are lying on paper towels inside the phone book. Lay two heavy bricks on top of the phone book and set it aside for 1–2 weeks to dry.

Pressed Herb Bookmarks

You can use the herbs and flowers you have pressed to create beautifully laminated bookmarks. They make excellent gifts! All you need is clear plastic, self-sticking paper, which is available at some craft supply stores. You can also use clear plastic shelf paper, which is available at hardware stores. Some craft stores also sell laminating sheets which require the heat of an iron to adhere to paper. These laminating sheets can be easily substituted for the self-sticking paper used in this project.

MATERIALS:

pencil and ruler
heavy white paper
pressed herb leaves and flowers
white craft glue (which dries clear)
paint brush
paper plate
tweezers
clear plastic, self-sticking paper
scissors
hole punch
ribbon

1. Use a pencil and ruler to lightly draw an outline of the bookmark shape you want to create on the paper. Pour some of the white craft glue onto the paper plate and use the paint brush to carefully coat the backside of some of the pressed

herbs with the glue. Position the pressed herbs within the bookmark outline in an attractive design. Gently press the leaves with your fingers. (You may need tweezers for the more delicate herbs.)

2. Continue gluing until your design is complete. Allow the glue to dry for a few hours.

3. Carefully cut out the bookmark along your penciled outline. Cut a piece of clear plastic, self-sticking paper approximately 1/2 inch larger than the bookmark. Carefully peel off the back and place it over the pressed flower bookmark. Smooth out any bubbles. Trim the plastic to match the bookmark edges.

4. Use the hole punch to make a hole in the top of the bookmark. Tie a ribbon through the hole.

Pressed Herbal Candle

Small, pressed herb leaves and flowers are used in this project to decorate a plain pillar candle. Choose a large candle (about 2–4 inches in diameter) so that you have enough surface to work on. Use very flat leaves, sprigs, and flowers such as salad burnet, dill, fennel, ivy, oregano, pansies, parsley, and thyme.

Paraffin wax can be found in the canning section or spice section of many supermarkets. Use extreme caution when melting paraffin wax. It is very flammable.

MATERIALS:

1 box paraffin wax
1 white pillar candle, circular or square
several different pressed leaves and flowers
2 paint brushes, one large and one small

1. In a double boiler, carefully melt the paraffin wax over very low heat. Watch the wax closely! It is very flammable!

2. When the wax is completely melted, remove it from the heat.

Use the wax as "glue" to adhere the pressed leaves and flowers in a decorative design on the sides of the candle. To do this, use the small paint brush to dab wax on the back of each leaf and then press the leaf to the candle. Continue until all the leaves are "glued" to the candle. (You can also use white glue to adhere the leaves to the candle.)

3. Use the larger paint brush to "paint" several layers of wax over the entire surface of the candle. This will seal in your leaves and keep them from falling off. Continue until the entire candle is covered with the paraffin wax.

Pressed Herb Wrapping Paper

For a dramatic effect, wrap a gift in plain white paper or brown postal paper and then decorate it with pressed herbs. (Postal paper is used for mailing packages and gives a country look.) Position your pressed herb designs in the corners of the package. Feverfew blossoms, oregano, rosemary, and sage work especially well on gift wrapping paper. Add a few pressed flowers such as pansies for color. Tie the package with raffia, lace ribbon, or twine so that you do not detract from the herbal design. It takes only a few minutes to spruce up a plain package in this way and the results are very romantic looking.

MATERIALS:

white craft glue (the kind that dries clear)
paper plate
paint brush
a gift wrapped in white or brown paper
pressed herb leaves and flowers
tweezers

1. Pour some of the white craft glue onto the paper plate and use the paint brush to carefully coat the backside of some of the pressed herbs with the glue. Position the pressed herbs

onto the wrapped package and gently press with your fingers. You may need tweezers for the more delicate herbs.
2. Continue gluing until your design is complete. Allow the glue to dry for a few hours.

Natural Herbal Gift Wraps

The pressed leaf wrapping paper described above is a great way to package a gift for a special person. But there are other ways to wrap and package gifts using herbs and other materials right out of the garden. Listed below are tips and design ideas for sprucing up your packages and making gift giving a garden experience.

- Tuck a small fresh or dried herbal bouquet under the bow of a wrapped package.
- Tie a fresh or dried herbal sprig onto a bottle of herbal vinegar.
- Dip dried bay leaves in gold paint and wire them onto jars of herbal jelly.

DRIED HERB AND SPICE CLUSTERS

After wrapping a package, tie it with something rustic such as twine, raffia, or paper ribbon. Then use a glue gun to attach air-dried herb sprigs in a mounding, cluster shape in the center of the bow. You can use bay, calendula blossoms, feverfew, lamb's ears, lavender, sage, or thyme. Next, glue on whole nuts (such as walnuts, almonds, and hazelnuts), spices (such as cinnamon sticks and whole star anise), and various dried pods. If necessary, you can add a few more herb sprigs to fill in any blank spaces. The result is a fragrant embellishment that makes the entire gift seem much more special.

FLORAL VIALS

Floral vials are tiny, pointed containers, with a plastic cap, that hold the stems of fresh plant material. They are used in floral design and act as tiny vases for flowers and leaves. You can purchase them from florists and floral supply stores. You can use these floral vials to make tiny bouquets of herbs which can be tucked into gift baskets or wired onto packages. They will allow the plant material to be used as a decoration for at least 24 hours. They are especially beautiful when used with lace ribbon on wedding presents or bridal shower gifts.

Source Guide

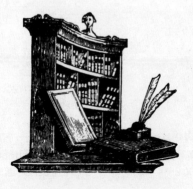

All the companies listed here offer mail-order services. Many of the companies charge nominal fees for their catalog. Since fees are constantly changing, they were not included in this listing. For availability and price information on any of these catalogs, you should send a self-addressed, stamped envelope.

Plants and Seeds

Carroll Gardens
P.O. Box 310
Westminster, MD 21157

The Cook's Garden
P.O. Box 535
Londonderry, VT 05148

The Flowery Branch
P.O. Box 1330
Flowery Branch, GA 30542

Goodwin Creek Gardens
P.O. Box 83
Williams, OR 97544

Heirloom Garden Seeds
P.O. Box 138
Guerneville, CA 95446

Logee's Greenhouse
141 North Street
Danielson, CT 06239

Nichols Garden Nursery
1190 North Pacific Highway
Albany, OR 97321-4580

Rasland Farm
N.C. 82 at U.S. 13
Goodwin, NC 28344-9712

Sandy Mush Herb Nursery
316 Surrett Cove Road
Leicester, NC 28748-9622

Shepherds Garden Seeds
30 Irene Street
Torrington, CT 06790

Territorial Seed Company
P.O. Box 157
Cottage Grove, OR 97424-0061

Well-Sweep Herb Farm
317 Mt. Bethel Road
Port Murray, NJ 07865

Organic Garden Supplies
(Fertilizers, natural pest management, etc.)

Bountiful Gardens
Ecology Action
5798 Ridgewood Road
Willits, CA 95490

Gardens Alive
5100 Schenley Place
Lawrenceburg, IN 47025

The Natural Gardener
8648 Old Bee Caves Road
Austin, TX 78735

**Peaceful Valley Farm
Supply**
P.O. Box 2209
Grass Valley, CA 95945

Worms Way Garden Supply
3151 South Highway 446
Bloomington, IN 47401

Antique Roses

**The Antique Rose
Emporium**
Route 5, Box 143
Brenham, TX 77833

**Roses of Yesterday and
Today**
802 Brown's Valley Road
Watsonville, CA 95076-0398

Vintage Gardens
2227 Gravenstein Highway
South
Sebastopol, CA 95472

Craft Supplies and Botanicals
(Essential oils, bulk botanicals, cosmetic-making supplies, bottles, cotton tea bags, etc.)

Aroma Vera
5901 Rodeo Road
Los Angeles, CA 90016-4312
*(Essential oils and
aromatherapy products)*

**Gabrieana's Herbal
Products**
P.O. Box 215322
Sacramento, CA 95821

*(Essential oils, bulk
botanicals, books, empty
"press 'n' brew" tea bags,
etc.)*

The Glass Pantry
231 Cherry Alley
Maysville, KY 41056
*(Small selection of unusually
shaped glass bottles for
vinegars and cosmetics)*

Lavender Lane

5321 Elkhorn Boulevard
Sacramento, CA 95842
(Big selection of glass and plastic bottles, everything you need for cosmetics, including essential oils, beeswax pearls, and heat-sealable tea bags)

LorAnn Oils

4518 Aurelius Road
P.O. Box 22009
Lansing, MI 48909-2009
(Essential oils, food crafting, candle-making supplies)

Mountain Rose Herbs

P.O. Box 2000
Redway, CA 95560
(Essential oils, lots of cosmetic supplies, beeswax, almond oil, bulk botanicals, cotton tea bags, books, bottles)

Nature's Herb Company

1010 46th Street
Emeryville, CA 94608
(Essential oils, bulk botanicals)

Jean's Greens Herbal Tea Works

RR1, Box 55J, Hale Road
Rensselaerville, NY 12147
(Tea, essential oils, bulk botanicals, miscellaneous herbal products)

The Scented Garden

P.O. Box 126
Anna, TX 75409-0126
(Miscellaneous herbal products, potpourri supplies, cotton tea bags, salve tins, teas, botanicals)

Sunburst Bottle Company

7001 Sunburst Way
Citrus Heights, CA 95621
(Big selection of glass and plastic bottles, vials, and jars which can be used for vinegar and cosmetics)

Tom Thumb Workshops

14100 Lankford Hwy. Rt. 13
P.O. Box 357
Mappsville, VA 23407
(Essential oils, bulk botanicals, craft and potpourri supplies, laminating sheets)

Herbal Books, Audiotapes and Videotapes

Country Thyme Productions
P.O. Box 3090
El Segundo, CA 90245
(Videos on home entertaining, cooking, and crafting with herbs)

The Herb Farm
32804 Issaquah-Fall City Road
Fall City, WA 98024
(Miscellaneous herb products, books, audiotapes of herbal instructors)

Jeanne Rose Aromatherapy
219 Carl Street
San Francisco, CA 94117
(Herbal books, lecture information)

Wood Violet Books
3814 Sunhill Drive
Madison, WI 53704
(Huge selection of books on herbal cooking, gardening and medicinal uses)

Floral Supplies

IFAR—Wreath Supply Company
2917 Anthony Lane NE
Minneapolis, MN 55418
(Wreath frames and supplies)

McFadden's Vines & Wreaths
Rt. 3, Box 2360
Butler, TN 37640
(Twig and moss wreath bases)

Bibliography

Allardice, Pamela. *Lavender.* London, England: Robert Hale, 1991.

Bremness, Lesley. *Herbs.* New York, New York: Dorling Kindersley, 1994.

Brinton, Diana. *The Complete Guide to Flower Arranging.* London, England: Merehurst Limited, 1990.

Brown, Alice Cooke. *Early American Herb Recipes.* New York, New York: Bonanza Books, 1966.

Cornell Plantations, U. Of California Botanical Garden & Matthaei Botanical Gardens. *Herb Gardening.* New York, New York: Pantheon Books, 1994.

Cox, Janice. *Natural Beauty at Home.* New York, New York: Henry Holt and Company, Inc., 1994.

Cox, Jeff. *Your Organic Garden.* Emmaus, Pennsylvania: Rodale Press, 1994.

Creasy, Rosalind. "Fennel". Loveland, Colorado: *Herb Companion Magazine,* April/May, 1995: 26–31.

DeBaggio, Thomas. *Growing Herbs From Seed, Cutting and Root.* Loveland, Colorado: Interweave Press, Inc., 1994.

Dinsdale, Margaret. *Skin Deep.* Buffalo, New York: Camden House Publishing, 1994.

Drury, Elizabeth. *The Butler's Pantry Book.* New York, New York: St. Martin's Press, 1981.

Facetti, Aldo. *Natural Beauty.* New York, New York: Simon & Schuster Inc., 1991.

Fox, Helen Morgenthau. *Gardening with Herbs for Flavor and Fragrance.* New York, New York: MacMillan Company, 1934.

Foster, Steven. "Aloe Vera". Loveland, Colorado: *Herb Companion Magazine,* Feb/March, 1995: 49–52.

Foster, Steven. *Herbal Renaissance.* Layton, Utah: Gibbs Smith Publisher, 1994.

Freeman, Margaret B. *Herbs for the Mediaeval Household.* New York, New York: The Metropolitan Museum of Art, 1943.

Garland, Sarah. *The Complete Book of Herbs & Spices.* New York, New York: Viking Press, 1979.

Genders, Roy. *Natural Beauty.* London, England: Promotional Reprint Company Ltd, 1992.

Hill, Madalene and Barclay, Gwen. *Southern Herb Growing.* Fredericksburg, TX: Shearer Publishing, 1987.

McDonald, Donald. *Sweet Scented Flowers and Fragrant Leaves.* New York, New York: Charles Scribner's Sons, 1895.

McLeod, Judyth A. *Lavender, Sweet Lavender.* Kenthurst, England: Kangaroo Press, 1992.

McVicar, Jekka. *Jekka's Complete Herb Book.* London, England: Kyle Cathie Limited, 1994.

Michael, Pamela. *All Good Things Around Us.* New York, New York: Holt, Rinehart and Winston, 1980.

Rohde, Eleanour Sinclair. *Herbs and Herb Gardening.* London, England: The Medici Society, Ltd., 1946.

Sanecki, Kay N. *History of the English Herb Garden.* London, England: Ward Lock, 1992.

Sedenko, Jerry. *The Butterfly Garden.* New York, New York: Running Head Books, Inc., 1991.

Siegler, Madeleine H. *Making Potpourri.* Pownal, Vermont: Storey Communications, Inc., 1991.

Simmons, Adelma Grenier. *Herbs Through the Seasons at Caprilands.* Emmaus, PA: Rodale Press, 1987.

Simmons, John V. *The Science of Cosmetics.* London, England: The MacMillan Press, Ltd., 1989.

Stokes, Donald & Lillian. *The Hummingbird Book*. New York, New York: Little Brown and Company, 1989.

Strauch, Betsy. "The Many Faces of Artemisia". Loveland, Colorado: *Herb Companion Magazine*, Oct/Nov. 1993: 24–29.

Tourles, Stephanie. *The Herbal Body Book*. Pownal, Vermont: Storey Communications, Inc., 1994.

Tucker, Arthur O. "Herbs vs. Bugs". Loveland, Colorado: *Herb Companion Magazine*, June/July, 1994: 44–47.

Tucker, Arther O. "Will the Real Oregano Please Stand Up?". Loveland, Colorado: *Herb Companion Magazine*, Feb/March, 1992: 20–27.

Willan, Anne. *La Varenne Pratique*. New York, New York: Crown Publishers, 1989.

Williams, Betsy. *Are There Faeries at the Bottom of Your Garden?* Andover, Massachusetts: Betsy Williams, 1994.

Young, Anne. *Practical Cosmetic Science*. London, England: Mills & Boon Limited, 1972.

Index

INTERNATIONAL NETWORKS OF BANKS AND INDUSTRY

STUDIES IN INDUSTRIAL ORGANIZATION

Volume 2

International Networks of Banks and Industry

by

M. Fennema

1982

Martinus Nijhoff Publishers

The Hague/Boston/London

Distributors:

for the United States and Canada

Kluwer Boston, Inc.
190 Old Derby Street
Hingham, MA 02043
USA

for all other countries

Kluwer Academic Publishers Group
Distribution Center
P.O. Box 322
3300 AH Dordrecht
The Netherlands

Library of Congress Cataloging in Publication Data

Fennema, M., 1946-
   International networks of banks and industry.

   (Studies in industrial organization ; v. 2)
   Includes bibliographies and indexes.
   1. Interlocking directorates. 2. International
business enterprises. 3. Banks and banking,
International. I. Title. II. Series.
HD2755.5.F46 1982   338.8'7   82-8243
ISBN 90-247-2620-4

ISBN 90-247-2620-4 (this volume)
ISBN 90-247-2434-1(series)

PRINTED IN THE NETHERLANDS

Acknowledgements

The idea of this study originated in 1971 when Robert J. Mokken and Frans N. Stokman released a first internal draft of their pioneering study on interlocking directorates in the Netherlands, which was finally published in 1975 under the title Graven naar Macht (Traces of Power).

A group of graduate students decided at that time to start with a similar study at the international level. It soon appeared, of course, that repeating a national study of interlocking directorates at the international level created many problems which are not included in the term 'repetition'. At the time I decided to carry the project to its end I was not aware of all of them, but fortunately I had the active and enthusiastic support of Frans Stokman, and especially Robert Mokken. Mokken worked through the different versions of the book with me, discussing many of the theoretical issues and shaping my thinking on them.
In 1974, I received a grant from the Netherlands Organization for the Advancement of Pure Research (ZWO), which enabled me to work that year full time on the project. In 1977 an additional grant from ZWO enabled me to profit from the invaluable assistance of Peter de Jong, who did most of the computer work. His critical mind and friendship helped me through several crises. In 1978 Willem Kleyn collected the 1976 data.
Of the many others to whom I am indebted I can only mention a few. Wladimir Andreff made me aware of theoretical problems involved in the institutional approach. His comments and exhortations helped me very much. Jac. M. Anthonisse was very helpful in the initial stage of the research, while he himself was engaged in writing a library of graph-programs. Frans J. van Veen helped me with GRADAP and also produced the manuscript. Henry W. de Jong read several drafts of the first three chapters and suggested useful solutions to awkward theoretical problems. With Huibert Schijf I wrote a survey of the research of interlocking directorates (Fennema and Schijf, 1979) which formed the basis of the Introduction. Helen M. Borkent-Richardson corrected the English. Leonie van Veen typed the final manuscript.
Finally, I want to mention Troetje Loewenthal, my companera de vida, without whom the book might have been finished long ago, and I with it.

M.F.
Baard, August 1981

Contents   page

INTERNATIONAL NETWORKS OF BANKS AND INDUSTRY

VIII

List of Tables

List of Figures

INTRODUCTION

Research into interlocking directorates and other organizational ties between large corporations dates back to the beginning of the century. In Germany and the United States interlocking directorates became an important means of coordination and control of large corporations and banks at the end of the nineteenth century and were, as a result, particularly subject to scientific investigation and public debate. Trusts were regarded with mistrust, especially in the United States, where John Moody's study from 1904 was significantly entitled The Truth about Trusts. In Germany much attention was paid to the role of the large Berlin banks in the economic development. The first large study in Germany carried the prolix title The Relationship between the Large German Banks and Industry with Special Reference to the Iron Industry (Jeidels, 1905).

The studies in the United States were predominantly induced and even carried out by committees of the Federal Congress. In Europe, on the other hand, the labor movement soon became interested in the patterns of interlocking directorates. In the Netherlands, for example, Wibaut, a socialist leader, carried out a study on interlocking directorates, copying the research design of Jeidels. Accordingly, two different schools can be distinguished from the start: the Marxian school which developed the concept of finance capital to explain the existing interlocking directorates, and the institutional economists who used the concept of economic power to explain the same phenomenon.

Three separate waves of research on interlocking directorates can be distinguished: between 1905 and 1915 five large investigations took place; between 1930 and 1945 again five large investigations were conducted; and between 1965 and 1980 more than thirty studies appeared. Between 1915 and 1930 and between 1945 and 1965 no research was done, except in rare cases outside the academic institutions. [1]
A similar wave-like movement is found in the number of antitrust cases in the United States. Between 1905 and 1920 there were actions against American Tobacco, Standard Oil, Du Pont, Corn Products, American Can, United States Steel, American Telephone and Telegraph, the 'meatpackers', American Sugar, United Shoe Machinery and International Harvester. In

[1] The figures are based on an extensive survey by Huibert Schijf and the author (Fennema and Schijf, 1979).

the second period, between 1937 and 1952, there were actions
against Alcoa, National Broadcasting Company, Pullman,
Paramount Pictures, again against American Can, Du Pont
(twice), United Shoe Machinery and American Tobacco; and
against United Fruit, Western Electric and IBM. Wilcox and
Shepherd (1975), from whom we have taken these figures, note
that in both periods the last cases were always won by the
companies. Finally, there is increasing antitrust activity
after 1969 with actions against Cereals, Xerox, and again IBM
and American Telephone and Telegraph (Wilcox and Shepherd,
1975: 203 ff.).

How should one explain these different waves, in which
scientific research seems to anticipate legal actions against
monopolistic firms in the United States? In my opinion these
waves coincide with political and economic crises in the
capitalist system. The first period is one of a series of
economic crises which began in 1873 and led up to various
depressions in the nineties and the famous 'rich man's panic'
in 1907. It was a period of trust formation, both in the
United States and in Germany. Although the crises in the
United States and Europe did not coincide (in Europe the
depressions in the nineties were shorter, while there was an
acute crisis in 1900), there was a strong similarity in
economic development. A rapid concentration in industry and
banking coincided with the development of a network of
interlocking directorates, especially between banks and
industry. In the United States this stimulated popular
antitrust movements. The Sherman Act of 1890, aimed at the
prevention of the 'abuse of economic power', enabled the
Federal Government to act against Standard Oil. In this
antitrust movement, interlocking directorates also came under
attack and the Interstate Commerce Act of 1887 made it
unlawful for any one person to hold a position as an officer
or director of more than one carrier, unless authorized by
the Interstate Commerce Commission after finding that neither
public nor private interests would be adversely affected (FTC
report, 1951: 9). In 1914 the Clayton Act was enacted to
supplement the Sherman Act of 1890. In speaking for the
proposed legislation before Congress, Senator Helvering
announced that "the practice of interlocking directorates
offends laws, human and divine" (FTC report, 1951: 3). The
Clayton Act did actually prohibit three types of interlocking
directorates: those between competing banks, those between
competing industrials and those between railroads and their
potential suppliers.

In Europe at the turn of the century, there is no such
popular antitrust movement. Here we find a marxist-inspired
social-democratic movement, which placed the struggle against

monopolies and trust in the perspective of a socialist
revolution. Rather than viewing monopolies as excesses of a
capitalist system which can be combated by legal action, the
social-democratic movement regarded them as a natural outcome
of capitalist development. Besides, socialist writers saw the
trustification not as a nefarious development but as a useful
planning system, which 'only' had to be socialized to
function perfectly (see Wibaut, 1903: 230, 231). The
development of monopolies and trusts was regarded as an
essential feature of capitalist development, heralding the
termination of the capitalist system. Thus, although there
was certainly great interest among marxist scholars for the
study of interlocking directorates, the socialist studies
were not aimed at legal antitrust measures. [2]

In certain business circles, however, there was uneasiness
about the concentration in banking. In England, the Treasury
Committee on Bank Amalgamations proposed "that legislation be
passed requiring that the prior approval of the Government
must be obtained before any amalgamations are announced or
carried into effect. And, in order that such legislation may
not merely have the effect of producing hidden amalgamations
instead, we recommend that all proposals for interlocking
directorates, or for agreements which in effect would alter
the status of a bank as regards its separate entity and
control, or for purchase by one bank of the shares of another
bank, be also submitted for the prior approval of the
Government before they are carried out" (cited in Westerman,
1920: 424). However, these proposals have not led to
legislation comparable to the antitrust laws in the United
States, either in England or in other European countries.

[2] Such measures were regarded as useless and harmful only
    to trusts whose control was already in jeopardy. As
    Hilferding argues, only a control relation in decay is
    characterized by overtly exercised power. A stable control
    relation does not show the exercise of power. But the most
    important argument of Hilferding is that the breaking up of
    trust is an attempt to turn the clock backwards and
    therefore a reactionary economic policy (Hilferding, 1914:
    149, 150). The latter argument is not of interest to us
    because it is outside the theme of the book. The former,
    however, is very relevant indeed. Because if it is true
    that control is only visible when in jeopardy, the research
    of control through interlocking directorates might show
    only those cases.

In antitrust perspective, interlocking directorates are particularly harmful in the financial sector of the economy. Here, it is assumed, a financial aristocracy enriches itself unduly, at the expense of the small shareholder. In 1905 Seno Pratt, an editor of the Wall Street Journal, identified "seventy-six men who make up the 'Business Senate' of the United States - what they control - their cliques and parties" (cited in Bunting and Barbour, 1971: 318). And, according to a more recent study of Bunting, "by 1910, the coterie of dominating corporations and individuals came to be collectively known as the "Money Trust" (...). Noyes dates concern over the Money Trust per se with the rapid ascendancy of holding companies "organized and floated" beginning 1899 (...). On the other hand, the assault on the Money Trust subsided with the advent of World War I" (Bunting, 1976: 8). In a sense it was a movement against the excesses of family capitalism symbolized by the families of such great 'tycoons' as Morgan, Rockefeller, and Vandebilt.

In a marxist perspective, one can also say that the movement was directed against the domination of money capital over productive capital. In many instances the bankers were the target of the popular movement. This movement subsided during and after World War I, but resurfaced in the Great Depression.
Roosevelt's New Deal also included stricter antitrust regulations as part of a program for more state intervention in business. The National Resources Committee started a series of studies in 1936, that were used as evidence in legal actions against several giant corporations. Some of the investigators, like Victor Perlo and Paul Sweezy, had a marxist inclination, but the popular -or populist- antitrust tradition remained dominant, as exemplified by the work of Lundberg (America's 60 Families, 1937).

An offshoot of the New Deal studies was the study on interlocking directorates published in 1951 by the Federal Trade Commission. By then, however, the Cold War had come to a head and the results of the study were never used for antitrust activities.

In Europe there were in the thirties also investigations on the relations between large corporations, again with special reference to the position of the banks. Prof. Verrijn Stuart, director of the Netherlands Economic Institute who was to become president of the Bank of the Netherlands at the end of the thirties, promoted a number of studies on the relationship between banks and industry in France, Switzerland, Belgium and Sweden. Surprisingly, no such study was conducted about the relationship between banks and

industry in the Netherlands. In Germany, there was an
extensive study done by Hagemann (1931). The end of the
Second World War was again a period of active research in
Germany, this time induced by the deconcentration measures
taken by the Allies, especially against the chemical and
steel concerns. In Japan the Americans proposed to break up
the old Zaitbatsu (see Hadley, 1970).

The Cold War brought these investigations and the policy
measures based upon them to an abrupt end. Capitalism was to
develop smoothly and rapidly for twenty years to come.
Marxism was eliminated from the universities and so was the
non-marxist school of institutional economists. And with
these two theoretical schools the research on interlocking
directorates disappeared. Only within the Communist Parties
was such research carried on, with small means and, as a
consequence, defective methodology (e.g. Perlo, 1957;
Aaronovitch, 1961; Baruch, 1962).

At the end of the sixties research on interlocking
directorates reappeared in the academic community. Grand Old
Lloyd Warner - of the Yankee City studies - conducted with
Unwalla an investigation which was pioneering in many
respects. But it was not until the seventies that a stream of
publications appeared, many of them making use of graph
theory to analyze networks of interlocking directorates in a
more sophisticated way than before (see for a summary Fennema
and Schijf, 1979).

All these studies were restricted to the national level.
While this is not surprising of the American studies, which
fit into the antitrust tradition and are aimed at legislative
actions of the Federal Government, it is surprising of those
studies which appeal to the marxist tradition. Indeed, from
Hilferding onward, marxist theory has proclaimed a direct
relationship between industrial concentration, interlocking
directorates between banks and industry, and
internationalization of capital. Nevertheless, no systematic
study on director interlocks between banks and industry at
the international level has ever been undertaken. Such a
study can shed light on the international organization of
capital, which is the central element in those theories of
imperialism for which Hilferding laid the foundation. The
differences between the theories of Kautsky, Bucharin and
Lenin can partly be traced back to different conceptions of
the international organization of capital. Analysis of the
international network of interlocking directorates can,
therefore, contribute to the theory of imperialism by
creating evidence for the theoretical positions in the still
ongoing debate.

The study presented here is new in three respects. First, it
is   a   quantitative   and   systematic   investigation   of
interlocking directorates based on application of the graph-
theoretical concepts   and an   organized set of computer
programs for the analysis of graphs, recently developed in
the Netherlands (GRADAP, 1980). Second, it is the first
monograph on the <u>international</u> network of interlocking
directorates. The   complete absence of an international
perspective has been noted, for example, by Andreff (1976:
231) who stressed its importance for the understanding of
global capitalism. Third, the results of this analysis will
be used to compare a number   of economic theories of
imperialism. I will proceed by deducing from several theories
the implications for the international structure of corporate
interlocks and comparing these "models" with the actual
networks of 1970 and 1976.

<u>Theoretical</u> <u>approaches</u> <u>in</u> <u>the</u> <u>research</u> <u>of</u> <u>interlocking</u>
<u>directorates.</u>

In   the   analysis   of   interlocking directorates several
theoretical approaches can be distinguished. The traditional
<u>sociological</u> <u>approach</u> considers interlocking directorates
primarily as an aspect of the economic elite cooptation.
Thus, Warner and Unwalla (1967: 121) ask questions like:
"(...) what kind of men are the directors of some of the
largest corporations in America? How many are managers and
how many are outside 'citizen directors', <u>i.e.</u> non-managers?
Where do these men come from - large, small or very small
companies?   How much and in what way are the boards
'interlocked' and how much are these boards connected with
small and large American firms?"

Related to the sociological approach is the <u>organizational</u>
<u>approach</u>, focusing on the impact of interlocks on
organizational effectiveness of corporations. A fine example
of such a study is that of Pennings (1980) who has paid
special attention to the impact of interlocking directorates
with financials on the performance of industrials in the
United States. The board of directors is considered as an
instrument for dealing with the organization's environment
(Pfeffer, 1972; Allen, 1974). The sociological approach is
personalistic,   while   the   organizational   approach   is
institutional, but both are <u>actor-oriented</u>; characteristic of
both is the frequent use of measures of association. Several
variables are isolated and correlated. In more sophisticated
studies a causal analysis is introduced; <u>e.g.</u> the question is
raised whether interlocking directorates is a dependent or an
independent variable <u>vis-a-vis</u> performance of corporations.

Thus both Warner and Unwalla and Pennings use aggregate data on interlocking directorates and associate these data – using conventional statistical techniques – with aggregate data on size, composition of the board, profits, etc. Such an approach, however, says little about the structure of the system of interlocking directorates. The focus on the structure is to be found in the network approach of interlocking directorates. In such an approach, data on interlocking directorates are not isolated and aggregated, but studied in terms of either the organization of organizations if the approach is institutional (Zijlstra, 1979b), or a social network if the approach is personalistic (Koenig and Gogel, 1981).

The network approach, however, lacks a methodological tradition outside the field of sociometric studies. Only recently has attention been paid to the application of graph theory to the study of corporate networks. When R.J. Mokken and F.N. Stokman introduced this type of analysis in the Netherlands, their first (internal) publication (Invloedsstructuren, 1971) created a public debate in which the big linkers of the Dutch network, especially the bankers, participated. In retrospect, it was not surprising that this debate broke out, because it was indeed the first publication of its kind. In the United States, with its long tradition of research on interlocking directorates, the application of graph-theory to this field of research was initiated by Sonquist and Koenig (1975) whose first publication appeared in the Insurgent Sociologist in the same year that the final publication of the Dutch study appeared in Amsterdam (Helmers et.al., 1975). Since then, other studies have been initiated. In the Netherlands, Mokken and Stokman continued their research and stimulated others. Zijlstra (1979a) has investigated the policy-field of nuclear energy in the Netherlands. The investigation presented here was initiated by the author in close contact with R.J. Mokken and F.N. Stokman. The train of research is still moving ahead. [3] In

[3] A large research project on intercorporate structures in different countries is being carried out by an ECPR research group headed by Frans N.Stokman and Rolf Ziegler. In this project the structure of the network of interlocking directorates between the 250 largest corporations of Austria, Belgium, Finland, France, Germany, Italy, the Netherlands and the United States will be compared. There are also historical studies in preparation that combine the network approach with more traditional historical analysis (Schijf, 1980).

the United States application of graph-theoretical concepts
has been further developed by Bearden, Bonacich, Mariolis,
Mintz and Schwartz, among others. Computer programs have been
developed in the United States (Alba,1973) and in the
Netherlands, where the first publication was that of
Anthonisse (1971) and where an extensive and organized set of
programs has just been completed (GRADAP, 1980). To
coordinate research activities the International Network for
Social Network Analysis now publishes a bulletin,
Connections, and in 1978 a scientific journal, Social
Networks, was founded to stimulate this interdisciplinary
field of research.

Nevertheless, in network studies of interlocking directorates
theory and methodology are still in their infancy. About the
meaning of indirect interlocks, for instance, very little is
known. And the problem of random graphs is still largely
unresolved. Such difficulties, however, should not be used as
an occasion to discard the network approach, as Pennings does
(1980: 44 ff). One should go ahead, with the frank admission
that many conclusions drawn from network analysis are
tentative. The research presented in this book builds on
previous studies, which often lack methodological rigor (for
an overview see Fennema and Schijf, 1979). Theoretically, a
lot of confusion is created because of the level-of-analysis
problem, already touched on when we distinguished the actor-
oriented sociological and organizational approaches from the
structural network approaches. Network studies focus on the
system-level. Here questions are raised about the density of
the network, the connectivity of the network and the
centrality of the network. Further, the position of different
types of firms is considered, often in terms of point
centrality. When the corporations are regarded as the actors
in the system, the analysis is institutional. Questions in
these network studies are: "What is the extent of
interlocking in the upper echelon of the (...) corporate
structure? Is every corporation connected to every other
corporation? If so, by how many steps? Are connections denser
in some parts of the network than in others? (...) Do
financial institutions tend to have a disproportionate number
of interlocks?" (Sonquist and Koenig, 1975: 201). One can
also apply the network analysis to a more personalistic
structural theory of elite-cooptation. As Koenig and Gogel
(1981: 37) argue, the "network can be visualized as a system
through which common norms, values, and a sense of "weness"
can flow. This sense of being part of a corporate
establishment would have significant effects on corporate
conduct" (italics in the original).

Whether institutional or personalistic, the network approach
should be clearly distinguished from the actor-oriented
approaches. The study of financial groups, for example, has
concentrated on the problem of the control of corporations.
Here questions have been asked such as: does unified control
exist in a group of corporations? If so, what role do
financial institutions play in such groups, and what is the
role of multiple directors within the groups (e.g.
Aaronovitch, 1961; Allen, 1978; Citoleux et.al., 1977;
Dooley, 1969; Sweezy, 1953)? Although these studies may
appear to be network studies, they are basically focused on
the structure and strategy of the actors in the corporate
system and, thus, actor-oriented. Confusion about the level
of analysis creates confusion about the significance of
interlocking directorates. At the actor-level they are often
regarded as channels of domination and control. At the
system-level they are generally seen as channels of
communication. Some authors have emphasized the first
interpretation, and others the second, without being aware of
this level-of-analysis problem. In this study the emphasis
will be on the system-level, and the analysis will be
predominantly institutional. Hence, the directorates will be
considered as a constitutive element of the international
corporate structure. Interlocking directorates are primarily
considered as channels of communication. Whether they are
channels of domination and control can only be demonstrated
at the actor-level by distinguishing different financial
groups. Our analysis will show that for the analysis of
financial groups, the study of interlocking directorates
alone will not suffice.

Another important, theoretical problem dealt with in this
monograph is whether the study of interlocking directorates
belongs to the field of economic theory, to that of
sociological theory or perhaps to the field of political
science. At first glance the question belongs to an academic
quibble. Interlocking directorates can be studied as part of
the market structure, in which case they belong to economic
theory. They can also be studied as an indication of the
structure of the business elite, in which case they belong to
sociological theory. Finally, they may be studied in terms of
decision-making arrangements, in which case they can belong
to political science.

These different disciplinary approaches emphasize different
aspects of the same phenomenon. In an actor-oriented approach
interlocking directorates certainly are strategic devices of
corporations to control their environment. But they can also
be strategic devices of individuals or families to accumulate
personal wealth or family fortune (see Zeitlin, 1974 and

1976). Turning from the actor-level to the system-level, the network of interlocking directorates can be considered as a system of personal interlocks between corporations or as a system of corporate interlocks between persons (see Levine and Roy, 1979). In other words, a network analysis can be carried out as a study of the structure of the corporate elite or as a study of the structure of the elite of corporations. [4] The main problem is that these different aspects of interlocking directorates are very seldom studied in relation to each other. There is no comprehensive theory, for example, on the relation between the economic structure (in terms of financial, commercial and industrial relations) and the structure of the business elite (in terms of regional or national affiliation, political affiliation, or family affiliation). Or, formulated in marxist terminology, there is no comprehensive theory relating the structures of capital to the structure of the bourgeoisie. An attempt to develop such a theory can be found in the economic theories of imperialism, but these attempts are often implicit and have an unpalatable general character.

Although this study focuses on the international structure of intercorporate relations, an attempt will be made to close the gap between the elitist or class-hegemony orientation and the institutionalist orientation by taking the structure of the international corporate elite also into account.

[4] Various authors, such as Sonquist and Koenig (1975: 199) and Ornstein (1980: 289), do not make the two-fold distinction between actor-oriented and system-oriented approaches on the one hand, and institutionalist versus personalistic approaches on the other. They wrongly set the studies focusing on interlocking behavior of singular firms against the class-hegemony orientation of other studies.

I THEMES AND PROBLEMS

1.0 Introduction

In this first chapter I will sketch the theoretical framework
of the two most important research traditions in the field of
corporate interlocks. The first is that of finance capital.
This theory is of German origin and has been developed
predominantly within the marxist tradition. The second is
that of (the abuse of) economic power. It is typically a
product of the U.S. antitrust movement and has been developed
within the school of institutional economics. The
contribution of each theoretical tradition to the development
of the empirical research will be assessed. [1] After that,
two fundamental problems of research on interlocking
directorates will be discussed: the theoretical and empirical
problems related to the concept of interest- or financial
group (Section 1.3) and the primarily theoretical problems
related to the concepts of capitalist class and economic
elite (Section 1.4).

1.1 The theory of finance capital

The first extensive and systematic study on interlocking
directorates was the dissertation of Otto Jeidels, Das
Verhaltnis der Deutschen Grossbanken zur Industrie mit
besonderer Berucksichtigung der Eisenindustrie (The
Relationship between the Large German Banks and Industry with
Special Reference to the Iron Industry), which appeared in
1905. This seems to have also been the first systematic
research on interlocking directorates. [2] Starting with the

[1] A detailed survey of all research on interlocking
directorates from 1900 to 1978 has been published elsewhere
(Meindert Fennema and Huibert Schijf, Analysing
interlocking directorates: theory and methods. Social
Networks, Vol 1,4: 297-332). Most of what will be said in
the first three sections is based on the evidence presented
in this article.

[2] In his 1894 study, The evolution of Modern Capitalism,
Hobson analyzed the relation between the London City and
some South-African mining companies by studying the
interlocking directorates. This analysis, however, is very
partial (see Hobson, 1906).

six biggest Berlin banks, Jeidels discovered 1350 interlocking directorates with German industry (see Table 1.1). He assigned great power to the big banks and regarded the interlocking directorates as an expression of the sphere of influence of these banks. The close and active relation between banks and industry was regarded as a new phenomenon caused by "the crisis of 1900 that enormously accelerated and intensified the process (of industrial concentration, M.F.), which for the first time transformed the connection with industry into an actual monopoly of the big banks, and made this connection much closer and more active" (Jeidels, 1905: 181). Jeidels related the network of interlocking directorates to a new phase in German industrial development caused by concentration and launched by the economic crisis of 1900. He also gave for this new development the theoretical explanation that "the bank to a certain extent embodies here the inner connection between a large number of enterprises which results from the development of large scale industry; it represents the community of interests existing between them" (Jeidels, 1905: 215). "By expansion of industrial combination, various directions of which can be seen in the electrical and large-scale iron and steel industries, the sphere of this consciously guided production can be considerably enlarged and in this unmistakable movement the big banks are an important factor" (Jeidels, 1905: 270; italics mine, M.F.).

The theoretical explanation comes close to the concept of finance capital, developed in 1909 by Hilferding, a marxist scholar, who defines finance capital as "capital at the disposition of the banks and used by industrials" (Hilferding, 1968: 309). Jeidels does not describe his research design in detail, but from his presentation it can be deduced that he started by selecting the largest German banks and looked for all interlocking directorates between these largest banks and industry. As a systematic empirical study on interlocking directorates Jeidels' study was an example for many scholars to come. In 1910 a similar study was published by Riesser and in 1931 Hagemann published a study which even carried the same title, but without special reference to the iron industry. The close relationship between banks and industry and the central position of the banks in the network of interlocking directorates were confirmed by these studies (see Table 1.1). The concept "sphere of influence" was used by Jeidels to describe the assumed domination of the banks over industrial firms. It was not only in Germany that such a close relationship existed between banks and industry. In the Netherlands, Wibaut (1913) copied Jeidels' research design and found 300 firms interlocked with the 9 largest banks.

Table 1.1 Interlocking directorates between banks and industry in Germany, 1902, 1910 and 1927

| | No. of industrials interlocked with | | | | No. of interlocking directorates | | | |
| | 1902 | | | '10 | 1902 | '10 | '12 | '27 |
	a)	[*]	[**]	[*]	a)	b)	c)	c)
Deutsche Bank	221	(101	120)	102	334	112	159	381
Diskontogesellschaft	92	(31	61)	71	194	101	143	351
Darmstädter Bank (Bank (für Handel und Industrie)	101	(51	50)	86	203	95	–	–
Dresdner Bank	133	(53	80)	79	233	94	120	371
Schaafhausenscher Bankverein	130	(68	62)	50	236	59		d)
Berliner Handels- gesellschaft	74	(40	34)	34	150	44	123	108
Mitteldt Kreditbank	–			–	–	–	–	70
Commerz u.Privatbank	–			31	–	34	–	195
National Bank für Deutschland	–			91	–	96	–	–
Total					1350	635		1785

[*]   through bankers
[**] through industrialists

a) Source: Jeidels, 1905: 170
b) Source: Riesser, 1910: Beilage IV
c) Source: Hagemann, 1931: 79
d) In 1914 taken over by Diskontogesellschaft

Lenin used Jeidels' empirical results for his study on imperialism, and through Lenin this type of research was introduced into the literature of marxism-leninism. [3] This has resulted in a number of studies in the United States

[3] Lenin misinterpreted the figures from Jeidels by adding the number of firms given in Table 1.1. He added the figures in the first column up to 751 and concluded that the 6 Berlin banks were interlocked with 751 industrial companies in 1902. Since the 6 Berlin banks may well have interlocks with the same firms, the total number of firms may be considerably less than 751 (Lenin, 1964: 221). The figure 751 gives the number of lines between the 6 Berlin banks and German industry. The overlap of bank-industry interlocks is neglected by Lenin.

(Rochester, 1936; Perlo, 1957; Menshikov, 1969), the United
Kingdom (Aaronovitch, 1961), the Netherlands (Baruch, 1962)
and Sweden (Hermansson, 1971) among others. All these studies
have relied heavily upon the theory of Hilferding. Because
Hilferding was the first to provide a systematic explanation
for the existence of interlocking directorates between banks
and large scale industry, and because his argument formed the
foundation of many - especially marxist - theories of
imperialism, we will summarize his argument.

Hilferding relates the development of finance capital to
monopolization in industry, which required ever-increasing
investment funds. The need for planning of production and
markets made the banks the focal points in the organization
of industry. Why? Hilferding's argument is based on the
distinction of two types of credit. The first type (credit
for circulation) results from commodity exchange, where
checks are used to facilitate the payment between regular
business relations. Endorsing a check meant an extension of
the dual credit-debt relation towards third parties, while
the intervention of a bank made the check a means of
extending the credit relations to a much larger network of
firms. At the end of the nineteenth century, however, credit
was no longer used solely for commodity exchange. Increasing
investment in fixed capital forced industrial firms to borrow
money to finance new investments. This put the lender in a
different position. No longer was he solely interested in the
solvency of the debtor in the short run; he now became
interested in the profitability of the firm in the long(er)
run. Thus banks became interested in industrial development
and required detailed knowledge of the structure and strategy
of the borrowing firm. Such a development was not restricted
to Germany. In 1914 an American railway tycoon testified
before the House Judiciary Committees on Trust Legislation:
  "Precise and detailed disclosures concerning the affair
   of the borrower are the recognized prerequisite of an
   application for credit, and constant information on the
   part of the banker is the desideration when the
   applications for credit frequently occur. The simplest
   and most natural provision to meet this necessity is
   representation of the banker on the corporate board"
   (quoted in Dixon, 1914: 940).
The need for regular and detailed information induced the
bankers to seek representation in the direction of their
debtor clients. A new institutional arrangement enabled them
to do so: the joint-stock company with its board of
directors. The joint-stock company had another very important
advantage over the private firms. By issuing shares it could
obtain new capital for investment not by entering into
liabilities but by extending its 'social capital', i.e., by

issuing claims upon future profits. The holders of such claims could exercise influence directly by appointing their 'representatives' to the board of directors of the firm (see Section 4.1). The foundation of joint-stock companies at the end of the nineteenth century required a new type of bank to handle the emission of shares: the investment bank, which obtained huge profits from these emissions by keeping blocks of shares temporarily in portfolio (Grundergewinn). The investment banks, therefore, not only felt the need to be represented on the board of directors because they required regular and detailed information, but they could actually demand seats on the board because of the shares they held in portfolio or in trust for their private clients. In other words, they were in a position to exercise control over many industrial firms. Banks assumed a mediating role between individual money-suppliers as private investors and the large industrial public companies. This led to a drastic increase in the banks' deposits during the first years of the twentieth century. In Figure 1.1 the development of deposits in leading English, French and German banks between 1890 and 1918 shows a sharp rise. German banks had a late start compared to French and British banks but seemed to have caught up by 1918, especially with regard to the French banks whose deposits dropped sharply at the beginning of World War I. But through this mediating role the banks also obtained a crucial position in the allocation of capital between different industries. The information necessary for an optimal allocation of capital was obtained through a network of interlocking directorates, which Hilferding called Personalunion. This Personalunion is, according to Hilferding, the result of the need for cooperation between organizations that belong together, but remain institutionally separated for other reasons. Finally, because banks and industry had a common interest, banks also became interested in maintaining industrial cartels and other 'barriers to entry' which were responsible for the monopoly profits obtained in the large-scale industry. Cartelization in the capitalist economy enhanced planning as a coordination mechanism. It repelled the market as such a mechanism, thus producing what Hilferding called 'organized capitalism' (Hilferding, 1927). Hilferding did not see any limits to a process which he felt could even end in the complete victory of planning in the form of a Generalkartell:

  "Die ganze kapitalistische Produktion wird bewusst geregelt von einer Instanz, die das Ausmass der Produktion in allen ihren Sphären bestimmt. Dann wird die Preisfestsetzung rein nominell und bedeutet nunmehr die Verteilung des Gesamtprodukts auf die Kartellmagnaten einerseits, auf die Masse aller anderen Gesellschaft mitglieder anderseits" (Hilferding, 1968: 321,322).

(The whole capitalist production is monitored consciously
from one locus of control, which determines the amount of
production in all industries. The price setting is purely
nominal and has only meaning for the division of the total
product between the corporate elite on the one hand, and the
rest of the population on the other.)

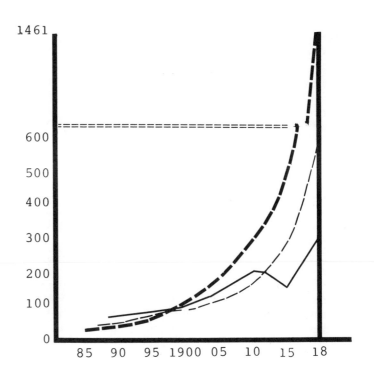

– – –	British banks
———	French banks
■■■	German banks

Figure 1.1 Increase of deposits in the three largest British,
French and German banks between 1885 and 1918
(1900=100; index based on local currency).
Recalculation of figures from Westerman (1920:
413, 414).

The above quotation stresses two aspects of the ownership of
the means of production: the right to dispose of capital
(usus) and a claim upon the revenues of its use (usus
fructus). These two aspects of ownership are separated at the
level of the individual joint-stock company (see Section 2.4)
but united again in the hypothetical Generalkartell. The
tendency towards unification of these two aspects of
ownership at a level beyond the singular corporation finds
its expression in the network of interlocking directorates:

> "Es bildet sich ein Kreis von Personen heraus, die
> vermöge ihrer eigenen Kapitalsmacht oder aber als
> Vertreter der konsentrierten Macht fremden Kapitals
> (Bankdirektoren) als Aufsichtsräte in einer grossen
> Anzahl von Aktiengesellschaften vertreten sind. Es
> entsteht so eine Art von Personalunion, einmal zwischen
> den verschiedenen Aktiengesellschaften untereinander
> und sodann zwischen diesen und den Banken, ein Umstand,
> der für die Politik dieser Gesellschaften von grösstem
> Einfluss sein muss, weil zwischen den verschiedenen
> Gesellschaften ein gemeinsames Besitzinteresse sich
> bildet" (Hilferding, 1968:157).

(A circle of persons is formed that by means of the power of
their own capital or as representative of the concentrated
power of the capital of others (bankers), sits upon the
boards of a large number of corporations. There thus arises a
kind of personal union, on the one hand between the different
corporations themselves, and on the other between them and
the banks, a situation which must have the greatest influence
upon the policy of these companies because a joint ownership
interest is being shaped between different companies).

The formation of joint ownership interests between banks and
industry is, according to the theory of Hilferding, of great
importance for the policy of these institutions. [4] Thus,
the network of interlocking directorates seems to be a
mechanism both for creating joint ownership interest and for
influencing the policy of large corporations in accordance
with this joint ownership interest. The two aspects of
ownership, usus and usus fructus, are not analytically

[4] Sweezy omits in his translation of the same text (1956:
    261) the ownership aspect of the Personalunion and speaks
    of "a community of interest". This omission makes
    Hilferding's remark fit more easily into his own theory of
    inside control of the large corporations (see for an
    empirical refutation of Sweezy's view: Norich, 1980).

separated by Hilferding, although his analysis focuses on the
former rather than on the latter. The analysis of Hilferding
has been questioned on several points by the French economic
historian Bouvier (1973: 115-120). To begin with, Bouvier
raises the question of whether the analysis of Hilferding,
however aptly it describes the development in Germany and
Austria, is applicable to countries like France and Great
Britain. (See for example, the somewhat slower increase of
deposits in France and Great Britain than in Germany (Figure
1.1)). Secondly, Bouvier argues that the structure described
by Hilferding may be more realistic in the case of merchant
banks than in the case of deposit banks. Thirdly, at the
level of personnel, the thesis of Hilferding does not apply
to everybody. Bouvier gives an example of a (deposit) banker,
Henri Germain, who sits on the board of an industrial
company, without having any control. The main problem here is
that the assumption that Germain exercises control is not
warranted a priori; but the opposite assumption is equally
unwarranted. As we lack more detailed empirical proof, the
plausibility of either assumption depends on the plausibility
of the theoretical framework from which the assumptions are
deduced. I do agree with Bouvier that the automatic
implication of bankers' control from the theory of finance
capital should be rejected. Indeed, a structure of finance
capital with industrial domination cannot be rejected a
priori. But here two interpretations of Hilferding's theory
are possible. The first and most common interpretation holds
that the interpenetration of bank and industrial capital
implies the domination of banks over industrial firms. This
interpretation is found in the theory of bank control which –
as will be shown later- reappears in the United States
studies on interlocking directorates. The second
interpretation, to which I will adhere, holds that the
interpenetration of bank and industrial capital does not
necessarily lead to control of banks over industrials. The
central thesis in the latter interpretation is that the
development of finance capital gives rise to joint ownership
interests of banks and industrial firms as expressed in a
network of interlocking directorates.

Finance capital and imperialism

Hilferding's theory of finance capital explained not only the
development of a network of interlocking directorates, but
also the capital export push which remained an integral part
of many economic theories of imperialism. The argument is
basically simple: to maintain monopoly profits it is
necessary to restrict investment in the cartelized
industries. Thus, restriction of investments leads to higher

investments funds which can only be invested in new
industrial sectors not yet cartelized, or - another
possibility - abroad. In the industrial sectors which are not
yet cartelized, investment is not very attractive either
because the profit rate in these sectors has been depressed
by the existence of cartelized sectors:

"So wächst einerseits rapid die Masse des zur
Akkumulation bestimmten Kapitals, während sich
anderseits seine Anlagemöglichkeit kontrahiert. Dieser
Widerspruch verlangt seine Lösung und findet sie im
Kapitalexport" (Hilferding, 1968: 321).

(Thus, on the one hand, the amount of investment funds
increases rapidly, while on the other hand, the investment
opportunities decrease. The solution for this contradiction
is capital export.)

The capital export push is strengthened because tariff walls
erected to protect the privileged and cartelized markets
prevent the export of commodities. According to Hilferding,
investment outlets are predominantly found in non-industrial,
colonial areas. This foreign investment necessarily leads to
imperialist rivalry, because finance capital from different
countries faces identical problems and tries to find the
same, but mutually exclusive, solutions. It is clear now that
Lenin's popular essay on imperialism, written in 1916, leans
heavily on the theory of Hilferding. Two citations must
suffice here:

"Thus finance capital, literally, one might say, spreads
its net over all countries of the world" and "The
capital-exporting countries have divided the world
among themselves in the figurative sense of the term.
But finance capital has led to the actual division of
the world" (Lenin, 1964: 245).

However, there are also elements in the theory of Hilferding
that are more in line with other variants of the economic
theories of imperialism to be discussed in Chapter 3. One
example is the idea that in spite of the rivalizing
tendencies, there are also tendencies leading to
international cooperation between finance capitalists from
different countries (Hilferding, 1968: 452, 453).

Unfortunately, Hilferding's analysis stops here. He does not
investigate the formation of finance capital at a global
level. The intergration of finance capital from different
countries is hardly considered. And although many writers -
marxist and non-marxist alike - have analyzed the
internationalization of capital more in detail, none of them
has tried to analyze international finance capital by

searching for a network of interlocking directorates at the
international level. Such a network of interlocking
directorates would - if it existed - also express the
international organization of ownership interests. Finance
capital is only truly international if such an international
organization exists. This study is an attempt to analyze the
joint ownership interest at the international level by
investigating the international network of interlocking
directorates.

1.2 Interlocking directorates and economic power

In the United States, research on corporate interlocks may
well have had the same economic background as in Germany.
Here we also find industrial concentration at the end of the
nineteenth century and a sharp economic crisis in 1900 and
again in 1907. The first studies of corporate interlocks,
however, had a very different social setting. Unlike the
detached, scientific studies by isolated scholars such as
Jeidels, Riesser and Hagemann, the research on interlocks in
the United States was a direct result of public debate. Thus
in 1913 the Pujo Committee conducted an official
investigation and found that the three largest New York
banks, J.P.Morgan and Company, First National Bank and
National City Bank, were represented through 341
directorships on the boards of 112 corporations. One hunderd
eighty persons held 746 directorships in 134 corporations.
The same 180 individuals held 385 directorships in 41 banks
and trust companies (cited in Bearden, et.al., 1975: 1).
Most interlocks existed between railway companies and banks.
The public debate centered around these two types of
companies (see Dixon, 1914). The results of the Pujo
Committee were used in the congressional debates which led to
the adoption of the Clayton Act in 1914, prohibiting
interlocking directorates between competing firms.
The Clayton Act specified three classes of prohibited
interlocks:
- interlocking directorates between banks;
- interlocking directorates between directly competing firms;
- interlocking directorates between railroads and their
  potential suppliers.

The research on corporate interlocks was stimulated by the
antitrust movement and sponsored or even conducted by the
government. Senator Sparkman, chairman of the Select
Committee on Small Business, writes in 1952:
  "It has long been the public policy of the United States
  to supplement the legal provisions of the antitrust
  laws with broad, fact-finding powers. The fundamental

purpose of fact-finding is to prevent the abuse of
power" (The international petroleum cartel, 1952: VI).
This strongly influenced the character of the research,
giving it a moralistic and legalistic bias. A theoretical
framework was either lacking or underdeveloped, whereas the
data were often extensive and reliable. The fact that
investigators were supposed not to take a stand in the
debate, but only to provide 'the facts' has undoubtedly
contributed to the theoretical poverty of the studies on
interlocking directorates in the United States. These
'official' United States studies, however, have contributed
enormously to the methodology of research on interlocking
directorates. They have elaborated different types of
interlocking directorates and clarified the meaning and
effects of these different types. Well known, for example, is
Sweezy's distinction between primary and secondary
interlocks:

"A primary interlock exists between companies X and Y if
a director of X, whose main business interest is with
X, sits on the board of Y. If the same person also sits
on the board of Z, then a primary interlock also exists
between X and Z. These two relations, however,
necessarily involve an interlock between Y and Z, and
this we call a secondary interlock. It goes without
saying that more weight should be given to primary than
to secondary interlocks and that the latter should be
interpreted only with caution" (Sweezy, 1953: 162).
Sweezy was invited to study interlocking directorates by the
the National Resource Committee, a New Deal agency which
undertook a large investigation into the structure of the
American economy in 1936 and published its results in 1939
(NRC, 1939). After World War II the Federal Trade Commission
published an investigation on interlocking directorates per
industry. The FTC report mentioned various factors that
determine the significance of interlocking directorates:

"Interlocking relationships among corporations through
persons associated with those corporations are of
various types, dependent upon the character of the
enterprises that are linked, the directness of the
linkage, the frequency of the linkage and the
responsibilities of the persons who constitute the
links" (FTC, 1951: 17).

Attention is drawn here to the fact that the significance of
interlocking directorates depends on four variables:
- the nature of the corporations that are interlocked
An interlock between a financial company and an industrial
company differs from an interlock between two financial or
two industrial companies. And an interlock between two
industrials that have identical market positions should be

interpreted differently from an interlock between industrials
that have different market positions.
- the directness of the linkage
Here we should not only mention the secondary interlock but
also the meeting line. Two companies may be indirectly
interlocked because they are represented on the board of
directors of a third company. The meaning of such an indirect
linkage may vary with the nature of the third company. If the
third company is a (potential) competitor of the two
indirectly linked companies, the interlock is "likely to be
at least as significant as a direct interlock between those
concerns. "(FTC report, 1951: 187). [5] If the third company
is a supplier, a customer, or a financial institution, the
meeting directors may act jointly on behalf of the companies
they represent. Here, however, the coordination between the
two indirectly linked companies may also be of a competitive
nature, as we will argue in Chapter 2. Furthermore, the FTC
report points to the possible business coordination through
persons who are not directors, but nevertheless represent the
interest of a company, such as large stockholders or officers
who are not member of the board of directors of the company
they represent. Finally kinship ties may be as important
corporate interlocks as interlocking directorates.
- the frequency of the linkage
Very often two companies are interlocked through more than
one person. Such multiple interlocks are evidently more
significant than single interlocks. The FTC report concludes
that "the more numerous the interlocks the stronger is the
presumption that they create unity of action" (see Section
4.4.1).
- the position of the interlocking directors in the companies
they interlock
It should also be clear that the character of the corporate
interlock may differ with the function and responsibilities

[5] A joint-venture is a special case of a potentially
    competing third firm. A joint-venture is a company founded
    by the two parent companies and fully owned by them,
    frequently on a fifty - fifty basis. Since the joint-
    venture often restricts its activities to a limited area of
    business, there is at least partial cooperation between the
    two parent firms. They may still be competing in other
    areas. If this is the case, no direct interlock between the
    two parent companies is expected. This is so because an
    interlocking directorate provides at least one of the
    companies with detailed information about areas of activity
    of the other company.

of the person who constitutes the interlock. Representation
by a president may mean more than representation by a lower
officer. An interlock based on an outside directorship in
both companies differs from an interlock based on an inside
directorship in one company and an outside directorship in
the other. Judgement of this kind requires insight into
division of authority between the board of directors and the
corporate management. In Chapter 4 I will compare the
division of authority between the decision-making bodies in
companies incorporated in different countries (see Sections
4.1 and 4.4.2).

More official investigations on interlocking directorates
followed that of the Federal Trade Commission. In 1965 the
Antitrust Subcommittee of the Committee on the Judiciary
published Interlocks in Corporate Management, a study which
was used by Dooley in his comparison of the network of 1935
and that of 1965 (see Section 1.3). In 1968 the so-called
Patman Committee published a study entitled Commercial Banks
and their Trust Activities, investigating interlocks between
commercial banks and major corporations (Patman Committee,
1968). Finally the Metcalf Committee also conducted research
and published it in Interlocking Directorates among major
U.S. Corporations in 1978 (Metcalf Committee, 1978).

Antitrust sentiments have also been a source of inspiration
for research on interlocking directorates outside Congress
and Federal Government committees. In 1973 a labor
organization, the Marine Engineer's Beneficial Association,
published The American Oil Industry. The commission of the
study was given to the consulting firm Stanley H. Ruttenberg
& Associates, and conducted by Norman Medvin, a former
government employee. In a second edition it was published
under his name (1974).

In conclusion we see that rather than providing a broad
theoretical framework which explains the development of
interlocking directorates, the antitrust investigations
provide us with a refined set of propositions about the
functioning of interlocking directorates. We will develop
these propositions further in Chapter 4 because they are
prerequisite for an empirical analysis of the network of
interlocking directorates. The results of this analysis will
be interpreted within the theoretical framework developed by
Hilferding. But we will have to elaborate on this framework
to suit our analysis of the network at the international
level.

1.3 Financial groups

Between the 'macro' theory of finance capital (Section 1.1) and the 'micro' propositions about the significance of different types of interlocks (Section 1.2) there are a number of studies on interlocking directorates using the concept of financial group as a starting point. While this concept is sufficiently broad to allow incorporation into the theory of finance capital, it should also permit operationalization in terms of (the different types of) interlocking directorates. In the theory of finance capital a group is a unit of capital consisting of financial and industrial companies which develops common policies, has elements of control in common and is connected by interlocking directorates (Soref, 1980: 67). This notion should be properly operationalized by stating which elements of control companies should have in common and by what types of corporate interlocks they should be connected to form an interest- or financial group. Unfortunately these concepts are too often rather loosely used to illustrate the theory of finance capital rather than to validate it by connecting it to the empirical findings.

The early studies of interlocking directorates concentrated on the relations between banks and industry and assumed that these relations indicated the sphere of influence of the banks (Section 1.1). In these studies the theory of finance capital was simplified into a theory of bank control. This can be seen, for example, in the study of Rochester (1936), who investigated the sphere of influence of the Morgan group and the Rockefeller group. Sweezy, when preparing a study for the National Committee in 1937 - although strongly influenced by the study of Rochester - did not use the concept of sphere of influence. Instead, he used the concept of interest group which he later defined as
"a number of corporations under common control, the locus of power being normally an investment- or a commercial bank or a great family fortune" (Baran and Sweezy, 1968: 30).
Here an attempt is made to specify the essence of belonging together by defining an interest group in terms of common control exercised from one locus of control. And the most important mechanisms of control are credit-relations, share ownership and interlocking directorates. Sweezy warned against the uncritical use of interlocking directorates as an indication for control and he emphasized the different meanings of the different types of interlocking directorates mentioned in Section 1.2. According to Sweezy, it is better to study the three mechanisms of control in combination (Sweezy, 1953: 161-164).

Twenty years later, Perlo (1957) used the same concept of interest group, although he combined it with the older concept of sphere of influence. Menshikov - still in the same tradition - used a slightly different concept of financial group, defining it as

"a sum total of companies managed independently. Each one is a commercial entity. Control (if it exists) is separated from management. The activities of such companies are coordinated at a higher level, outside the companies themselves" (Menshikov, 1969: 205,206).

Menshikov's concept is looser than Sweezy's, but neither Sweezy nor Menshikov tried to operationalize the concepts they used. The results are therefore difficult to compare, and the investigators avoid any rigorous comparison. Thus, while quoting the study of Perlo with approval, Menshikov distinguishes at least nineteen groups in comparison with Perlo's eight. He does not explain the difference anywhere. And the results of Sweezy, Perlo and Menshikov are indeed hard to compare. This is partly due to the fact that no clear distinction is made between different types of corporate interlocks. Thus, for one firm its belonging to a group is demonstrated by the existence of interlocking directorates, while for another firm the financial linkages are taken as evidence. Furthermore, the link between the theory of finance capital and the propositions explaining the meaning of different types of corporate interlocks is nowhere explicit in terms of financial groups. Besides, a methodological problem concerning the detection of corporate interlocks remains. Like Jeidels, Perlo and Menshikov seem to start with a selection of large banks or large industrials which are presumed to be the core of some financial group. Behind the investigating of interlocking directorates between these firms and other firms circularity between hypothesis and evidence lurks: if one starts investigating the network from a specific firm and works snowball-wise, it is not surprising that the starting point is found to be the center of the network.

Table 1.2 Interest groups according to Sweezy, Perlo,
       Menshikov and Dooley

1935 (Sweezy)   1956 (Perlo)

1. Morgan - First National   1. Morgan
2. Rockefeller   2. Rockefeller
3. Kuhn, Loeb   3. First National City
4. Mellon   4. Mellon
5. Du Pont   5. Du Pont
6. Chicago   6. Chicago
7. Cleveland   7. Cleveland
8. Boston   8. Bank of America

1962 (Menshikov)   1965 (Dooley)

New York groups   Tight-knit groups Nr. of corp.
1. Morgan Guaranty Trust   1. New York   38
2. Chase Manhattan/Chemical   2. Chicago   14
   Bank/ New York Trust   3. San Francisco   13
   (Rockefeller)   4. Pittsburg   8
3. First National City   5. Los Angeles   6
4. Manufacturing Hanover   6. Cleveland   5
5. Sullivan and Cromwell   7. Detroit   4
   Marine Midland
6. Lehman-Goldman, Sachs
7. Harriman-Newmont
   Mining
8. Dillon, Read and Co.

Regional groups   Loose-knit groups

 9. Mellon-First Boston Corp   8. Milwaukee   7
10. Du Pont   9. Hartford   6
11. Boston   10. Philadelphia   4
12. Cleveland, of which   11. Portland, Ore.   4
    Cyrus Eaton
    Humphrey-Hanna
    Kirby group
13. Chicago, of which   12. Minneapolis-St.Paul 3
    Crown-Hilton group
14. Texas, of which   13. Boston   3
    Greatamerica
15. California, of which   14. Dallas   2
    Giannini heirs
    Western Bancorporation
    Crocker-Wells Fargo-
            Securities
16. Minneapolis-St.Paul   15. Houston   2
17. St.Louis
18. Hartford
19. Detroit

Recent research on corporate interlocks has tried to avoid
such pitfalls by studying different types of corporate
interlocks separately and by selecting a sample of firms
rather than choosing the presumed center of the groups as a
starting point. Dooley (1969) defined a group by the number
of times its members were interlocked. He found seven tight-
knit groups, in which corporations interlock four or more
times, and eight loose-knit groups, in which corporations
interlock two or three times (see Table 1.2). Comparison of
the results of Sweezy, Perlo, Menshikov and Dooley makes
clear that they depend heavily on the definition and
operationalization of the concept of group. Sweezy and Perlo,
using the same concept of interest group and similar
operationalization, obtain comparable results. The eight
groups they find are either defined by a dominant bank
(Morgan), or by a family fortune (Rockefeller, Du Pont) or by
region (Chicago, Cleveland, Boston). Only slight changes have
taken place between 1935 and 1956. Two groups have
disappeared (Kuhn, Loeb and Boston), while two new groups
appear in 1956 (First National City and Bank of America) (see
Table 1.2). Menshikov makes a distinction between New York
groups and regional groups. All New York groups have their
locus of control in a bank. Of the regional groups some have
the locus of control in a bank (Mellon-First Boston Corp.) or
in a family (Du Pont) but the majority is simply labeled
according to region. Dooley finds fifteen groups, all
regionally defined. In Dooley's study no distinction between
the Morgan and the Rockefeller groups is found. In Dooley's
study, however, although a group is solely defined by
interlocking directorates, the operationalization of the
concept is somewhat hazy. Since the study of Dooley (1969)
more sophisticated attempts have been made to analyze the
network of interlocking directorates in the United States in
terms of groups. Sonquist and Koenig (1975) used an
application of graph theory to search for clusters, defined
as a set of corporations all of which are linked to one
another in such ways that the number of interlocks in the set
is high, while the number of interlocks with firms outside
the set is low. They base their analysis directly on the
concepts and computer programs of Alba (1973), in which the
structural unit is the N-clique. The reader is referred to
Alba's paper and that of Mokken (1979) for more detailed
information. The analysis yielded thirty-two clusters ranging
in size from three to fifteen corporations. Although some
regionalization appears from the analysis, these clusters
bear little resemblance to the groups identified by either
Sweezy, Perlo, Menshikov or Dooley, if only because some of
the banks which seem to be the center of the clusters defined
by these authors appear in two of the cliques found by
Sonquist and Koenig. Mariolis used on the same dataset a peak
analysis by defining a peak as a corporation that interlocks

only with corporations less central than itself. Centrality
is measured in terms of the intensity of the lines with
neighboring firms and of the centrality of these neighbors.
[6] Although the correlation between this sophisticated
centrality index and the number of interlocks is .91,
Mariolis (1975: 430) argues that the differences can be
substantial for local firms (see Section 5.0). Each peak
defines a cluster: any other corporation is in the cluster
defined by the peak if and only if all the more central
corporations with which it is interlocked are also in that
cluster (Mariolis, 1977: 11).
A peak analysis on the centrality score of the 797
corporations results in three peaks: Chemical Bank,
International Harvester, and U.S. Smelting, Refining, and
Mining. Only one of these peaks is a bank; what is more the
three peaks define three clusters of only 13, 2 and 3 firms
respectively. The vast majority of the 797 corporations
cannot be assigned to a cluster, although only 61 of these
are isolated, while 84 corporations have more than 24
interlocks each (Mariolis, 1975: 430).
According to Bearden et.al. (1975) this is due to the fact
that two-thirds of all interlocks in the network are weak
ties, i.e., interlocks carried by a person who is an outside

---

[6] Mariolis uses a modification of the centrality measure
    developed by Bonacich (1972) based on overlapping
    memberships of groups. The centrality of a firm depends on
    the centrality of its neighbors (a) and on the intensity of
    the lines with these neighbors (b). The intensity $r(i,j)$ of
    a line is defined by:

$$r(i,j) = \frac{d(i,j)}{\sqrt{d(i) * d(j)}}$$

    where $d(i,j)$ is the number of interlocks between i and j
    and $d(i)$ is the number of directors on the board of
    corporation i and $d(j)$ is the number of directors on the
    board of corporation j. The centrality of i is defined in
    terms of the centrality of its neighbors, which, in turn,
    (partly) depends on the centrality of i:
    $c(i) = r(i,1)*c(1) + r(i,2)*c(2) + \ldots + r(i,n)*c(n)$
    This represents a system of n linear equations. This linear
    problem has, generally, no (non-zero) solution. By
    modifying this equation to $C = R * C$, however, Bonacich
    shows that an approximate solution, which gives the
    required centrality scores, can be found (Mariolis, 1975:
    30n).

director in both companies. These weak ties are communication
lines rather than control lines and form manifold overlaps
between different groups. Due to these overlaps many
corporations cannot be assigned to any other group in the
cluster analysis used by Mariolis. Therefore, Bearden et.al.
take only those interlocks into account which are carried by
an inside director in one of the firms. They call these
officer-interlocks or strong ties (see Section 4.4.2). The
peak analysis now results in five peaks: Continental Illinois
defines a cluster of 131 firms, Mellon Bank one of 12, Morgan
one of 10, Bankers Trust one of 5 and United California Bank
one of 4. Although Bearden et.al. are able to assign 162
firms to a cluster, they again find one large cluster (of 131
firms) and a number of small ones. They warn the reader as
well that the results of the peak analysis are unstable
because of the problems of calculating the Bonacich
centrality measure in a directed graph with a skewed
distribution of multiplicities of the lines [7] in the
network (Bearden et.al., 1975: 36,45). They conclude that the
use of peak analysis does not enable one to distinguish
different interest groups. The results (or the lack of
results) from the peak analysis of Mariolis and Bearden
et.al., however, go in the direction of those of Mokken and
Stokman [8] who in 1970 found in the Dutch network of 86
largest firms a central core of highly connected
corporations, without a trace of separate clusters. [9]

[7] The multiplicity of a line is defined by the number of
    interlocks between the two firms connected by the line (see
    Section 4.4.1).

[8] The study of Mokken and Stokman is based on research
    which they initiated in 1970. A first publication of the
    results was in Dutch (Helmers et.al., 1975). After that,
    the investigation continued and the results were reported
    in a series of papers, used here as a source. A monograph
    is being prepared, comparing the network of interlocking
    directorates in the Netherlands between 1969 and 1976.

[9] Elsewhere I have shown that it is possible to separate
    this core into two clusters around the two largest
    commercial banks ABN and AMRO. The core is separated by
    searching for two sets of firms so that the density within
    the two sets is maximal while the density between these
    sets is minimal. However, the density of the separate
    clusters is 90 percent, but the density between the two
    clusters is still 64 percent (see Fennema, 1976).

Finally it should be noted that the results of a peak
analysis depend in part on the density of the network. Thus
any comparison of the results from two or more networks with
different densities are likely to be confounded by the
methodological artifacts. For this reason Mariolis has
dropped peak analysis altogether. [10]

Other techniques, such as multidimensional scaling and factor
analysis, have been used to detect different forms of
clustering in the network. An application of the former has
been used by Levine (1972) in what he called a 'smallest
space analysis'. Originally this technique was developed by
Guttman and Lingoes to recover the 'joint space' from the
preference order of individuals responding to stimuli
(questions). Levine has transferred this procedure by
identifying banks as 'individuals' and industrial
corporations as 'stimuli'. An interlocking directorate is
accordingly interpreted as a 'preference' of a bank. He
applied this technique to a subset of the Patman data on
interlocking directorates in 1965. Levine chose seventy
industrials and fourteen banks from New York, Pittsburg and
Chicago. As expected, he found regional clusters. In Chapter
7 a similar procedure will be followed, using a stochastic
scaling model developed by Mokken (1970), to analyze
interlocking directorates between banks and industry and
compare them with the international bank consortia.

Allen has continued the search for the groups in the network
of interlocking directorates by using factor analysis for
clique detection. By comparing the network of the 250 largest
corporations in 1935 with that in 1970 the changes are
investigated. In both years, the factor analysis results in
ten separate groups of firms but in 1970 the groups are
smaller, less dense and show a more regional character than
in 1935 (Allen, 1978). The results of Allen's study differ
again from the preceding results. [11]

[10] Personal communication in 1980.

[11] I do not understand how Soref can possible conclude that
     "research on interest groups yields roughly the same
     picture of interest group structure" (Soref, 1980: 68).

The problem with all these studies is that the amount of
technical elaboration of the empirical investigation is not
matched by an equally extensive theoretical elaboration of
the concept of interest group. On the contrary the more
sophisticated the research techniques, the less these
techniques seem to be related to a systematic elaboration of
the theoretical problems. In Chapter 2 I will deal with some
aspects of these theoretical problems of detection of groups
through the analysis of interlocking directorates. In Chapter
3 I will elaborate the international aspects of the theory of
finance capital. Part of the problem is whether we expect
financial or interest groups to be predominantly national -
as is implicitly assumed in the American investigations
mentioned in this section - even though they may have an
international strategy (see Pastre, 1979), or whether there
also exist international groups. This latter assumption seems
particularly relevant for smaller countries and has been
suggested by the results of the analysis of corporate
interlocks in the Netherlands, where the largest
multinationals have a marginal position in the network of
interlocking directorates (see Helmers et.al., 1975).

1.4 Corporate elite and capitalist class

In Section 1.1 it was argued that Hilferding assumed the
network of interlocking directorates to express common
ownership interests both in terms of the collection of the
revenues and in terms of strategic control. The revenue
aspect of the interlocking directorates was already glimpsed
by Marx when he wrote about the stock companies producing
   "(...) a new financial aristocracy, a new variety of
   parasites in the shape of promotors, speculators and
   simply nominal directors; a whole system of swindling
   and cheating by means of corporation promotion, stock
   issuance, and stock speculation" (Capital, III: 438).
Hilferding, on the other hand, placed more emphasis on the
aspect of strategic control, an emphasis also found in the
more recent studies on financial groups (Section 1.3). In
this book emphasis will also be on this aspect. The
international network of interlocking directorates will be
analyzed to detect international strategic control over
capital rather than international division of the spoils
through an international rentier class. This distinction is
related to another equally important distinction between the
concepts of corporate elite and capitalist class. The
capitalist class consists of all those who own, control
and/or manage (at a senior level) all corporations, including
their families (Clement, 1977: 25). It also includes those
who obtain a major part of their income from the ownership of

capital, without having any controlling or managing position
in a corporation. The corporate elite, on the other hand, is
a much more restricted concept. It is empirically more
restricted because it is defined as those persons who hold
the top positions in the largest corporations. The corporate
elite forms a subset of the capitalist class, a subset of
persons who collectively exercise strategic control over
large corporations. But also, the concept of corporate elite
is theoretically more restricted than the concept of
capitalist class. The latter presupposes a theoretical
framework in which capitalism is defined and a class theory
elaborated. In Marxist theory, for example, it is assumed
that the capitalist class is hegemonial in the economic as
well as in the political sphere. [12] Hence, part of the
political elite is also defined as belonging to the
capitalist class. (In my definition only those members of the
political elite who obtain a major part of their income from
the ownership of capital are part of the capitalist class.)
Furthermore, the concept of capitalist class also refers to
ideological domination and to those persons who control the
"ideological apparatuses." Many marxist and elitist scholars
have studied the overlap between the corporate elite and the
political elite. Recently some sophisticated attempts have
been made to study the overlap of their networks (Useem,
1979, Mokken and Stokman, 1979a, Domhoff, 1980).

In nearly all definitions of class it is implicitly assumed
that a class reproduces itself intergenerationally.
Nevertheless, very little attention has been paid to the
feminine half of the capitalist class. [13] Furthermore, most

[12] "If not all entrepreneurs, at least an elite amongst
     them must have the capacity to be an organiser of society
     in general, including all its complex organism of services,
     right up to the state organism, because of the need to
     create the conditions most favourable to the expansions of
     their own class, or at least they must possess the capacity
     to choose the deputies (specialised employees) to whom to
     entrust this activity of organising the general system of
     relationships external to the business itself" (Gramsci,
     1971: 5,6).

[13] For an exception see Domhoff, The Higher Circles (1970).
     Domhoff is a pioneer in other aspects of structural class
     analysis as well.

of the studies on class reproduction focus their research on
the reproduction of that part of the capitalist class which I
defined as the corporate elite. They show that the corporate
elite receives a large share of their income from ownership
of capital. Through 'stock option plans' and other devices,
even the 'mere managers' obtain a large part of their income
from capital gains revenue and stock dividends. Llewellen's
(1971) study of the top executives of fifty large
manufacturing companies during the early sixties showed that
their after-tax incomes from stock-based compensation
schemes, capital gains, and stock dividends were more than
six times as large as their salaries (cited by Useem, 1980).
The reproduction of the capitalist class, however, cannot be
equated with the reproduction of the corporate elite. Most of
the research in this area concentrates on the
intergenerational reproduction of the corporate elite. Bendix
(1956), for example, studied the corporate elite in the
United States between 1835 and 1955. He found an increasing
part of the corporate elite descending from upper class
families (65 percent in 1835, 74 percent in 1955), while
noting a decreasing part coming from working class families.
This change occurred between 1865 and 1925. At the same time
the career pattern of the corporate elite changed: the
entrepreneurial career pattern disappeared, while the
bureaucratic career pattern spectacularly increased. Also,
the percentage of 'heirs' doubled between 1835 and 1855. In
Europe the social background of the economic elites have not
been studied over such a long period. Nevertheless, the
little evidence available points in the same direction.
Bourdieu and de Saint Martin (1978: 46) found that of the
presidents of the 100 largest firms in France in 1952, 31
were sons of bankers and industrialists. In 1962 this number
increased to 45, while in 1972 it was still 44. At the same
time the number of presidents from working or middle class
origin remained fairly stable between 1952 and 1972: in 1952
11 presidents had a working or middle class origin; in 1972
this number was 13. In post-war France, the number of heirs
has increased, while the number of social climbers has
remained fairly stable. Research on Italy seems to yield
similar results (see Martinelli, Chiesi and Dalla Chiesa,
1981).

Whitley has done research on the social background
characteristics of the British economic elite in relation to
their network connections. His results show that the boards
of industrial companies are not nearly as integrated into the
traditional upper status groups as those of the large
financial institutions. However,
    "a considerable degree of connection between many large
     companies and financial firms does exist through the

aristocracy. This may well have increased over the last
30 or so years as the management of large sums of money
has become of increasing concern to the very large
firms, and the need for sophisticated financial advice
correspondingly increased in conjunction with the
growth of institutional investment" (Whitley, 1974:
75).

Whitley's observation reminds us of the fact that
sociological studies of the economic elite tend to
concentrate on the social composition of the elite and to
neglect its structure. How the members of the economic elite
are related to each other and whether there are different
cliques or groupings within the elite are typically questions
that are tackled in the structural approach. Because I have
assigned the function of strategic control to the corporate
elite, it is legitimate for the purpose of this study to
restrict the concept of corporate elite to those who have at
least a top position in two large firms. By doing so, the
organizing aspect of the corporate elite is stressed. The
structure of the corporate elite can be studied by analyzing
the interlocking directorates. Studying interlocking
directorates is not the only way to study the structure of
the corporate elite. One could also study family linkages or
linkages through social clubs, as is done by Lupton and
Wilson (1973). A study of the corporate elite through
interlocking directorates, however, is - more than any other
structural analysis - linked to the problem of the
fractioning of the capitalist class. Just as the social
background and compositions of the corporate elite are
related to the reproduction of the capitalist class, so is
the structure of the corporate elite related to the
fractioning of the capitalist class. Class fractions are
defined as all those who share an owning, controlling or
managing relation to a specific fraction of capital, such as
industrial, commercial or bank capital (see Poulantzas, 1974:
189-196). A fraction of the corporate elite can accordingly
be defined as a set of people holding multiple senior
executive or directorship positions in a specific type of
firm, such as industrial, commercial or financial firms.

Since the interpenetration of industrial, commercial and bank
capital has given rise to a new fraction of capital (finance
capital), it can be assumed that this development has led to
an interpenetration of correspondent segments of the
corporate elite through Personalunion between firms from
different fractions. Accordingly, the corporate elite has
changed and now consists partly of persons who are
simultaneously directors of banks and industrial firms. They
are neither "financiers" extracting interest at the expense

of industrial profits nor "bankers" controlling corporations; rather they are finance capitalists "presiding over the banks' investments as creditors and shareholders, organizing production, sales, and financing and appropriating the profits of their integrated activities" (Zeitlin, 1976: 900). These finance capitalists should be regarded as the core of the corporate elite. Their role in the international network will be investigated in Sections 4.3.1 and 8.3.1.

While most studies on finance capital have studied the interpenetration of industrial and bank capital, this book will concentrate on the interpenetration of the industrial and financial fraction of the corporate elite. And while most studies on the internationalization of finance capital have studied the interpenetration of national finance capital (in terms of direct investment, for example), this study will concentrate mainly on the resulting interpenetration of the national corporate elites. The international corporate elite, however, will not be studied as a social category (by analyzing its social background and composition) but in relation to the firms it represents.

The approach is structural as well as institutional: structural, because it focuses on the network of relations within the corporate elite; and institutional, because these relations are considered as relations between firms. I also do not intend to study the economic relations between corporations, but will concentrate instead on the personal relations between them. On the other hand, the persons are considered solely as channels or media of communication and control between firms. The unit of analysis is not the persons who constitute a corporate elite, but the firms that are connected by these persons into a network of communication and control. I hope thereby to bridge the gap between the purely economic analysis, based on the structure and composition of capital, and the purely sociological analysis based on the social composition of the economic elite(s).

In the analysis of personal ties between corporations I will not consider the family relations. As a result the centralization of the network(s) may be underestimated. There are, however, good reasons to do so. For historical reasons, families seem to be of declining importance in corporate relationships. But even if this were not the case, as is for example argued by Zeitlin (1974), it is not easy to take them systematically into account. There are at least three reasons for this. First, family relations are not easy to detect because members of a family do not all have identical surnames. Looking only for identical names would create a patrilineal bias. Second, it cannot always be said that a

family tie involves coordinated control of the share-holding
possessed. There may be feuds in the family, often with
economic origins. This was the case with the Rothschilds in
the nineteenth century (see Gille, 1967 and Bouvier, 1967).
The splitting up of the Empain empire in 1934 was, according
to Baudhuin (1946: 146), mainly due to "incompabilite de
caractere". In other cases, different branches of a family
may simply act independently without such feuds. This seems
to be the case with the Du Pont family (Kotz, 1978: 18n).
But, and this is another problem, it may also be that the
blood relationship does not involve a family fortune. Such
seems to be the case with the brothers Baumgartner. Wilfrid
Siegfried is president directeur general of Rhone-Poulenc,
administrateur of Pechiney and member of the international
Advisory Board of Chase Manhattan. His brother, Richard Paul,
is administrateur of the Compagnie Général d'Electricité and
of Elf-ERAP. There is no indication, however, that these
typical managers behave in a way that would warrant their
being regarded as one unit of (family) control.

Finally, one can even wonder whether network analysis does
underestimate family control. One can just as well argue that
the more pertinent forms of family control do take the form
of financial control, i.e. strategic control through
financial institutions. Bankers may then represent family
control, acting as a trustee. Even members of the controlling
family may act as such. It is therefore possible that the
network analysis of interlocking directorates does not
underestimate the amount of family control, even though it
does not make family control apparent either.

For these - different - reasons I decided not to go into the
problem of family relations. I do not want to suggest,
however, that family relations are unimportant for the
network of corporate interlocks.

1.5 Summary

In this chapter the most important previous research has been
reviewed according to important theoretical themes. In
Section 1.1 the German studies were presented within the
framework of the theory of finance capital as developed by
Hilferding. In his view the basic cause of the rise of
finance capital is to be found in the socialization of
production and the cartelization of markets, especially in
the heavy industries. The development of finance capital
leads in turn to an interpenetration of ownership interest
expressed in the network of interlocking directorates between
banks and industry. The development of finance capital also

creates an export push, which leads to imperial rivalries. This latter aspect, however, has been largely neglected by Hilferding and also by the subsequent research on interlocking directorates in which the theoretical framework developed by Hilferding was used.

In the United States studies on interlocking directorates have not induced general theories comparable to that of Hilferding. They were often carried out by government agencies to support antitrust legislation. The focus was more restricted to propositions about the exact meaning of interlocking directorates and, consequently, about the differences between various types of interlocking directorates (Section 1.2). A promising road to bridge the gap between the general theory of finance capital and the detailed propositions about the different types of interlocking directorates is the study of interest- or financial groups. Here the network of interlocking directorates is broken down into components, cliques or clusters which can be interpreted as concrete examples of the interpenetration of financial and industrial ownership interests. The structure of the components, cliques or clusters may indicate the locus of control in a specific community of ownership interests. Unfortunately, there is a rift between the application of general and potentially fruitful theories and the application of sophisticated models and procedures to detect groups in the network (Section 1.3). Besides, it is implicitly assumed that the groups are national groups.

In Section 1.4 attention was drawn to different elite studies and a distinction made between the concept of capitalist class and the concept of corporate elite. The concept of capitalist class is wider than that of corporate elite. Not only is the corporate elite but a part of the capitalist class, it also refers less to the intergenerational reproduction and to the revenue aspect of the capitalist mode of production and more to the aspect of strategic control of societies' economic resources.

This book is a study of the international corporate elite. However, this elite will not be investigated according to the personalistic approach commonly used in elite studies. Our investigation is institutional rather than personalistic: persons are considered solely as representatives of economic institutions and particularly as channels or media of communication and control between firms. Hilferding's theory of finance capital provides us with a theoretical framework within which the origin and development of national networks of interlocking directorates can be explained. In Chapter 3 I

will summarize contending economic theories of imperialism
because they provide alternative explanations of the
international networks of interlocking directorates. From
these alternative explanations different models of the
international structure of interlocking directorates will be
deducted. First, however, I will present in Chapter 2 an
entirely different explanation of the existence of
interlocking directorates and discuss some conceptual
problems.

II BETWEEN MARKET AND HIERARCHY

2.0 Introduction

In Section 1.1 the development of an intricate network of
interlocking directorates was explained in terms of
Hilferding's theory of finance capital. In this theory, which
firmly stands in the classical marxist tradition,
interlocking directorates are explained by reference to the
changing relations in the production process. According to
historical materialism, the ownership relations follow suit.
In the following section another explanation will be
presented, based on the neo-classically inspired 'new
property-rights approach'. This approach differs
fundamentally from that of Hilferding. While Hilferding
explains the behavior of individuals from the economic
structures, the neo-classical theorists explain the economic
structures as resulting from the (economic) behavior of
individuals.
It is surprising that theories developed from such different
starting points provide similar and - for the explanation of
networks of interlocking directorates- compatible conclusions.

2.1 The organization of firms and markets: a neo-classical
    explanation

According to Hilferding, the development of finance capital
is directly related to the need for planning of the
production process in large scale industry and for
cartelization of the market. Planning and markets are
implicitly assumed to be antagonistic forms of allocation of
resources and of coordination of productive activities. Why
is this so? To answer this question it is necessary to
develop a theory of the relation between economic
organization through planning and organization through the
market. Such a theory has not only been developed by
Hilferding and his marxian colleagues, but also by a number
of neo-classical economists who, because of their critique of
certain aspects of neo-classical theory itself, are often
called the 'new economists'. [1] They criticize neo-classical
theory because it lacks a proper theory of the firm. Their
argument begins with the following question. If it is true,

[1] See for a critical treatment of the 'new economists',
    Andreff, 1982.

as neo-classical theory assumes, that the market is the
optimal allocation mechanism for the economic resources, why
do firms exist at all? Why are not all economic resources of
individuals allocated through the market? This question is
answered by Coase (1937) who assumes that markets do not
operate costlessly. The higher the costs of transaction
across markets, the greater will be the comparative advantage
of organizing resources within the firm. A new question
arises immediately. Under what circumstances are costs of
market transactions high? To answer this question it should
be remembered that according to neo-classical theory,
resources are distributed according to marginal productivity.
However, in some forms of economic organization it is very
difficult (and thus costly) to determine each individual's
marginal productivity. Those forms of economic organization
in which marginal productivity of individuals is difficult to
measure are called team production by Alchian and Demsetz
(1972). Team production is therefore effected through the
firm which they define as "a team use of inputs and a
centralized contractual agent in a team productive process"
(Alchian and Demsetz, 1972: 778).

Central to this concept of firm is that in a firm the output
of individuals is neither measured nor controlled by the
market. By consequence other devices of measurement and
control of output are used that are apparently less expensive
than measurement and control through the market would have
been. What the team offers to the market can be taken as the
marginal product of the team, but not of the team members.
Measuring and controlling the individual's contribution to
the team product requires new organizations and procedures.
For a variety of reasons, elaborated by Alchian and Demsetz,
efficiency of team production requires a certain degree of
centralization of measurement and control, which in the
classical firm was the function of the entrepreneur. The
entrepreneur paid the owners of the inputs and 'monitored'
the members of the team. The basis of this payment cannot be
the marginal productivity of each worker. But what is it, if
not that? Marx solved this problem by relating the payment of
the worker to the cost of reproduction of the laborpower of
the worker. The entrepreneur received the residual rewards of
the team production, which are determined on the one hand by
the market and on the other by the efficiency of the team.
The efficiency of team production depends on the
possibilities of measuring and controlling the individual's
contribution to the team production and these possibilities
therefore determine the costs of team production. A number of
technological innovations at the end of the nineteenth
century induced an increasing amount of team production,
which could only be realized through a more complicated

system of measurement and control of individual output introduced under the name of scientific management. Hilferding called this process socialization of production. [2]

Since these new forms of production required investments on a much larger scale than before, the advanced forms of production had to be accompanied by advanced forms of organizing financial inputs. Institutionally this was made possible by the introduction of the joint-stock company. Two aspects predominate in the new form of organizing financial inputs. The first is the parcellization of the investment by selling shares which are infinitesimally small in relation to the new investment. The second is the fact that such a share is no more, and no less, than a promise of future returns. The importance of this new arrangement had already been noticed by Marx in 1864:

> "The world would still be without railways if it had had to wait until accumulation had got a few individual capitals far enough to be adequate for the construction of a railway. Centralization, on the contrary, accomplished this in a twinkling of an eye, by means of the joint-stock company" (Capital I: 628).

And more than a hundred years later the joint-stock company is still regarded as one of the greatest innovations in human history. According to De Jong (1979: 21) the advantages of

---

[2] Both Hilferding and Alchian and Demsetz argue that the socialization of production (i.e., team production) stems from technical necessity, given the level of technological development. Control and measurement of individual output stems logically from these requirements. Others, such as Marglin (1976), tend to argue the other way around. According to Marglin technological development is primarily induced by the need to control and discipline the worker, and scientific management is primarily a method of increasing exploitation rather than of increasing efficiency. The thesis of Marglin is a fundamental attack on the conception of class struggle current in communist parties and upon the dominant view in the labor unions that technological innovation is somehow 'class neutral'. For the explanation of the network of interlocking directorates the discussion has no direct relevance.

the joint-stock company can be summarized in the fundamental
possibility of the permanent existence of the corporation
apart from individual persons, which makes a continuous
accumulation of wealth possible. [3]

This time aspect of the joint-stock company is not without
relevance for the study of interlocking directorates. Persons
with directorships in several corporations do in general have
an executive position in one of these. They represent their
company at the boards of directors of other companies rather
than their own -private- blocks of shares. The joint-stock
company marks the beginning of an era in which institutions
rather than individuals or families are the main actors in
the accumulation process. The corporation rather than the
family becomes the historical agent bridging the gap between
generations. Several studies have shown that most of the
largest firms in 1900 still belonged to the largest firms in
the seventies. Of the 20 largest British firms in 1905, seven
appeared in 1976 under the same name on the Fortune list of
the 500 largest industrials outside the United States (see
Paine, 1967: 539; and Fortune, August 1977). For United
States firms there is the same historical continuity. Of the
20 largest firms in 1905 eight still belonged to the 500
largest American industrials in 1976. This historical
continuity has certainly contributed to the corporation's
success.

But the immediate cause of the success of the joint-stock
company was the enormously increased need for financial
inputs. For several reasons, capital can be obtained more
cheaply if many investors contribute small portions to a
large investment. And since the marginal productivity of each
'bit of investment' cannot be measured, the investors are
rewarded according to the total output of the team production
in proportion to the share they have had in the initial
investment. However, this 'sharing system' makes information
about and control over the total investment very costly for
the individual investor. These costs are reduced by
transferring decision authority to a smaller group (the board
of directors) who is to 'represent' the investors vis-a-vis

[3] Colonial enterprises like the Netherlands-chartered East
    India Company were also organized as joint-stock companies
    and are often regarded as the first modern corporations
    (see De Jong, 1979: 21). However, because these are not
    industrial enterprises, they will not be considered here
    (see Section 2.2).

the entrepreneur who monitors the team production. The stockholders retain the authority to revise the membership of the board of directors and over major decisions that affect the structure of the corporation or its dissolution (see Section 4.1). Apart from this, the individual stockholder has been secured against abuse of the privileged information position and the resulting power of the board of directors by limited liability and the right to sell his or her shares without approval of any other stockholder. For the large stockholders representation on the board is a means of monitoring the use of the investments. And if these large stockholders are firms themselves, representation on the board of directors constitutes interlocking directorates.

Theoretically, the question arises of why stockholding firms do not invest in their own organization. The theoretical framework developed by Alchian and Demsetz provides a simple answer: the costs of measurement and control of team production based on the new investment are apparently lower within the investee firms than within the investing firm. Interlocking directorates can be assessed theoretically as a means of avoiding the cost of measurement and control through the market, without taking up all the costs of measurement and control through the (own) firm. The argument is nearly identical to that of Hilferding when he describes Personalunion as the result of the need for cooperation between organizations that belong together, but are separated institutionally because of the additional costs that would be incurred from their unification. Finance capital is the merger between bank-, commercial- and industrial capital, but this merger has not led to a unification of banks, commercial companies and industrial companies. Rather, these different types of firms are systematically linked through a network of interlocking directorates. The interlocking directorate is halfway between market and hierarchy. The market relationships of the interlocked firms are not nullified, yet interlocks impose some hierarchy (Pennings, 1980: 192). It therefore implies competition and cooperation as well as control. The ways in which the interlocking directorates are related to competition, to cooperation and to control depend, as has been shown in Section 1.2, upon the character of the firms that are linked, the directness of the linkage, the frequency of the interlocks and the responsibilities of the persons who constitute the interlocks. Some general propositions can be made here.

a. Between two firms of which a representative of the one sits on the board of the other, competition has been excluded. This is so because at least one of the firms has direct access to all information concerning the financial, commercial or industrial strategy of the other. Whether

competition is also excluded when two firms are directly related through an interlocker who is outside director in both firms remains to be seen. This depends on the function of the outside director. It is possible that the strategies of the two firms are coordinated by the third firm and competition has given way to cooperation.

b. If an inside director of firm A and an inside director of firm B are both directors of firm C, then firms A and B meet in firm C. Now competition may or may not be excluded. The firms may cooperate, as is the case if the third firm is a joint-venture, but they may also compete, each trying to dominate the firm in which they meet.

c. Domination is typically associated with interlocking directorates that are directed, i.e., if the interlocking director is an executive of one firm and an outside director of the other. Furthermore, control relations often give rise to multiple interlocks.

d. Multiple interlocks indicate a strong relationship between firms. Thus, if the interlocks are associated with competition, multiple interlocks should be considered as indicating strong competition; if cooperation, then intensive cooperation; if dominance, then control. The possible interpretation of different types of interlocking directorates can be clarified by taking distance-two relations systematically into consideration. Following Zijlstra (1979b), we distinguish three types of distance-two relations: meeting lines, coordination lines and hierarchical lines.

Distance-two relation   Meaning
(dotted line)

Meeting line

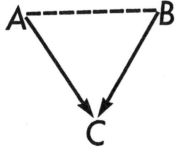

Executive directors of A and B meet in C. There is confrontation or cooperation between A and B. If confrontation, the position of C vis-a-vis A and B is relatively strong. If cooperation, the position of C is relatively weak.

Coordination line

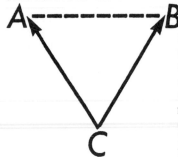

Executive directors of C are outside
directors of A and B. There is
exchange of information between A
and B managed by and in the interest
of C. This situation becomes even
more clear when the same is an
outside director of A and B. In the
latter case there exists a secondary
but direct interlock between A and
B, which is nevertheless comparable
to the coordination line.

Hierarchical line

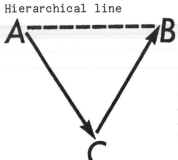

An executive director of A is an
outside director of B. An executive
director of B is an outside director
of C. If A controls C and C controls
B, then A controls B.

Figure 2.1 Meeting, coordination and hierarchical lines

What is clear from these three types of distance-two
relations is that the meaning of the interlocking
directorates depends strongly on the position of those who
carry the interlocks. But not only that. An interlock can
hardly be meaningfully interpreted when it is considered in
isolation. For example: the interlocking directorate between
A and C is in the first and in the third case identical.
Nevertheless, it should be interpreted differently because
the relation between A and C is influenced by the relation
between B and C, and B and A. Given the extreme simplicity of
the three models, it is also clear that a precise
interpretation of each singular interlock is very difficult
indeed, the more so because the meaning of each interlock is
heavily dependent on other relations between the interlocked
firms, such as markets or financial relations.

2.2 Some definitions of firms

For a consistent set of concepts related to the different
forms in which team production is organized, three different
criteria should be used: the historical specificity of the
organization, the legal structure of the organization, and
the amount of financial centralization within the
organization.
According to the first criterion it is necessary to restrict
these concepts to a specific historical epoch. The phenomenon
of interlocking directorates is typical for the era of
corporate capitalism beginning at the end of the nineteenth
century. My concepts will be somewhat broader but still
restricted to the era of industrial capitalism, which in most
countries did not begin until the nineteenth century. If we
define an undertaking as any organization engaged in
production, trading or financial activities, then these
undertakings already exist in ancient Greece and still exist
in Soviet Russia. The definition of Alchian and Demsetz of a
firm as "a team use of inputs and a centralized contractual
agent in a team productive process" coincides with the
concept of undertaking. A firm is defined as a capitalist
undertaking. The definition of Alchian and Demsetz can still
be used if it is assumed that the contractual agent operates
in a capitalist economy. Although I have resticted the use of
the terms to the era of industrial capitalism, this does not
mean that a capitalist firm is necessarily an industrial
firm. It can also be engaged in trading or financial
activities, in which case, however, it operates in a market
together with industrial firms.

For the second criterion, which focuses on the legal
structure of the firm, we distinguish two concepts: a company
refers to any firm which has a separate legal existence; and
a joint-stock company is a share company with limited
liability. Most of the firms under investigation are joint-
stock companies. There are of course many more statutory
forms than the joint-stock company, but they differ from
country to country and cannot be caught in a general
definition.

Turning to the third criterion we can distinguish different
types of industrial firms according to the distance that
exists between the level of production and the ultimate
control in the firm. The larger this distance, the more the
locus of control becomes a purely financial center. We can
thus define a plant, a corporation, a concern, a holding and
a financial group as follows:
A plant is a manufacturing establishment that is part of a
company. Such a company, which consists of a number of plants
tied together through financial control in one locus of
control, is called a corporation.

If the different plants (or groups of plants) have a separate legal existence, but there exists a mother company who controls the daughter companies through <u>majority</u> ownership of the shares, we speak of a <u>concern</u>. If the mother company of a concern has no productive activities of its own but is a purely administrative financial center, it is a <u>holding</u>.

Finally, we can define a <u>financial group</u> as a group of companies in which there exists a locus of control through <u>minority</u> ownership of the shares and/or other forms of control such as interlocking directorates, credit relations etc.

The distinction between concern and financial group is thus a rather formal one: if control is exercised through the majority ownership of the shares, we speak of a concern. If control is exercised through the minority ownership of the shares plus other means of control, we speak of a financial group. From this formal difference we nevertheless may draw a tentative conclusion that there will in general also exist a difference in <u>degree of control</u> between financial group and concern.

The definition of financial group is empirically more ambiguous than the other concepts because neither minority share ownership nor interlocking directorships nor credit relations are in themselves necessarily control relations. Often these relations only become control relations if they exist simultaneously. And even then one needs rather detailed information to identify a financial group. If the locus of control of such a financial group lies in a financial institution, we speak of a financial group proper. If, on the other hand, the locus of control lies in an industrial company, we speak of a financial group under industrial domination. According to Pastre (1979: 261) the essential characteristic of a financial group is the capacity to mobilize the necessary investments funds <u>autonomously</u>. This characteristic follows logically from our definition since there cannot be an independent locus of control within a group of firms if investment funds cannot be raised autonomously. In fact, the criterion of internal financing normally used at the level of the individual corporation is by Pastre adapted to the level of a set of firms. The implication that the locus of control is located in a firm does not follow from our definition of financial group. There may well be a locus of control outside the firms that form the financial group. We agree with Allard in this respect:

> "Le centre financier, société mere ou ensemble de holdings, est le lieu où se nouent les liens determinants d'appropriation des moyen de production, c'est aussi le lieu où sont prises les décisions de réaffectation, à chaque cycle de production, des profits et, par la meme, ou est determinée la stratégie

de valorisation du capital pour les cycles futurs:
choix industriels, spécialisation, diversification,
internationalisation, etc. Le centre financier est du
moins en moins constitué par une société continuant à
exercer des activités industrielles (....); c'est de
plus frequemment une holding ayant un petit nombre de
salariés. Ce centre financier peut également entre le
relais d'une famille (....) ou d'un capitaliste
individuel (...)" (Allard et.al., 1978: 7,8).
(The financial center, be it the mother company or the sum of
the holdings, is the place where the control lines through
which the appropriation of the means of production is
determined come together. It is also the place where
decisions are taken about the (re)allocation of profits after
each production cycle and also about future strategy, e.g.,
choices of industry, of specialization, of diversification
and internationalization etc. The financial center is less
and less a company that is itself engaged in industrials
activities (....); it is more and more often a holding with a
tiny number of employees. The financial center may also be a
family (....) or a single capitalist (....)).

The weakness of the position of Allard et.al. lies in the
fact that they confuse the problem of institutional locus of
control with the problem of who controls the corporation.
This is the problem area of the debate on the managerial
revolution. I would therefore prefer as an example of an
outside locus of control the private foundation rather than a
family or an individual.

Using the third criterion, we can distinguish financial
institutions according to their distance from the level of
production. [4] This distinction is different from the former
ones because it is not based on determination of the locus of
control in a particular firm, but on the distance between
production and financial activities in general. The holding
company has already been discussed as part of a concern.
However, the links between the holding company and its
industrial companies may be too loose to warrant their
consideration as a concern. In that case, the holding company
is a separate financial institution, which of all financial
institutions is the most directly linked to production. A
classical example of such a holding company is the Société

[4] This typology of financial institutions has been
suggested by R.J. Mokken.

Général de Belgique. [5] Next to the holding company we find the _investment bank_, which owns large blocks of shares in a number of industrials, providing a number of links to the level of production that are sometimes short of control. _Investment companies_ also hold blocks of shares in industrials companies, but they do so mainly for reasons of stable and safe investment rather than for reasons of control. The same is true for _insurance companies_ and _pension funds_. The latter are in many cases tied to, and controlled by, one industrial corporation. Finally, a _commercial bank_ normally does not have large blocks of shares but specializes in credit provision. It maintains client relations with many industrials and the distance between production and financial activities may remain very large indeed.

2.3 _Power and control_

In the foregoing section I used the terms power and control without a formal definition of the concepts. [6] The concept of economic power is widely used in the field of industrial economics, which is concerned with the structure and functioning of markets. Economic power is conceived as market power, i.e. "(...) the ability of a market participant or group of participants (persons, firms, partnerships, or others) to influence price, quantity, and the nature of the product on the market place" (Shepherd, 1970: 3). From the definition of Shepherd, we can deduce that market power only exists when there is no perfect competition. Accordingly, the concept of economic power is closely tied to theories of oligopoly and concentration. Lerner, for example, developed an index of the degree of monopoly power for the $\underline{k}$ largest firms based on the divergence between price and marginal costs, a divergence that does not exist in the case of perfect competition (Jacquemin and De Jong, 1977: 82). A common measure of market power is based on market share and

[5] See for example Daems, 1978.

[6] Many economists have given attention to the problem of economic power and control: Böhm Bawerk,(1914); Berle and Means, (1932); Brady, (1943); Machlup, (1952); Bain, (1956); Houssiaux, (1958); Perroux, (1961); Lhomme, (1966); Larner, (1966); Jacquemin, (1967); Shepherd, (1970); De Vroey, (1973); and Arndt, (1974).

entry barriers (see Wilcox and Shepherd, 1975: 199). This concept of power has been elaborated in the field of antitrust investigation in the United States. Here the discussion centers around the relation between the (dominant) market position of a firm, the amount of market power stemming from that position, and the actual exercise of that power ("monopolistic abuses"). The association of economic power with monopoly is common among classical and neo-classical economists. It is revised by Arndt (1974) who argues that the exercise of economic power is compatible with competition when this latter concept is not defined according to the familiar models of the neo-classical economists as an equilibrum beyond time and space. Competition, then, refers to a process of economic development in which an innovation gives a temporary monopoly, which – and in this sense Arndt is not different from the neo-classical economists – is associated with power. Most economists use the concept of power in relation to a firm's position and behavior in the market, thus referring to relations between actors with equal status (e.g., companies) even though the actors may differ in size.

At the level of the individual firm the concept of power is hardly used. Here we find the concept of control, which refers to the decision-making process in the firm. Berle and Means (1932: 69) define control as "the actual power to select the board of directors (or its majority)". Thus, control refers to the locus of decision in a hierarchical organization in which the actors explicitly have no equal status. In the firm labor is subjugated to capital (or to management as Berle and Means try to argue) and – formally at least – it is up to the board of directors to decide in what way the production process is structured. This difference between power between firms and power within firms has been stressed by Max Weber in his Wirtschaft und Gesellschaft (1925: 604). He distinguishes two opposing types of Herrschaft (domination). One is based on a constellation of interest; the other is based on 'authority'. The purest form of the former is, according to Weber, a monopolistic market position; the market as a constellation of interest is a system of power within which relations of domination (Herrschaft) are generated. The purest form of the latter is sovereign or bureaucratic power. Giddens concludes from this passus that according to Weber the market, being a power structure,

> "is not a normatively defined system of authority in which the distribution of power is, as such, sanctioned as legitimate. The rights of property, and of the sale of labour are rights of the alienation or disposal of goods (commodities in the Marxian sense), which

underpin the system of power, not in spite of, but
because of the fact that they are specified in terms of
freedom of economic exchange" (Giddens, 1973: 102;
italics in the original).

The power structure within the firm is, on the other hand, a
normatively defined system of authority. The obligation to
obey is based on the exchange of labor power and enforced by
law, i.e., ultimately by force. No wonder that market power
has been defined in terms of bargaining position, while
control has been defined in legal terms (cf. the definition
of control by Berle and Means). Weber rightly stresses the
fact that the two types of Herrschaft can shade into another.
As an example of such a shaded area in the economic field he
mentions interlocking directorates:

"Jede   typische   Art   von   Herrschaft   kraft
Interessenkonstellation,   insbesondere   kraft
monopolistischer Lage, kann aber allmählich in eine
autoritäre Herrschaft übergeführt werden. Zur besseren
Kontrolle verlangen z.B. die Banken als Geldgeber
Aufnahme   ihrer   Direktoren   in   den   Aufsichtsrat
kreditsuchender Aktienunternehmungen: der Aufsichtsrat
aber   erteilt   dem   Vorstand Befehle kraft dessen
gehorsamspflicht (Weber, 1925: 605).

(Each type of domination based on a   constellation of
interests, especially the one based on a monopoly position,
can shade into authoritative domination. For example, to have
better control the banks require their directors to be
accepted on the supervisory boards of corporations in search
of credit: the supervisory board, however, is able to give
orders to the executive committee (Vorstand, see Section 4.1,
M.F.)).

We may conclude from the economic literature that the concept
of power is used at the level of the market structure, i.e.,
the level of the economy as a whole, while the concept of
control is used at the level of the individual firm. The
definitions of the terms, however, are not very precise.
Berle and Means define control in terms of power ("the actual
power to select the board of directors") while Shepherd
defines power in terms of influence ("the ability....to
influence price, ...").

Because the concept of power is a central concept in
sociology and political science, it has been more frequently
debated and defined. Part of this debate has been summarized
by Mokken and Stokman (1976) who also propose definitions for
power and influence that are more precise than those to date.
Leaning heavily on Weber, the authors define power as "the
capacity of actors (persons, groups or institutions) to fix
or change (completely or partly) a set of action alternatives
or choice alternatives for other actors."

Further "influence is the capacity of actors to determine
(partly) the actions or choices of other actors within the
set of actions or choice alternatives available to those
actors" (Mokken and Stokman, 1976: 37). Thus power refers to
fixing or changing a set of action alternatives, whereas
influence does not affect the set of alternatives, but the
choice to be made within this set of alternatives.

According to Weber: "Macht bedeutet jede Chance, innerhalb
einer sozialen Beziehung den eigenen Willen auch gegen
Widerstreben durch zu setzen, gleichviel worauf diese Chance
beruht" (quoted in Mokken and Stokman, 1976: 34).
(Power is the chance that one actor within a social
relationship will be in a position to carry out his own will
despite resistance, regardless of the basis on which this
chance rests.)
The definition of Mokken and Stokman differs from Weber's in
three respects. According to Mokken and Stokman, power and
influence can be exercised unintentionally; yes, even against
one's will. Second, the concept of actor not only refers to a
person but may also refer to an organization. Third, Mokken
and Stokman emphasize the relational framework in which power
is exercised: "the power or influence of actors as a capacity
is inherent in the particular position or configuration. We
shall designate that place or configuration as a power
position or influence position" (Mokken and Stokman, 1976:
42).
Power position should be distinguished from the power base
which is the specific combination of resources at the command
of an actor in a specific power position.

Of the three differences, the most important is the first.
Indeed, the exercise of economic power is often
unintentional: the intention is to affect "price, quantity,
and the nature of the product on the market place"; the
result is that a set of action alternatives or choice
alternatives is changed or fixed for other actors. The
exercise of economic power, however, need not be
unintentional. When a firm has the "actual power to select
the board of directors (or its majority)" of another firm,
the exercise of that power will have the purpose of fixing or
changing the action or choice alternatives for the other
firm. Control can now be defined as the intended exercise of
power over the other actors, and the intended exercise of
influence will be called domination. Power, then, is the
general concept, while control is a special case of power.
How can we reconcile the concepts of power and control
derived from economic literature with those derived from the
social sciences? As we have seen, in economic literature the
concept of power generally means the capacity to fix or
change market variables, and the concept of control refers to

a person-to-company or a company-to-company relation. Since
the social sciences define the concept of power as a relation
between actors, the exercise of market power will mostly be
unintended power. On the other hand, Berle and Means'
definition of control - while rather formalistic - does
correspond with the definition of Mokken and Stokman and is
related to Weber's concept of authority. Control seems to be
an appropriate concept to describe those relations in the
network of interlocking directorates where exercise of power
can be assumed to be intentional. Control is typically
exercised within a financial group, either through voting
rights in the board of directors or through the exclusive
possession of resources. Domination, on the other hand, is a
more appropriate concept in a network of interlocking
directorates in which the information aspect predominates.

2.4 Ownership and control

In contrast to the emphasis on interlocking directorates in
the antitrust investigations, there are many American
economists who belittle their importance. The theoretical
basis for this is the theory of management control, launched
by Berle and Means in 1932. According to this theory, a
growing separation of ownership and control enables
management to appoint most members of the board of directors.
At best, the board then serves as an advisory board, but
directors are often chosen solely for reasons of prestige. In
the Encyclopaedia of the Social Sciences, Gardiner Means
stresses the positive contributions of interlocking
directorates in terms of channels of communication, increase
in experience and knowledge, and even "insuring business on
profitable terms and with a minimum of selling costs."
However, even Means has to acknowledge that they can also
serve as channels of control: "Where a combination of
competitors has been achieved, with the enterprises still
retaining their corporate identity, the device of
interlocking directors is used to unify policy and
administration within the combination" (Means, 1932: 148,
149; emphasis added).
Separation of ownership and control was noticed long before
the publication of The Modern Corporation and Private
Property in 1932 by Berle and Means. In the third volume of
Capital Marx argued that by means of the joint-stock company
it becomes possible to control much more capital than
actually is owned. At the same time the joint-stock company
induces the "transformation of the actually functioning
capitalist into a mere manager, administrator of other
people's capital, and of the owner of capital into a mere
owner, a mere money capitalist" (Capital III: 436).

Strangely enough, the separation of ownership and control has
been regarded as evidence of the obsolescence of marxian
theory. In the debate between marxist and managerialists the
fact that social production is dominated by a few is
undisputed. The discussion, initiated by Berle and Means,
centers around the question of who exactly control social
production. According to Berle and Means, the managers
increasingly obtain control over the large corporation. Their
research led to the theory of managerial control, which has
been further developed, in different forms, by Burnham
(1941), Dahrendorf (1959) and Galbraith (1967). They maintain
that the loss of control by the majority of shareholders
tends to increase the power of the management. Their argument
may be summarized as follows:
a. The development of the joint-stock company disperses legal
   ownership and separates it from control over the
   corporation.
b. A new social group replaces the outdated capitalist-
   entrepreneur.
c. The interests of the managers differs from those of the
   shareholders; since it is the managers who set the goals
   of the firm, these goals can change from profit
   maximization to continuity of the organization, to growth
   or enhancement of the welfare of the community.
d. From the former propositions it follows that capitalism
   has been replaced by a new form of industrial society.

However, as De Vroey has demonstrated, the managerialists do
not realize that the notion of separation of ownership and
control can be understood in two different ways:
   "on one hand, it refers to the dispersion of shares
   among a large public in large corporations. Its
   consequence is a new type of owner - the absentee
   stockholder - who, in contrast with the traditional
   owner, no longer holds effective control over the
   corporation. On the other hand, the notion points to a
   shift of the power base within the corporation. In this
   second case one speaks of a separation of ownership and
   control whenever the basis for the controlling power is
   no longer ownership but rather something else, as in
   the case of expertise" (De Vroey, 1975: 1).
If we survey the research based on the first meaning of
separation of ownership and control, we begin with Berle and
Means. Taking as their example the largest non-financial
corporations in 1929, they classified the firms according to
the following five types of corporate control:
1. privately owned, 2. controlled through the ownership of a
majority of the voting stock, 3. controlled through the
ownership of a dominant minority of the voting stock, 4.
controlled by means of legal device [7] and 5. management
controlled.

A firm is considered privately owned if an individual, a
family, or a group of business associates holds 80 percent or
more of its voting stock. Stockownership between 50 and 80
percent   is   regarded   as   majority   controlled,   whereas
stockownership between 20 and 50 percent is regarded as
minority controlled. Berle and Means assigned corporations in
which no base of control in stockownership could be found to
management   control   on   the   belief   that   no   group   of
stockholders would be able under ordinary circumstances to
muster enough votes to challenge the rule of management (see
Larner, 1966: 79). Eighty-eight out of 200 firms were found
to be management controlled. Larner repeated the research of
Berle and Means in 1963 and found that management control had
increased considerably: from 44 percent in 1929 to 84.5
percent in 1963 (Larner, 1966: 781). Finally Palmer (1972:
57) , who compared the years 1965 and 1969 with a research
design slightly different from that of Larner, confirmed the
trend towards management control. On th other hand, a host of
empirical research has convincingly shown that many of the
firms regarded as management controlled by Berle and Means
were on closer examination controlled from outside. Such
evidence was first provided by Ann Rochester (1936) and
Ferdinand Lundberg (1937), followed by the TNEC-report
(1940), the NRC study of 1939 (Sweezy 1953), Perlo (1957) and
Villarejo (1961/62).

Re-analysis of the Berle and Means data by Burch suggests
that the extent of management control has indeed been
exaggerated. Burch estimates that between 37 and 45 percent
of the top non-financial companies in 1929 were family
controlled; many of these were classified as 'managerial
controlled' by Berle and Means (Burch, 1972: 114, 115). In
the classification of Berle and Means 'management control'
was not conceptually defined but introduced as a residual
category. Lack of data placed a firm automatically in the
'management controlled' category. Other important counter-
evidence to the findings of Berle and Means was provided by
the Temporary National Economic Committee, commissioned by
the federal government under F.D. Roosevelt to investigate
the ownership of the 200 largest firms in America. It found
the following distribution of stock in the year 1937: 20

[7] Control by legal device was found in forty-one
     corporations. In other countries, such as the Netherlands,
     control by legal device is even more common (see Helmers
     et.al., 1975: 90).

largest stockholders held 32 percent of the voting rights;
980 large stockholders held 18 percent of the voting rights;
and 35,000 small stockholders held the remaining 50 percent.
It is clearly impertinent to speak about "the shareholders"
as a unified category. Lampman (1959) has demonstrated
considerable increase in the unequal distribution of shares
in the United States: one percent of American citizens held
61.5 percent of all shares in 1922, 69 percent in 1939 and 76
percent in 1953. Since a firm can be controlled by owning far
less than 51 percent of the stock, it is clear that these
large stockowners can control much more capital than they
actually own. Another kind of counter-evidence results from a
closer examination of financial institutions, which were left
out of the study of Berle and Means. Especially Perlo (1957)
and Villarejo (1961/62) have stressed the importance of
financial institutions as stockowners. The share of their
holdings in total amount of securities rose from 23 percent
in 1900 to 26 percent in 1929, but jumped to 58 percent in
1949. "The huge wartime rise in federal debt, mainly held by
the banks, contributed to this, but the post-1929 rise in the
bankers' share of corporate securities was almost as
dramatic" (Perlo, 1957: 24; emphasis added).

However, such evidence hardly touches upon the two most
important findings from the managerial point of view:
a. an increasing separation between ownership and control
   resulting in an increasing amount of management-controlled
   firms. Even Chevalier, who opposes the management control
   thesis, cannot exclude the possibility that the number of
   management-controlled firms could have increased between
   1937 and 1965 (Chevalier, 1970: 203).
b. a positive correlation between size and management
   control. Of the top 50 United States industrials 30 are
   management controlled, while of the top 200 eighty are
   management controlled (Chevalier, 1970: 65).
The basic tenets of the management control thesis so far have
hardly been challenged. This can only be done by an
investigation from a different angle into the mode of control
of large corporations. The basic weakness of the research on
ownership and control is not empirical but theoretical. All
managerial research focuses on the individual corporation
viewed in isolation. Most of the writers who dispute its
results take the same starting point and, as a result, only
show that the managerialists stretch their point a bit too
far, without proving them wrong. However, just as the
corporation does not operate in isolation, it cannot be
controlled in isolation. From the perspective of the overall
corporate sector, it may well be that a firm is controlled
from the outside, even though there is no specific group of
shareholders exercising "actual power to select the board of
directors."

Scott (1979) speaks in this situation of a <u>constellation</u> <u>of</u>
<u>interests</u>. In fact, his interpretation of the findings of
Chevalier, Burch, and others leads him to conclude that the
trend has not been towards management control, but towards
control through a constellation of interests. "What seems to
have occurred is a transition from 'personal' to 'impersonal'
forms of possession and control. Direct family control
through majority ownership has given way to control through a
constellation of interests" (Scott, 1979: 73).
I largely agree with these conclusions of Scott. However, two
important remarks should be made. <u>First</u>, Scott does not give
an explanation for the trend towards control through a
constellation of interests. The explanation, in my opinion,
can be found in the emergence of the joint-stock company,
through which ownership loses its individual character
(individual ownership of a firm), without losing its private
character (private appropriation of the revenues). Hence we
come to the paradoxical conclusion that private property
still continues, but without the existence of 'private'
firms, which are going 'public'. This may result in control
of industrial corporations by financial institutions to
maximize the revenues for the financial group as a whole.
Second, the debate with the managerialists is more than just
a quarrel about empirical findings. It involves a level-of-
analysis problem. The managerialists study the (industrial)
firm in isolation. In my opinion, one should study the firm
as a part of the business system that exists as a network of
personal and financial linkages between firms. This implies
that the empirical results of the managerialists on the level
of the individual firm are not necessarily incompatible with
the results of the research of their opponents on the level
of the business system. One cannot confirm the conclusions of
either one as long as one cannot demonstrate that the firm's
external relations are more important than its internal
relations for the locus of decision in the firm. This will
not be attempted here. [8] Our study will exclusively deal
with the external relations of the large corporations, not to
refute the theory of Berle and Means, but to complete it by
examining the field that they have wrongly neglected. Our
critique, then, is not aimed directly at the theory of
management control in the narrow sense, but at all those
theories in which conclusions about <u>interc</u>orporate power are

[8] It is noteworthy, though, that the theory of management
    control was launched in a period in which internal
    financing increased and was generally considered as a
    lasting feature of monopoly capitalism in the United States
    (Lintner, 1972).

based on a theory and evidence based at most on
intracorporate power. Such a structural approach to the study
of the control of corporations has been suggested by Zeitlin,
who stated in 1974 that
  "confining our attention to the single corporation may,
  in fact, limit our ability to see the pattern of power
  relationships of which this corporation is merely one
  element: and it may restrict our understanding of the
  potential for control represented by a specific block
  of shares in a particular corporation. An individual or
  group's capacity for control increases correspondingly,
  depending on how many other large corporations
  (including banks and other financial institutions) in
  which it has a dominant, if not controlling, position"
  (Zeitlin, 1974: 1091).

2.5 Competition, cooperation and control

2.5.1 Concentration and centralization redefined

The network of interlocking directorates is part of the
market structure. This can easily be demonstrated at the
level of the individual firms. If, for example, the five
largest firms in a market are connected by a network of
interlocking directorates, the concentration of economic
power may, in fact, be higher than if this were not the case.
If , for example, this network ties three of the five largest
firms into one financial group, the concentration ratio is
higher if it is defined as the market share of the x largest
financial groups. Such an extension of the traditional
definition of concentration ratio is suggested by Jacquemin
and De Jong (1977: 44) who state that "it is becoming more
and more necessary to ask whether the concept of company
should be replaced by that of the group, that is a set of
distinct legal entities controlled by a central economic unit
calculating on an overall basis."

A similar argument can be developed for the market as a
whole: if the measures of relative concentration (which take
the market share of all firms into account) are based on
groups rather than companies, concentration will ceteris
paribus be higher when there exists a network of interlocking
directorates between the companies than when no such network
exists.

Karl Marx, who was the first to integrate a theory of
economic concentration into a general theory of capitalist
development, made a distinction between concentration and
centralization. According to Marx, concentration, being akin
to capital accumulation, takes place because surplus value

derived from variable capital is invested in fixed capital, i.e., in means of production. Through the process of concentration the amount of means of production in capitalist society increases. This process raises the scale of the companies, but the increase is limited by the overall economic growth. The scale of the companies can be increased much more rapidly by centralization: "(...) concentration of capitals already formed, destruction of their individual independence, expropriation of capitalist by capitalist, transformation of many small into few large capitals" (Capital I: 625). Concentration is thus used by Marx to indicate an increase in productive capacity, while centralization is used to indicate a redistribution of productive capacity over fewer units of control. The economies-of-scale argument - implicit in marxian accumulation theory - would suggest that centralization in itself can lead to further concentration. Institutionally, centralization was facilitated by the introduction of the joint-stock company and the extension of the credit system at the end of the nineteenth century.

Although contemporary Western economists owe more to Marx's concentration theory than most of them acknowledge, the terminology has changed somewhat. The concept of centralization has been dropped and the concept of concentration has been given a meaning that comes close to the concept of centralization developed by Marx. Concentration now generally refers to the process by which a few large companies come to dominate a given market. This is called juridical- or firm concentration. As such, the concept is related to different measures of concentration. Two types of concentration measures can be distinguished: absolute and relative.
Absolute concentration measures consider a certain number of firms and the share of each in a certain economic quantity. Such a measure is the concentration ratio measuring the share of the market or industry held by the m largest firms ($m = 1$, 2, 4, 8, 20, etc.) (see Jacquemin and De Jong, 1977: 42 $\overline{ff}$.). Relative concentration, on the other hand, measures the share of all firms in an economic quantity in relation to each other. Measures of relative concentration are in fact indices of inequality. They measure the size distribution of a population, without paying special attention to the largest firms.

Subscribing to the Western usage of the concept of concentration, I will restrict the term centralization to a phenomenon that has been almost totally neglected in the study of industrial concentration: the network of interlocking directorates. This can be argued in the following way. If concentration refers to the distribution of

assets (or employees, or market shares) over a number of firms, it indicates a certain amount of centralization of decision power over productive capacity. However, not every company is necessarily a unit of capital with an autonomous locus of control. A firm can be brought under the control of another company - be it an industrial or a financial company - without losing its juridical independence. The emergence of 'financial groups' discussed in Section 1.3 and defined in Section 2.2 is a special case in point. By means of (often minority) shareholdings and interlocking directorships these groups are able to control larger amounts of human and financial resources than the concentration measures would suggest (Jacquemin and de Jong, 1977: 44).
The economic concentration that results from this process underlying and generating interlocking directorates can now be called centralization, and centralization measures can accordingly be associated with the centrality measures developed in social network theory (see Freeman, 1979 and Hoivik and Gleditsch, 1970).

In this section I will not define any such centralization measures, because the empirical meaning of their application to networks of interlocking directorates has still to be developed. However, a distinction should be made between the measures indicating the compactness of the networks, to the degree that the distances between pairs of firms are short, and those indicating the centralization of the network based on the difference between the centrality of the most central firm(s) and that of others (Freeman, 1979: 227). [9] Centralization measures indicating the compactness of the network of interlocking directorates could thus be compared with relative concentration measures, while centralization measures based on the most central firms in the network could be compared with the absolute concentration measures. Concentration and centralization are related concepts in that they both indicate the amount of centralization of decision-making power over the means of production, i.e., over human and financial resources. [10]

[9] These concepts are derived from the graph theory and will be defined in Section 5.0.

[10] The new definition of the concept of centralization has been suggested to me by H.W. De Jong. It can easily be used within a marxian conceptual framework when the term accumulation is reserved for what Marx defined as concentration, and the term concentration for what Marx defined as centralization.

2.5.2 The level-of-analysis problem

As a planning- and information structure the network of interlocking directorates is opposed to the market principle. The market implies economic coordination ex-post, while the network of interlocking directorates implies economic coordination ex-ante. Ex-ante coordination refers to behaviour of actors, ex-post coordination refers to the structure of a social system. The metaphor of the Invisible hand expresses the ex-post coordination of the market: behavior of economic actors responds to market stimuli which results — unintentionally — in a coordination of their economic activities. The concept of organized capitalism, on the other hand, refers to the ex-ante coordination of economic activities. The two mechanisms of coordination seem to exclude each other.

However, in a capitalist economy, the planning structure is always part of a market structure. In this market structure, there exists a dialectical relation between competotion on the onde hand and cooperation and control on the other. The latter not only seek to exclude competition, they also induce it. Returning to the example from Section 2.5.1, let us assume that there are no interlocking directorates between the five largest firms in a market, but a tight network between a number of smaller firms, which creates a financial group equal in size to the five largest firms. If the financial group thus formed does not collude with the largest firms, competition in the market has increased, because the number of oligopolistic groups has increased. Competition and cooperation are not only alternative forms of economic coordination; they can also be complementary. To give another example: antitrust legislation is designed to suppress cooperation and control and enhance competition. Sometimes, however, certain forms of cooperation and control are supported for the sake of competition. In 1963 the Director-General for Competition of the EEC Commission said at a conference: "It would be absurd, for instance, to prevent the creation of an enterprise which would dominate the market of a small country, when such an enterprise would need its size to be competitive on the export markets" (Verloren van Themaat, 1963). Here control seems to be essential to competition. Such a policy of enforced economic cooperation for the sake of competition was pursued in the nuclear energy industry in the Netherlands: joined together in Neratoom the two Dutch reactor builders RSV and VMF tried to maintain a competitive position in the national and international markets. Their strategy failed. Subsequently, the RSV joined the United States company General Electric and VMF the German company Siemens. By means of these two consortia they tried

to hold both a national and an international place on the
market for light water reactors (see Zijlstra, 1979a: 365).
This example also makes clear that the question of
competition or monopoly depends on the scope of the
investigation. Regional monopoly may well be part of a
nationally competitive economy (Pennings 1980: 97). In turn,
a monopolistic market structure at the national level may
become part of a competitive structure at the international
level. When the scope of the investigation is the
international level, a similar problem has to be faced: an
integrated network of interlocking directorates at the
national level may well be part of an international network
of interlocking directorates with a completely different
structure.

Focusing on the network as a whole, one faces another
problem, which is often overlooked in social research. Social
structure is hardly ever the result of purposive action of an
actor or a set of actors to create that structure. It is
rather the unintended outcome of a series of purposive
actions of actors in the structure, each striving to attain
its own ends, while creating a structure which none of them
has designed or even foreseen. This seems to be the case with
the network of interlocking directorates: each firm strives
for a singular set of interlocks with other firms according
to its own strategy. In aggregation, however, these sets of
interlocks form a network of interlocking directorates that
functions quite independently from the strategy of each of
the firms in the network. [11] One can go even further and
assume that the structure of the network has in turn an
impact on the strategy of each firm to create a specific set
of interlocks. This can be illustrated with an example from
Chapter 7. In that chapter it will be shown that banks seek
cooperation with banks from other countries. In doing so,
they try to avoid cooperation with banks that already have
friendly relations with their national competitors. This
strategy leads to a specific structure of international
consortia which, in turn, restricts the strategic options for
each individual bank. This complicated relation between
strategy and developing structure lies at the heart of the
level-of-analysis problem: one cannot study the interlocking
directorates from the point of view of the single corporation
or even the single financial group without taking into
account the structure of the network as a whole and vice
versa. Nevertheless most of the research so far has been

[11] The argument is also valid if the interlocking directors
     are regarded as the main agents in the network.

either on the level of the strategy of the singular firm, as
in the study of financial groups (e.g., Knowles, 1974,
Menshikov, 1969), or on the aggregate level of the network as
a whole (e.g., Allen, 1974, Pennings, 1980, and Warner and
Unwalla, 1967). In this book I attempt to study the network
of interlocking directorates at both these levels.

2.6 Summary

According to the neo-classically inspired theory of the firm
developed by Coase, Alchian and Demsetz, the existence of
firms should be explained by comparing the cost of
information and control within centralized organizations and
within a market organization. Interlocking directorates is a
device used to avoid the costs of information and
coordination through the market, without taking up the costs
of information and coordination that would result from a
complete unification of the two firms. This theory of the
'new economists' does not contradict the marxian theory of
Hilferding presented in Section 1.1 Both theories explain why
the joint-stock company has become a dominant form of
business organization and why it, rather than the individual
entrepreneur or the family, should be regarded as the central
agent in capitalist development. In both theories an
institutional interpretation of the network of interlocking
directorates is more relevant than a personalistic
interpretation (Section 2.1). After providing the reader with
a set of concepts of the firm based on historical
periodization, legal forms and the amount of financial
centralization (Section 2.2), I have tried to distinguish
more precisely between the concepts of power and control.

The survey in Section 2.3 of the use of the concepts of power
and control in economic and political theory led to the
conclusion that the concept of power is more precisely
defined in political science while the concept of control is
more precisely defined in economic theory. Seldom are the two
concepts related. Using the concepts of power and influence
defined by Mokken and Stokman (1976), we defined control as
the intended exercise of power, and domination as the
intended exercise of influence. In Section 2.4 I argued that
the debate between marxists and managerialists on the problem
of managerial control misses the point in so far as both
sides confuse the theory of intracorporate power (as
developed by Berle and Means) with a theory of intercorporate
power. In my opinion the managerial control thesis holds true
when the corporations are studied in isolation but does not
need to be correct when the external relations with other
firms are systematically taken into consideration. Although
this study is not aimed at refuting the theory of Berle and

Means, the results may constitute an   important   element in a fundamental reconsideration of it.

Following these conceptual clarifications I set out to relate the phenomenon of interlocking directorates to that of economic concentration. Economic concentration as defined   in modern economic theory   refers   to centralization of decision making in a given   market   due to a decrease in the number of (dominant) firms. This concept neglects the centralization of decision making resulting from the network of interlocking directorates.   Therefore,   the   concept   of   economic centralization was used   to   indicate   the   centralization of decision   power   in   a   market   due   to   the   existence   of interlocking   directorates.   Just   as   concentration   can   be measured   by   concentration   measures, centralization can   be measured   by centralization   measures.   These   centralization measures still have   to   be developed. Finally, it was argued in   Section   2.5.2   that   concentration   and   centralization enhance   the   coordination   in   the economy through   planning rather than through the market. These different mechanisms of economic coordination are, however, dialectically related. On the   one   hand   competition   gives rise   to   cooperation   and control,   but on the other hand cooperation and   control   may induce   competition   'at   a   higher   level'.   Interlocking directorates,   therefore,   not   only   express cooperation and control, they   may   also   express (new) forms of competition. The interpretation of this depends on the level of analysis.

III IMPERIALISM IN THE SEVENTIES: two models

3.0 Introduction

Preceding the emergence of industrial capitalism, the international economic order was based on mercantile capitalism. In this economic order there already existed an international financial network which found its summit in the internationally organized European merchant banks such as the Rothschild House, with its major branches in Paris, London and Vienna.

When in the nineteenth century the American railroads became an important field of investment for European capital, the United States investment banks such as Drexel, Morgan and Company, Peabody and Company, and Kuhn, Loeb and Company owed their supremacy for a large part to the contacts they had with these European merchant banks. And these ties were more often than not based on family relations: the 'Yankee' banks had contacts with English capital, the Jewish houses with German capital (Kotz, 1978: 26, 27). In this early period of industrial capitalism, industrial expansion was confined to the national borders, while internationalization of capital was restricted to the export of industrial products, in which the United Kingdom had an incontestable advantage. Apart from investment in railways and mining, the international financial network was based on trade rather than on capital export. It was internationalization of money capital without internationalization of productive capital.

In the twentieth century, a new form of internationalization took place, based on the direct foreign investment of emerging corporations. Interlocking directorates between banks and industry were typically a sign of the emerging corporate capitalism, with its internationalization of production. The new era, therefore, was to become characterized by the simultaneous and related internationalization of money and productive capital in the form of finance capital. This development was initiated at the national level. The new system of interlocking directorates developed at the end of the nineteenth century within a national framework, especially in the then industrially backward nations, Germany and the United States. It was the rapid increase in industrial concentration – both cause and effect of the development of finance capital – which enabled these countries to make up for arrears.

It has been argued in Chapter 1 that finance capital is the interpenetration of bank- and industrial capital, relating the decisions about money capital directly to the decisions

about production. These structural changes between firms were
accompanied by structural changes within firms. Within firms
the financial decision became centralized, while the
decisions about production were decentralized. This
development, which I have described elsewhere (Fennema, 1975:
ch.2), allowed for an enormous increase in direct foreign
investment. No longer restricted to portfolio investment in
the extractive and transportation industries, international
investment - especially after 1945 - appeared in
manufacturing. The motive was no longer solely the
appropriation of raw materials but increasingly the
utilization of foreign laborpower. This meant no longer an
internationalization of capital for the sake of market
outlets, or for the sake of securing inputs of production at
home, but an internationalization of production proper (see
Aglietta, 1979). The internationalization of production
required a far greater decentralization of decisions over
production, given the fact that each country had its specific
conditions of production and of reproduction of its laborpower. Centralization of financial decisions and
decentralization of decisions over production were essential
to the development of international finance capital.

Even if such conditions are met, the internationalization of
finance capital can take different forms: the centralization
of financial decisions can take place at a national level; it
can also take place at an international level. The question
can be put as follows: given the internationalization of
production, is the centralization of financial control
contained within a national framework or does financial
control itself become international? Different economic
theories of imperialism have provided different answers to
this question. Relating the question of internationalization
of finance capital to the network of interlocking
directorates, one can ask whether or not there exists at the
international level a cohesive network of interlocking
directorates indicating an internationalization of ownership
and control. In the next section we will look at these
different answers and in Section 3.3 deduce their possible
implications for the structure of interlocking directorates,
with the purpose of constructing different 'models'.

3.1 Theories of imperialism

3.1.1 Their origins

Since Adam Smith's The Wealth of Nations, international
economic relations have been a focal point in the debate on
economic policy. The free traders assumed that free exchange
of commodities between nations would bring maximal welfare to
all of them. [1] Towards the closing of the nineteenth
century, however, a new phenomenon called for attention: the
export of capital. Imperialism became an overriding concern
of liberal and marxist scholars, who started to reflect upon
the relation between the international economic structure and
the problem of peace and war. The liberal scholar J.A.
Hobson, writing in 1902, saw capital export as "the taproot
of imperialism."

> "Aggresive Imperialism, which costs the tax-payer so
> dear, which is of so little value to the manufacturer
> and trader (..) is a source of great gain to the
> investor (...)" and even worse:

> "In large measure the rank and file of the investors
> are, both for business and for politics, the cat's paw
> of the great financial houses, who use stock and shares
> not so much as investments to yield them interest, but
> as material for speculation in the money market"
> (Hobson, (1902) 1938: 62, 63).

Hobson saw the underconsumption of the English working class
as the basis of the need for foreign investment and proposed
for England a conscious and voluntary abandonment of its
imperialist policy as an alternative to inevitable and tragic
disintegration of its hegemony. He saw in a free exchange
between equal nation-states a prerequisite for world peace
(see also Arrighi, 1978: 87). Although Hobson referred
especially to nineteenth century England, viewing the
nationalist reaction of the dominated nations (such as the
Boers in South Africa) as the main threat, he also pointed to
the possibility of a dangerous rivalry between different
imperialist powers.

Although Hobson's analysis has a superficial similarity with
that of Hilferding, it is basically different. Whereas
Hilferding sees imperialism as a result of the
internationalization of finance capital, Hobson regards it as

[1] This liberal paradigm has been challenged, but I will not
    discuss that here.

a phenomenon caused by the internationalization of money
capital. In Hilferding's view international investment is
investment of productive capital. For Hobson it is the
international investment of speculative money capital. It is
not difficult to relate these theoretical differences to the
actual differences of the economic structure in Germany and
Great Britain at the turn of the century. Whereas German
foreign investment was predominantly direct investment of the
chemical and electrial-engineering companies, British foreign
investment was predominantly portfolio investment in railways
and mining. Before 1914 the United States and continental
European companies had established, respectively, 122 and 167
manufacturing subsidiaries abroad, while companies from the
much more industrially developed United Kingdom had
established no more than 60 manufacturing subsidiaries abroad
(Franko, 1976: 10). This is the reason why Hobson, in the
above quotation, regards imperialism as having "so little
value to the manufacturer and trader." In The Evolution of
modern Capitalism (1906), for example, Hobson analyzes the
domination by the financial elite in South Africa of the
diamond and gold mining companies like De Beers, Premier
Diamond Company, Consolidated Goldfields and Rand Mines
through financial houses like the South African Chartered
Company which linked the mining companies in a network of
interlocking directorates:
  "Following these illustrative lines of connection we can
  perceive the close union of management between all the
  chief gold groups, and between gold and diamonds and
  the speculative finance of the Chartered Company, while
  the railroads, banks, collieries, telegraphs,
  exploration companies and newspapers are seen to be
  appendages of this central cluster" (Hobson, 1906:
  271).
The corporate elite carrying this network is, according to
Hobson, essentially a cosmopolitan financial elite. Of
course,
"in the acquisition of the material bases of finance the
services a class of adventurous explorers and consession-
mongers were essential," but the main work of building the
structure of the network is "attributable to the presence of
a group of 'pure financiers' (...)."
And, Hobson continues, "most of the abler and more succesful
members of this class are Jews, originally from the European
continent, though assimilating with ease and fervour to the
British sentiment, which is helpful to their financial
designs." Nevertheless, this elite admitted a few members of
the British aristocracy to the inner financial circle, mainly
"for the slower and more delicate work of constructing
political and 'social' supports (...)" (Hobson, 1906: 268).
Thus, although the corporate elite in South Africa consisted

of three sub-elites: the mining entrepreneurs, the 'pure financiers' and the British aristocracy, it is the group of 'pure financiers' that dominates the system and is mainly concerned with the international division of the spoils within the international <u>rentier</u> class.

As we indicated in the first paragraphs of Section 1.4, Hilferding places more emphasis on the aspect of strategic control of corporations, assuming a more direct relation between financial management and productive activity. Hobson's analysis of the financial system in South Africa makes clear that this distinction, which in Section 1.4 was made on logical grounds, also has a historical dimension. The mode of internationalization of capital analyzed by Hobson creates a business system in which holding- and investment companies strongly interlock with foreign mining companies abroad. Correspondingly, a group of internationally recruited 'pure financiers' forms the core of the corporate elite. Such a business system is typical for the period of classical imperialism (1870-1914). The mode of internationalization foreseen by Hilferding creates a business system in which banks interlocked with national industrial firms are the core. Correspondingly, a group of nationally recruited finance capitalists will form the core of the corporate elite. Such a business system, we assume, is typical of the period of modern imperialism, which developed at the beginning of the twentieth century in Germany and the United States, but only became dominant at a global level after World War II.

In the remainder of this section we will discuss several theories of imperialism which are based on the theoretical foundations laid by Hilferding. In 1914 Kautsky published an article on imperialism in the theoretical journal of the German Social Democratic Party (SPD). In it he argued a tendency in the international economy towards one gigantic world trust. Thus on a global level, cooperation between international firms would dominate competition and this cooperation could eventually be extended to the political sphere. A peaceful imperialism would be within reach:
  "From a purely economic point of view it is not
  impossible that capitalism will yet go through a new
  phase, that of the extension of the policy of the
  cartels to foreign policy, the phase of ultra-
  imperialism" (Kautsky (1914) 1970: 46).
In other words, according to Kautsky, the development of international finance capital tends to contain international competition and forms the economic basis on which a superstructure of peaceful alliances between capitalist states can be built.

Kautsky's position was challenged by his opponents in the Second International. The first attack from the left-wing social democrats (later communists) was launched by Bucharin. In a book written in 1915 but not published until 1918, Bucharin argued that there was no such tendency towards international economic cooperation between firms from the different countries. Bucharin saw a growing world economy, which he defined as "(....) a system of production relations and corresponding exchange relations on a world scale" (Bucharin, (1918) 1972: 26). The growth of this world economy was both <u>extensive</u> - including more and more geographic and social areas - and <u>intensive</u> - involving a "thicker network" of international economic relations (Bucharin, 1972: 28; see also Picciotto and Radice, 1973). The intensive growth of the world economy can be conceived as the development of finance capital at an international level. However, Bucharin saw not only a tendency towards internationalization but also a tendency towards nationalization, which <u>dominated</u> <u>the</u> <u>former</u>:

"The centralization process proceeds apace. Combines in industry and banking syndicates unite the entire national production, which assumes the form of a company of companies, thus becoming a state capitalist trust. Competition reaches the highest, the last conceivable state of development. It is now the competition of state capitalist trusts in the worldmarket" (Bucharin, (1918) 1972: 119).

In Bucharin's theory the capitalist world system is divided strictly along national lines. Each of these national financial groups (if they are strong enough to keep foreign influence outside their boundaries) has the state apparatus at its disposal. War is a prolongation of competition by other means. Under imperialism, Bucharin argued against Kautsky, competition on the international level must increase in scope and intensity. On the national level a state capitalist trust is formed as a coalescence of the nation-state and the national monopolies. It is this very coalescence which gives the international competition its violent character and results in wars like World War I. In terms of our concepts: <u>formation</u> <u>of</u> <u>finance</u> <u>capital</u> <u>at</u> <u>a</u> <u>global</u> <u>level</u> <u>is</u> <u>prevented</u> <u>by</u> <u>the</u> <u>specific</u> <u>form</u> <u>which</u> <u>international</u> <u>competition</u> <u>assumes</u> <u>in</u> <u>the</u> <u>imperialist</u> <u>rivalry</u> <u>between</u> <u>state</u> <u>capitalist</u> <u>trusts</u>.

In <u>Imperialism,</u> <u>the</u> <u>Highest</u> <u>Stage</u> <u>of</u> <u>Capitalism</u>, written in 1916, Lenin also attacks the position of Kautsky, siding with Bucharin's conclusion that imperialism increases the rivalry between imperialist states and creates the danger of world wars. Lenin does not argue - as Bucharin does - that at the economic level international capitalism is divided strictly along national lines. He explicitly mentions the formation of

international cartels (Lenin, 1964: 251). And although he
speaks frequently about the role nation-states play in the
division of the world between the capitalists, he never
assumes national capital to be unified, as Bucharin does.
Lenin's view about the international corporate structure
comes very close to that of Kautsky, but he does not believe,
as Kautsky does, that the economic structure under
imperialism ever will be a stable structure:
> "the capitalists divide the world, not out of any
> particular malice, but because the degree of
> concentration which has been reached forces them to
> adopt this method in order to obtain profits. And they
> divide it 'in proportion to capital', 'in proportion to
> strength', because there cannot be any other method of
> division under commodity production and capitalism. But
> strength varies with the degree of economic and
> political development" (Lenin, (1917) 1964: 253).

A more explicit formulation of Lenin's theory would include
the following statements:
- international cartels come into existence;
- between international cartels competition is growing;
- within national boundaries competition is not eliminated,
  but can only be analyzed within the framework of
  international competition;
- uneven development leads to a constant rearrangement of the
  international cartels, to an increase in size and power of
  some financial groups and a decline in size and power of
  others; and
- the constantly shifting power balance between financial
  groups leads to a redivision of the world by violent means.

Lenin's position is somewhat vaguer than those of Kautsky and
Bucharin, but it is clear that he foresees some form of
finance capital on the global level, which increases
international competition and the danger of war. The
international competition is not necessarily between national
syndicates or financial groups. These groups become
international and the war becomes a world war. Although it
may seem that Lenin stands just in the middle of the
theoretical road between Kautsky and Bucharin, there is in
fact a sharp division between Kautsky on the one hand and
Bucharin and Lenin on the other. Kautsky does envisage a
possibility of elimination of competition under capitalism,
while Lenin and Bucharin maintain that competition will
increase or - at the very least - appear on a higher level,
i.e., on the international level. The difference between
Bucharin and Lenin on the one hand and Kautsky on the other
lies not so much in their analysis of the economic structure,
but in the political conclusions drawn from it. According to
Kautsky, the economic tendency towards international rivalry

and conflict may be contained by political action, supporting
the peace-oriented segments of the capitalist class (see also
Salvadori, 1979: 181 ff). Lenin and Bucharin maintain, rather
deterministically, that imperialist rivalry cannot be
contained unless capitalism is abolished. The question,
however, lies outside the scope of this study.

Their vehement political debate notwithstanding, in terms of
the international network of corporate relations, Lenin and
Kautsky both expect an internationally integrated network,
whereas Bucharin does not. The difference between Lenin and
Kautsky lies in the amount of competition to be expected
within the internationally organized business system. History
seems to have proved the position of Bucharin and Lenin as
against Kautsky's. World War I was a classic example of the
prolongation of competition by other means (Bucharin) or the
redivision of the world by violent means (Lenin). On the
other hand, the period after 1945 has shown a marked tendency
towards internationalization of the economy together with
peaceful and stable relations between the major capitalist
countries. Yet another, theoretical, argument against the
position of Bucharin and Lenin is that they tried to explain
the outbreak of World War I with a theory based on an
economic development only just begun: the
internationalization of finance capital. In other words, they
explained the outbreak of World War I, which can only be
related to classical imperialism, in terms of modern
imperialism. It is characteristic, in this respect, that
Lenin, who used Hilferding's theory of finance capital as a
starting point for his analysis, incorporated the theory and
conclusions of Hobson without realizing that Hobson's theory
differs fundamentally from that of Hilferding. In my opinion,
the theories of Kautsky, Bucharin and Lenin are better
applicable to the period following World War II than to the
period in which they were developed.

3.1.2 After World War II

No wonder that after 1945, and especially during the sixties,
the debate broke out again. Again three positions can be
distinguished. The first theoretical stand is that of
super-imperialism put forward by Sweezy, Magdoff, Jalée and
others. The capitalist world is dominated by the United
States, who acts as the organizer of world capitalism,
preserving its unity in the face of the socialist countries
and the nationalist and anti-imperialist movements in the
Third World. The economic and political world order is
conceived as a pyramid with the United States at the top and
the Third World at the bottom.

A corrolary of this view is elaborated by those who see the
capitalist world order maintained by a coalition of dominant
capitalist states, who by a rapid proliferation of
supranational institutions resolve the antagonisms between
national capital and preserve the unity of imperialism. This
position is taken by the Soviet economist Varga (1968). A
similar view is found in the reports of the 1980's Project of
the Council on Foreign Relations and the allied Trilateral
Commission. Although neither of these institutions is engaged
in developing marxist theories of imperialism, the object of
study is the same and so are some of its conclusions. The
1980's Project was initiated in 1974 with the publication of
The Management of Interdependence: A Preliminary View by
Miriam Camps, senior research fellow at the Council. In this
book, Camps challenged the traditional balance of power
paradigm in which the rivalry between the United States and
the Soviet Union was the principal source of international
conflict and had to be contained in some sort of balance of
(super) power. Instead, she argued that the international
order should be managed collectively by the United States,
Western Europe and Japan. According to Camps,
  "the rules, goals and processes that the advanced
   countries adopt to govern economic relations with
   another should be the norms of the global system"
   (Camps, 1974: 45).
The Soviet Union, Eastern Europe and the Third World
countries should eventually become integrated into the new
Trilateral World Order. In this perspective, which is
disseminated by the Trilateral Commission, the major
potential for world conflict is no longer the rivalry between
the United States and the Soviet Union, but the strains
between the advanced capitalist countries. "The overall goal
of the Commission is thus to minimize the friction and
competition within the Trilateral World, unifying it as much
as possible" (Shoup and Minter, 1977: 268).

The views of Varga, Camps and the Trilateral Commission are
essentially Kautskian because they express the possibilities
of containing imperialist rivalries through international
cooperation. They even show a resemblance in their
explanation of historical events. Kautsky pointed to the arms
race between capitalist countries and the revolutionary
movement in the 'agrarian zones' to explain the urgent need
for international cooperation (Kautsky, 1970: 44, 45). Varga,
Camps and the Trilateral Commission emphasize the danger of
the popular movements in the Third World for global stability
and mention the heavy burden of the arms race on the
capitalist countries, even though this race is predominantly
between the Soviet Union and the United States.

A different position is taken by those who foresee a growing
imperialist rivalry. Competition between national capitals
becomes so strong that neither the United States nor a
coalition of capitalist states can any longer perform the
necessary organizing role. Serious conflicts arise between
them, and the unity of the system is threatened. This
position, which is very close to that of Bucharin, has been
put forward by Mandel (1970) and Rowthorn (1971). Mandel, in
his Europe versus America? sees a growing competition between
American, Japanese and European capital, forcing each to rely
on its own national state, especially in times of crisis. The
European big capital needs a European state to survive in
international competition. Rowthorn, although largely
agreeing with Mandel's analysis, stresses the possibility of
a discrepancy between the strength of a national capital and
the state. For Britain, Rowthorn sees a strong and highly
internationalized capital and a relatively weak nation state.
He continues:
  "Paradoxically, the weakness of the British state is to
  be explained not by the simple decline of British
  capitalism as such, but by the very strength of the
  cosmopolitan activities of British capital (..)"
  (Rowthorn, 1971: 46).
This may also be the position of the Dutch state, given the
strong international position of the Dutch multinationals and
the weakness, or at least smallness, of the Dutch nation
state. Such conclusions may cast doubt on the direct relation
between national capital and the state but they do not attack
the presumption on which the analyses of both Bucharin and
Mandel are based: the unity of national finance capital.
Poulantzas, for example, attacks Mandel on this very point.
And this brings us to the third position. According to
Poulantzas, there is no autonomous European business system.
He speaks about a "bourgeoisie interieure", which is in many
ways dependent on the American bourgeoisie because of its
place in the international division of labor, but at the same
time maintains its own accumulation base. Central to the
conception of Poulantzas is the idea that capital forms no
unity, and accordingly, different fractions of the
bourgeoisie exist:
  "En effet, la dépendance du capital par rapport au
  capital américain traverse les diverses fractions du
  capital autochtone: d'ou précisément sa desarticulation
  interne, les contradictions entre capital americain et
  bourgeoisies interieures constituant souvent la forme
  complexe de la reproduction, au sein des bourgeoisies
  interieures des contradictions propres au capital
  americain" (Poulantzas, 1974: 81).
And De Brunhoff pushes the argument to its logical end by
criticizing Poulantzas for considering American capital as
one block with a sole interest (De Brunhoff, 1976: 97).

More recently, this position has been taken as a starting
point for a class analysis of the Atlantic community by Van
der Pijl (1979). It is this position which comes closest to
the position taken by Lenin; there exists, according to this
view, an integrated business system, but the system is
characterized by sharp cleavages, which do not necessarily
run along national lines.

The theories discussed so far are primarily concerned with
the relations between the economic and the political world
order. The network of interlocking directorates derives its
significance, if any, mainly from the developments in the
economic world order. What relevance does the analysis of
networks of interlocking directorates then have for these
theories? There are two answers to this question. In the
first place, it has been argued in Section 1.4 that an
analysis of the network of interlocking directorates is not
concerned with economic structures in the strict sense of the
word. In fact, we argued there, it is at the same time an
analysis of the structure of joint-ownership interests of the
corporate elite as part of the capitalist class <u>and</u> an
analysis of the intercorporate structures associated with the
strategic control of these corporations. Therefore the
analysis of the international network of interlocking
directorates is on the one hand an analysis of international
class formation and international class alliance and on the
other hand an analysis of the international structure of
strategic control of corporations.
Second, even if one were to maintain that this has very
little to do with the political world order, which consists
of nation states and the relations between them, our analysis
should still be regarded as relevant. Since most of the
authors claim to follow the method of historical materialism,
it is implicitly - or explicitly - assumed that the political
structure is, whether or not 'in last instance', determined
by the economic structure. Therefore, the analysis of the
economic structure is basic to the analysis of the political
structure. This does not mean that the political structure
can be directly inferred from the economic structure. It <u>does</u>
mean, however, that if the analysis of the economic structure
is deficient, the whole theory falls apart.

In the next section we will analyze the implications of the
different theories of imperialism for the international
network of interlocking directorates by constructing some
models by which the actual network will be compared. From
each of these models, we will also deduce some implications
for the structure of the corporate elite.

3.2 Two models

The theories of Kautsky and Lenin, and all those who were
called Kautskian and Leninist respectively, assumed an
international network of corporate relations between the
largest firms from the advanced capitalist countries.
According to the first basic model, one would expect a
cohesive network of interlocking directorates between these
firms. Such a network would be in accordance with the
theories of both kautsky and Lenin. From the theory of super-
imperialism and the Leninist theory of Poulantzas, it can be
deduced that control exercised by means of interlocking
directorates is predominantly directed from the American
firms to the firms from other countries.

The theory of Bucharin, on the other hand, assumes a tight
network of corporate relations at the national level,
cementing the state capitalist trust in each country. In the
second basic model, therefore, there exist tight networks of
interlocking directorates at the national level, which are
not connected internationally, and which cannot be separated
into different international groups, cliques or clusters. In
other words, in this model, few international interlocks
exist, and the international cohesion of the network is
accordingly weak. The models derived from the Bucharinist
theories of Mandel and Rowthorn deviate only slightly from
this second basic model. Accordingly to Mandel, there exists
a growing network of economic relations between firms from
EEC countries, indicating the integration of the Common
Market. The theory of Mandel would imply tight national
networks except for the continental Common Market countries,
which are integrated into a Common Market of interlocking
directorates. Rowthorn's theory would also leads us to
believe that there are tight national networks connected by
interlocking directorates of Dutch and British corporations.

We have thus deduced two basic models of international
networks of interlocking directorates, the first derived from
the theories of Kautsky and Lenin, with some specifications
derived from the theories of super-imperialism and of
Poulantzas, and the second derived from the theory of
Bucharin, with two deviations derived from the theories of
Mandel and of Rowthorn.

It is now necessary to introduce the dynamic aspect of these
theories, because all of the authors discussed so far have
presented their theories in a development perspective. Rather
than presenting a picture of an economic structure, they have
tried to portray imperialism as a result of economic
tendencies. The theories of imperialism are typically
theories of crisis. Lenin and Bucharin, especially, assumed

an immanent tendency in the economic world order towards
economic and political breakdowns, caused by imperialistic
rivalry between the capital exporting countries. Although
there is permanent conflict between these countries, economic
crisis 'sharpens' these 'contradictions', economically as
well as politically, meaning that economic reality comes
closer to the structure they portray and political reality to
the disaster they predict. If the structure of the network of
interlocking directorates resembles one of the basic models
in 'normal times', it should do even more so in times of
crisis. The two years I have chosen to investigate are 1970
and 1976, the one occurring just before and the other just
after the economic recession of 1974. By 1976 the effects of
the economic world crisis should be visible in the network of
interlocking directorates.

The difference between the theory of Lenin and that of
Kautsky, which is not reflected in the models constructed
here, lies in the question of whether or not the economic
world order is inherently unstable. Large changes in the
structure of interlocking directorates would lend support to
the theory of Lenin.

Although the use of the term model may give rise to the
expectation that the economic theories of imperialism will
undergo a procedure of rigorous testing, this is certainly
not the case:
first, because the economic theories of imperialism are more
than theories of the economic aspects of imperialism. And
only an economic aspect is considered here;
secondly, because even if they were theories of the economic
aspects of imperialism, only one of these aspects - the
international organization of the economic elite - is
considered here;
thirdly, because the 'models' that I have constructed are far
too general to allow any testing procedure;
fourthly, because the sample of firms will be relatively
small, providing but a first impression of the complicated
structures of interlocking directorates, both nationally and
internationally; and
finally, because we are considering only the small span of
time, whereas theories of imperialism focus on a historical
epoch, comprising at least several decades. This study can
only lend some credibility to one of the theories. More often
still, the contending theories of imperialism are used as a
general background for describing and analyzing the data.

What implications can be drawn from these models of networks
of interlocking directorates for the structure of the
corporate elite carrying the network? First, the fact that
both models are based on theories of modern imperialism, in

which the relations between banks and industry are
predominant, implies that the corporate elite will
predominantly consist of finance capitalists. That is, most
members of the corporate elite will have a position in at
least one bank and one industrial firm. Few members will have
a position in financial institutions only.
Secondly, according to both models, the international
interlocks will be significantly more carried by finance
capitalists than by other members of the corporate elite.
Since in the model derived from the Bucharinist theories few
international interlocks exist, it follows logically that few
members of the corporate elite will carry an international
interlock. In the model based on the theory of Mandel those
few members of the corporate elite who do carry international
interlocks are nationals from continental Common Market
countries. And in the model based on the theory of Rowthorn,
they are British and Dutch nationals.

According to the model derived from Kautskian and Leninist
theories, there are more members of the corporate elite who
carry an international interlock. So far, however, it is
difficult to specify the proportion and thus discriminate
between the two models. Only from the theory of super-
imperialism can a prediction be made: the members of the
corporate elite carrying an international interlock will be
preponderantly American.

3.3 Research design

To study the international network of interlocking
directorates and especially the integration of different
national networks into an international network requires a
selection of firms from different countries. The selection of
the years 1970 and 1976 allows comparison of the network
before and after the entrance of the United Kingdom into the
Common Market. It also allows comparison of the network
before and after the economic recession of 1974. Our source
was the Fortune Directories. Given the theoretical
perspective of this book, the largest firms of the world
should be included in the sample because these are the firms
most likely to be central in the network of interlocking
directorates. Furthermore, since a high correlation exists
between size and foreign investment, these companies are also
likely to be the most internationally oriented. Because banks
have a very central position in the national networks, they
should certainly be included in the sample.

Because of financial and computer limitations, the sample could not exceed 200 firms. [2] Therefore, we decided to select a maximum of 150 industrials and 50 banks.

There appeared, however, one great problem: out of the 150 largest industrials 92 were American firms in 1970 and 74 were American firms in 1976. Thus, a selection of the 150 largest industrials would seriously hamper an international comparison of the national (sub)networks, because so few firms from the other advanced capitalist countries would be included. We therefore chose a stratified sampling method instead. Because in many economic theories of imperialism a distinction is made between the United States, the Common Market, and Japan as geographical cores of capitalist development and expansion, we decided to distinguish the largest firms of the world accordingly, adding the United Kingdom as a fourth hypothetical core. Using the category 'other countries' as a residual one, it was now possible to select an equal number of firms from each category, say the 30 largest. Although this would have provided 150 firms whose selection was based on the size as well as on the geographical criterion, there remained one problem. Of the old EEC countries, France and Italy would hardly be represented in the sample and Belgium/Luxembourg not at all. Since the structure of the networks of interlocking directorates in the Common Market and its changes after the entrance of the United Kingdom are focal points in the analysis, more firms from the old EEC countries had to be included. It was finally decided to select the 26 largest industrial firms from the United States, from the United Kingdom, from Japan and from the category 'other countries', along with the 41 largest firms from the old EEC countries.

After elimination of those firms for which no information on the composition of the boards of directors could be obtained, we ended up with 135 industrial firms from 14 countries. Two countries, Belgium and Luxembourg, were regarded as one because their economic structure is strongly integrated and because they often appear together in official statistics. Table 3.1 gives the distribution of the 135 industrials over 13 countries. (For the list of firms and a detailed description of the selection procedure see Appendix A.)

[2] In the course of this research many computing problems have been solved by a new program package called "Graph Definition and Analysis Package" (GRADAP, 1980).

Table 3.1 Number of firms per country in the sample 1970.

	Industrialists	Banks
United States	25	8
United Kingdom	25 [*]	5
Japan	22	8
West Germany	15	4
France	14	4
Canada	7	4
Switzerland	7	3
Sweden	7	-
Italy	5	3
Netherlands	4 [*]	2
Belgium/Luxembourg	3	-
Australia	2	-
South Africa	1	-

[*] The Dutch-British firms Unilever and Shell are counted twice.

For the selection of banks a similar procedure was followed. From the United States, the United Kingdom, Japan and the category 'other countries' the eight largest banks were selected. To this number, five were added from the old EEC countries to give a total of thirteen. The criterion for size was not, as with the industrial firms, sales. In accordance with Fortune's "fifty largest commercial banks outside the U.S." and "fifty largest commercial banking companies", we used assets as an indicator of size. Of course the disadvantage of using assets as an indicator of the size of banks is the same as with industrial firms. However, to arrange the banks according to deposits would not change the order much. Using deposits as an indicator of size would bias our selection in favor of deposit banks.

In the case of British banks only five were selected. Smaller banks did not appear in the Fortune list or in the Banker's Almanac. Besides, two of the top five banks were a result of a merger in 1969: Barclays Bank Ltd. and Barclays Bank DCO formed Barclays Bank, and Standard Bank and Chartered Bank formed Standard and Chartered Banking Group. After elimination of the banks for which no information could be obtained regarding the composition of the boards of directors, forty-one banks from nine countries were left (Table 3.1).

Four countries have no banks represented in the sample. Given
the crucial role played by the banks in the network of
interlocking directorates, this may cause serious problems.
This is not the case for Australia and South Africa, since
they are hardly represented at all and will be marginal in
the analysis. For Sweden and Belgium-Luxembourg, however, the
lack of banks in the sample seriously hampers comparison with
other countries. On the other hand, Canadian, Italian and
Dutch banks seem to be overrepresented in relation to the
number of their countries' industrials in the sample.
We should not forget, however, that within each nationality
group, selection is based on size. Belgian and Swedish banks
do not even appear on the Fortune list of top fifty banks.
The non-representation of Swedish and Belgian banks in the
sample does not result from an arbitrary selection procedure,
but from the application of a general and objective selection
criterion. By using this criterion, ten countries are
represented in the sample in such a way that allows for
further analysis. The representation of Belgian, Australian
and South African firms is too small for further analysis.

The network of interlocking directorates between these 176
selected firms will first be analyzed to see whether or not
there exists a cohesive international network in which the
firms from different nationalities are firmly integrated.
Secondly,the analysis will determine whether there exist
clusters in the network corresponding with the concept of
financial group. Thirdly, the position of the banks in the
network will be analyzed in greater detail and compared with
the network of international bank consortia. Finally, the
networks of 1970 and of 1976 will be compared to see whether
the extension of the Common Market and the economic world
recession has had an impact upon the networks of interlocking
directorates.

3.4 Summary

In this chapter we have been in search of a theoretical
framework within which to interpret the international
structure of the network of interlocking directorates. This
theoretical framework, though at a much more general level,
is found in the economic theories of imperialism, most of
which are based on the conceptions of Hilferding (see Chapter
1). These theories are on the whole consistent with
Hilferding's explanation of the development of a network of
corporate interlocks, thus allowing us to concentrate upon
the international aspects of this network. There exist,
however, a great many different economic theories of
imperialism, not always spelled out in sufficient detail and

certainly not developed for the purpose of explaining
networks of interlocking directorates. Three main theories
stand out at the beginning of this century: that of Kautsky,
that of Bucharin and that of Lenin. And most of the theories
after World War II can be classified as either Kautskian,
Bucharinist or Leninist in their outline and emphasis. For
the purpose of this book some conclusions have been deduced
from each of the three theories regarding the structure of
the network of interlocking directorates. We have constructed
two basic models, the first inspired by the premises of the
theories of Kautsky and Lenin, the second by those of the
theory of Bucharin. Furthermore, deviations of each of the
basic models have been elaborated to fit the different
theories developed after World War II (Section 3.2). Finally,
in Section 3.3, the research design was presented. In the
sampling of the firms the theoretical perspective as given in
the first three chapters was taken as a starting point, but
practical and technical considerations restricted the
possibilities. The selection resulted in 176 firms. A
detailed description of the selection procedure can be found
in Appendix A. In Chapter 4 the selection of the
international corporate elite is presented and the most
important network characteristics of this elite and of the
interlocks it carries are discussed. After that, the network
will be analyzed, taking the following questions into
account:

- Does a cohesive network of interlocking directorates exist
  at a national level and how are the national networks
  integrated in the international network (Chapter 5)?
- Are there internationally organized financial groups in the
  network and what type of interlocking directorates is
  particularly relevant to the detection of such financial
  groups (Chapter 6)?
- What role do the banks play in the network of interlocking
  directorates and how does their position relate to other
  intercorporate networks (Chapter 7)?
- What are the changes in the international business system
  in the period 1970 to 1976. What conclusion can be drawn as
  to the two models of networks of interlocking directorates
  constructed in Section 3.2 (Chapter 8)?

IV THE INTERNATIONAL CORPORATE ELITE

4.0 Introduction

Even though the study of interlocking directorates is basically a study of intercorporate power which cannot be based on theories and evidence of intracorporate power, the structure of the corporation is important for the position of the directors, especially for their position as interlocking directors. If, for example, the internal function of the board of directors is regarded as insignificant, the function of interlocking directorates will also be considered of minor importance. [1] In Section 4.1 the development of the decision-making structure of the large corporation and the main functions of different boards will be sketched. Furthermore, an international survey is necessary to compare national differences and to assign an identical meaning to corresponding positions. Since it is well known that formally similar positions may differ in content from one company to another within the same country, it is obvious that the idiosyncratic differences in companies from different nations will be even greater. For this reason the goal of Section 4.1 is very modest: only some major distinctions will be made to enable us to select the most important positions (Section 4.2) and to construct a simple typology of interlocking directorates according to the character of the position held in each of a pair of interlocked firms (Section 4.4.2).

4.1 The organization of the supervising and executive function in different countries

The separation of ownership and control was accompanied by important changes in the organizational structure of the large firms. Such changes first appeared in the American railroad companies. The size of these companies was very large indeed and most of them expanded rapidly in the second half of the nineteenth century. In an early railroad company, the key decisions were usually made by the so-called general manager who acted in close consultation with the representatives of the large investors. After the Civil War, the railroad system, rather than the individual railroad, became the dominant operating organization, and a more explicit overall structure was needed. A central office was

[1] For a defense of this position see Gordon (1966) and more recently, Mace (1971).

created to guide and coordinate the separate operating units. This central office was run by the heads of the functional departments responsible for transportation, sales, finance etc. Thus, an executive committee was formed out of the functional specialists.
Consultation with the representatives of the large investors also needed a more formal arrangement. Thus, a board of directors was formed, consisting of the (most important) members of the executive committee and the representatives of the (most important) investors, who in the emerging joint-stock companies were the large stockholders. Here key decisions could be discussed and long-term objectives determined.

In the nineteenth-century stock company, stockholders were still regarded as co-owners of the firm. In the twentieth century, the stockholders gradually came to be regarded as mere shareowners. Legally, it is the corporation that owns the assets and not the stockholders. The stock company is a legal entity endowed with property rights. Although shareholders have lost these property rights, they have the right to participate in the decision-making process of that legal entity by voting in the meeting of shareholders, which includes in many countries the right to vote for the nomination of the board of directors. In legal terms, the shareholder has lost juridical ownership, but, at least formally, she or he still has economic ownership (Valkhoff, 1941: 34). Besides, the shareholders own their shares, which provides them with a claim on the remunerations of the company. In other words, usus and usus fructus have been separated. Share ownership has become revenue claim (usus fructus) and is only indirectly related to usus because it provides the owner with a right to participate in the decision-making process. This right has become dissociated from individuals and can only be exercised collectively. Therefore, the stock company was seen by Marx as the abolition of private ownership of capital and the introduction of social capital. A similar idea was expressed by Keynes when he wrote in 1926 about
"(...) the trend of joint stock institutions, when they
have reached a certain age and size, to approximate to
the status of public corporations rather than that of
individualistic private enterprise. One of the most
interesting and unnoticed developments of recent
decades has been the tendency of big enterprise to
socialise itself" (Keynes, 1972: 289).
And Berle puts it another way: "the capital is there, and so is capitalism; the waning factor is the capitalist" (Berle, 1954: 39).
The central question in this section is the relation between

two pivotal institutions of the 'socialized' stock company:
the general meeting of shareholders and the board of
directors. Formally, the highest authority of a joint-stock
company is vested in the general meeting of shareholders.
Individually, the shareholders have no possibility of
exercising the economic property rights, as Valkhoff called
it; only in the general meeting of shareholders can these
rights be exercised. And even then, most of these rights can
only be exercised indirectly, through the nomination of
directors. Throughout the history of the joint- stock company
there has been a continuous trend towards domination of the
board of directors over the meeting of shareholders. The
dominant position of the board of directors was legally
acknowledged in the Netherlands when in 1971 the cooptation
of the board was legalized, leaving the meeting of
shareholders with a qualified veto power. Before 1971,
however, the shareholders had been deprived of their economic
property rights through the device of priority shares, which
gave their holders (in many cases the board directors) the
right to nominate the directors.
In other countries no such legal devices are available, but
there are other methods of controlling the meeting of
shareholders. In particular, voting by proxy, which enables
certain persons to vote on behalf of the (small)
shareholders, is used both in the United States and in
Germany. In the United States, however, the proxy committee
is generally controlled by the board of directors, while in
Germany the banks exercise the voting rights for the shares
belonging to their clients. Other devices to eliminate the
control of the shareholders are the 'fiduciary institutions'
which hold shares in trust for their owners, and investment
companies, which hold blocks of shares, while issuing their
own shares to the public. In practice the difference between
fiduciary institutions, investment companies and other
financial institutions is of little significance with respect
to the problem of control (see Scott, 1979). But who control
these financial institutions? The answer lies in the
mutualization of control by crossing the holdings. It
reinforces the group in control through interlocking
directorates and a 'self-perpetuating board of directors'
(Perlo, 1957: 82).

Rather than representing the shareholders, the board of
directors has come to represent the stock company. Through
the board of directors arose the possibility of
institutionalizing consultation with large stockholders. The
consultations with important suppliers of raw materials, with
important clients and with those who controlled financial
resources could also be institutionalized by inviting their
representatives on the board. And it was again the American

railroad companies who were the first to develop an intricate
network of intercorporate relations through interlocking
directorates. This led to the investigations of the
Interstate Commerce Commission, published in 1908 under the
title "Intercorporate Relationships of Railways in the United
States."

Although it can be said that the board of directors as a
whole represents the corporation towards third parties, this
is not true for the individual director. Many directors
represent large blocks of shares that are owned by cohesive
groups of individuals such as families, or by institutional
investors. Others represent their 'own' companies, which may
have specific commercial interests to be defended.
This duality of the board of directors always exists. On the
one hand the board has to supervise the executive officers on
behalf of the financial interests represented on the board,
and on the other hand it has to act as a unified body
representing the company. The duality can explode into a
proxy fight over the nomination of directors. In continental
European firms this duality has been solved by a two-board
system. In this system there is an executive board
representing the company as a legal entity towards third
parties and a supervisory board representing the (large)
shareholders. The supervisory board meets three to six times
a year. Members of the executive board cannot be on the
supervisory board.
In fact, the situation in continental European is even more
complicated because there are both a 'German' and a 'Latin'
version of the two-board system. In Germany and in the
Netherlands the supervisory board (Aufsichtsrat and Raad van
Commissarissen) tends to become involved in executive
functions as soon as important decisions are to be taken.
This is the case when the articles of association require
that certain basic decisions only be taken with the consent
of the supervisory board. In emergency cases the supervisory
board can even nominate one of its members to take over the
management of the company (Delegationsrat in Germany and
Gedelegeerd Commissaris in the Netherlands). Finally, the
supervisory board nominates the members of the executive
board (see De Boer, 1957: 141). In the German two-board
system the supervisory board is often in control of the
corporation although the situation varies from company to
company and depends heavily on the specific structure and
history of the corporation. Sometimes the supervisory board
is controlled by the executive board rather than the other
way around.
The Latin variant of the two-board system can be considered
the purest form of separation of the executive and
supervising function. The supervisory board has in fact only

an auditing function as indicated by its name: <u>commissaires</u>
<u>aux</u> <u>comptes</u> in France and Belgium; <u>syndaci</u> in Italy.
A portion of the membership of these boards must be chosen
from a national list of certified accountants; [2] the others
can be chosen freely at the meeting of shareholders. The
supervisory board in the Latin variant is by no means
comparable to the German <u>Aufsichtsrat</u>, if only because this
board does not nominate the members of the executive board
and is not able to interfere with policy making.
Subsequently, in the Latin variant of the two-board system
the position of the meeting of shareholders is stronger than
in the German variant. We find the Latin variant in Belgium,
France and Italy. In France, however, the German variant has
been optional since 1966.

In the Anglo-Saxon structure both the supervisory <u>and</u> the
executive functions are entrusted to the board of directors,
which meets more frequently than the supervisory board in the
continental European system, normally once a month. However,
in this one-board system a separation can be made between
<u>inside</u> and <u>outside</u> directors. The inside directors are
employed by the company and often form an executive
committee, which has some resemblance to the executive board
in the two-board system. The outside directors have a more
supervisory function, representing large shareholders and
other financial interests (see Frommel and Thompson, 1975).
But again, in many instances the inside directors may well
dominate the outside directors on the board, in which case
the outside directors become representatives <u>towards</u> third
parties rather than <u>of</u> third parties.

To summarize our survey so far, there are always two
functions to be performed by the top organs of a joint-stock
company:
1. the supervising function related to the representation of
   the (large) shareholders and other financial interests;
   and
2. the executive function related to the management of the
   firm and to the representation of the firm towards third
   parties.

[2] The <u>commissaires</u> <u>aux</u> <u>comptes</u> and the <u>syndaci</u> are not
    comparable to the accountants in the Netherlands ·and
    Germany and the auditors in the Anglo-Saxon countries. The
    latter cannot be regarded as part of the company; they
    represent the 'public interest' rather than the
    shareholders.

In continental Europe these two functions are performed by two separate boards, while in the United States, the United Kingdom and Sweden these functions are performed by one board, within which a separation can be made between inside and outside directors.

4.2 Selection of the international corporate elite

From the two-board corporations members of both boards were selected. From the one-board corporations all members of the board of directors were selected. Members of the executive committee in the one-board corporations who were not on the board of directors were also selected, as were the highest officers in the two-board corporations who were not members of either of the two boards. This was done to determine whether or not interlocking directorates between the corporations in the sample are also carried by officers outside the board of directors.

Members of advisory boards or committees were selected as a special category. These boards have no formal authority in the company. Most of them have been set up by banks to satisfy the need for (international) consultation. Such is the case, for example, with the international advisory boards of Chase Manhattan and Chemical Bank (New York) and the European advisory boards of AMRO and Midland Bank. These latter boards were created to coordinate the activities of the European Banks' International Company (EBIC).

In toto 6,054 persons and 6,523 positions were selected for 1970, i.e., a mean of nearly 37 positions per firm. Of the persons, only 372 had a position in two or more firms in the sample. Only 6 were not a member of the board of directors in a one-board corporation or of the supervisory board or the executive board in a two-board corporation. From this it can be concluded that very few officers outside the board of directors carry interlocks between the very large firms and that the term interlocking directorate remains an appropriate term for the interlocks investigated here.

We regarded the 372 persons who carry the international network as the international corporate elite. In the remainder of this chapter we will present some network characteristics of both the international corporate elite (Section 4.3) and the interlocks they carry (Section 4.4).

4.3 Network characteristics of the international corporate elite

4.3.0 Introduction

In Section 1.4 we said that the analysis presented in this book would be structural and institutional: structural, because the members of the elite are only considered in relation to each other; and institutional, because the firms are regarded as the main actors, while the members of the elite are regarded as channels of communication and control between these firms.

Does it not seem illogical, then, to start with a description of the characteristics of individual members of the elite? Indeed, the categorization of individuals according to specific variables seems neither structural nor institutional. The objection is partly warranted. To make a distinction between members of the corporate elite who are finance capitalists and those who are not, between those who carry many interlocks and those who carry few, is certainly not an institutional approach. But it is structural in so far as the variables used in this section are network variables: individuals are distinguished according to the positions they have in the network of interlocking directorates. Later on, these distinctions will be used to analyze certain network characteristics more in detail (Chapter 6).

4.3.1 The finance capitalists

If the theory of finance capital is correct, the interlocking directorates of the sample are predominantly carried by persons who have a position in at least one bank and at least one industrial company. These persons are called after Zeitlin (1976) finance capitalists (see Section 1.4). Of the 372 persons who carry at least one interlocking directorate, 262 are finance capitalists in this sense. Only 3 persons exclusively carry interlocks between banks. These three (L. Medugno, F. Persegani and U. Tabanelli) carry interlocks between Banco di Roma, Credito Italiano and Banca Commerciale Italiana, three out of four Italian banks in the sample. They constitute an exceptional case, also because Persegani and Tabanelli are both members of the board of auditors (Collegio Sindacale) of Credito Italiano and of Banco di Roma (see Section 4.1). [3] The remaining 107 persons in the sample have only functions in industrial corporations. This does not imply that they are not affiliated with financial institutions. They may be affiliated with financial institutions other than banks, such as insurance companies or

pension funds, or they may be affiliated with banks that are not included in the sample. This is particularly serious for those who are directors of Belgian or Swedish industrials, because the sample includes no banks from these countries. As a consequence, three members of the Swedish Wallenberg family, the late Jacob, Marcus, and Marcus junior, are counted as non-finance capitalists, although it is well known that the center of their financial empire is the Enskilda Bank (Hermansson, 1971: 238 ff). If we exclude all those affiliated with Belgian and Swedish industrials, the number of persons with only industrial affiliations drops to 95. Thus, roughly three-quarters of the interlocking directors in the sample can be defined as 'finance capitalists', while only one-quarter cannot. If we compare this with previous research, the number of finance capitalists in the sample is high. In the network of 86 Dutch firms in 1969 there were 248 interlocking directors. Of these, 140 were finance capitalists, 55 carried only interlocks between financial firms, and 53 carried only interlocks between non-financial firms (Helmers et.al., 1975: 22).

These results are in accordance with those of Soref (1980) who has done extensive research on the finance capitalists in the United States. Studying 196 directors of a much larger sample of firms, Soref found that 62 of these were finance capitalists. The finance capitalists were found to be significantly more affiliated with the larger companies. [4] Another conclusion from Soref's study can also be confirmed. Soref found that finance capitalists have significantly more directorships than non-finance capitalists in the United States. Of the 95 non-finance capitalists studied here, only 7 have more than 2 directorships and only 1 has more than 3 (F.H. Ulrich). Of the 262 finance capitalists 62 have more than 2 directorships and 18 of these have more than 3 directorships. Thus, while less than 10 percent of the non-finance capitalists has more than two directorships, 24 percent of the finance capitalists has more than two

[3] Medugno is a director of Banca Commerciale Italiana and of Banco di Roma.

[4] It is not true, as Soref maintains, that his study is the first systematic study on finance capitalists. The Dutch study of Helmers et.al. in 1970 was the first (Helmers et.al., 1975).

directorships. Finally, we want to know whether the
international interlocks are also predominantly carried by
finance capitalists. Of the 113 international interlocks
(i.e., an interlocking directorate between two firms of
different nationalities), 97 are carried by finance
capitalists, while 16 are carried by non-finance capitalists.
The finance capitalists, being three-quarters of the
international corporate elite, carry 86 percent of the
international interlocks. [5]

Table 4.1 Distribution of international interlocks

| | | interlock carried by a finance capitalist | | |
		yes	no	total
international interlock	yes (row pct)	97 (85.8)	16 (14.2)	113 (18.8) (100)
	no (row pct)	383 (78.5)	105 (21.5)	488 (81.2) (100)
	total (row pct)	480 (79.9)	121 (20.1)	601 (100) (100)

But do finance capitalists carry significantly more
international interlocks? This question can only be answered
by calculating the possibility that a random distribution of
all interlocks would result in a distribution in which at
least 97 of the international interlocks were carried by
finance capitalists. According to a hypergeometrical
distribution this possibility is less than 4 percent. Of the
interlocks carried by finance capitalists, 20 percent is
international, while of those not carried by finance
capitalists only 13 percent is international.

[5] Two international interlocks are carried by two non-
    finance capitalists affiliated with a Belgian and a Swedish
    firm. If we regard them as finance capitalists, the
    percentage increases to 84.

4.3.2 The big linkers

In the former paragraph it was mentioned that the finance capitalists hold more directorships than the non-finance capitalists. In this paragraph the total distribution of positions will be discussed and compared with the results from previous research. The theoretical relevance of the distribution of positions lies in the fact that persons who hold a large number of directorships carry an even larger number of interlocks. A person holding directorships in n firms carries $n(n-1)/2$ interlocks. These n firms form a completely connected subgraph. [6] And since all interlocks are carried by one person, it is called a person-clique (see Figure 4.1a).

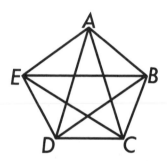
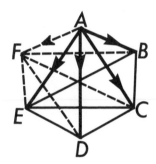

Figure 4.1a   Figure 4.1b

Now if the person carrying $n(n-1)/2$ interlocks is an executive of, let us say, firm A, then all interlocks between other firms and firm A are called primary, while the interlocks among the other firms are called secondary. When n increases, the number of secondary interlocks increases more rapidly than the number of primary interlocks. The number of primary interlocks is n-1, while the number of secondary

[6] A completely connected subgraph is defined as a collection of firms, in which each firm is adjacent to all other firms in the collection.

interlocks is (n-1)(n-2)/2, increasing quadratically with n.
If, for example, n goes from five to six, then the number of
primary interlocks increases with one, while the number of
secondary interlocks increases with four (see Figure 4.1b).
Since it has been argued (Section 1.2) that secondary
interlocks are less likely to be control lines, we can
conclude that large person-cliques increase the potential for
communication more than the potential for control.
In Table 4.2 the distribution of directorships of directors
over the members of the corporate elite is given, and the
number of interlocks is calculated per person and in total.

Table 4.2 Distribution of directorships among the
international corporate elite

a number of persons	b number of directorships	c number of interlocks per person [n(n-1)/2]	d total
1	7	21	21
1	6	15	15
1	5	10	10
16	4	6	96
53	3	3	159
300	2	1	300
5682	1	0	0
6054			601

As can be seen from Table 4.2, half of all interlocks (300)
are carried by a person who holds only two directorships.
Nearly a quarter of all interlocks are carried by a person
holding four or more directorships, even though these
nineteen persons constitute only 5 percent of all multiple
directors. We will call these nineteen persons the big
linkers. Their contribution to the network will be analyzed
in this section.
Is the proportion of big linkers in the international network
high or low when compared to the different national networks?
To answer this question, we must compare the distribution of
positions over the corporate elite in different nations with
the distribution of positions over the international
corporate elite. Zijlstra (1979b) has summarized the
different national studies for this aspect, making the task
of comparing their results with ours on the international
level much easier (see Table 4.3). The proportion of big
linkers (fourth row in Table 4.3) is much smaller in the

international network than in the national networks. This is
also   true   when   the   big   linkers   are   considered   not   in
proportion to all directors (fifth row in Table 4.3),   but in
proportion to the total number of multiple directors. In the
latter comparison the big linkers constitute 5 percent of the
multiple directors in the international network, whereas they
constitute   between   11   and   24   percent   in   the   national
networks.

Table 4.3 Distribution of positions over the   populations   of
          persons in interlock networks [*]

Networks of financial and industrial corporations

USA		USA		Belgium		Scotland		Nether-lands		Internat-ional net-work	
[a]	[b]		[c]		[d]		[e]		[f]		
	1935		1965		1975		1973		1972		1970
	n	%	n	%	n	%	n	%	n	%	n	%
1	2234	82	2602	82	48202	73	1178	90	690	78	5682	93
2	303	11	372	12	9706	15	79	6	102	12	300	5
3	102	4	123	4	3453	5	31	2	44	5	53	.9
>3	83	3	67	2	4687	7	28	2	45	5	19	.3
	2722	100	3165	100	66048	100	1316	100	882	100	6054	100

[a] Number of positions held by one person
[b] Dooley (1969)/US National Resources Committee (1939)
[c] Dooley (1969)
[d] Vessière (1978)
[e] Scott (1978)
[f] Mokken and Stokman (1978)

[*] Adapted from Zijlstra, (1979b)

Although the figures from Table 4.3 are not comparable in all
respects,   since   the   number   of   firms   and   the   selection
criteria   for the directors vary in   the   different   samples,
some general conclusions can safely   be   drawn. First, in the
international   sample of 1970 the   percentage   of   selected
persons who do not carry an interlock is higher than   in   any
of the national networks presented in the table. It is   even
higher   than   that   of   the   Scottish   selection,   which   is
exceptionally   high   in   relation   to   the   'truly   national'
samples. Secondly, among the multiple directors, the number

of persons who carry just one interlock is exceptionally high
as well. While in all national networks the percentage of
persons carrying just one interlock is between 55 and 65
percent, for the international network in 1970 this
percentage is 80. Conversely, the number of big linkers is
smaller in the international network than in different
national networks. Consequently, the number of large person-
cliques is smaller in the international network than in the
national networks previously studied.

Since the big linkers preponderantly carry weak ties, we
assume that they carry the system of business communication
rather than the specific control and domination network.
Their position in many different firms can provide them with
information from many different sources and, since they are
often 'grand old man', their prestige in the business world
is such that they may well represent large parts of the
business world. As Barrat Brown aptly stated, they are
"trying to supply some order and coordination in place and
anarchy" (Barrat,Brown, 1973: 103).This is especially true
for those big linkers who are not tied to one firm, i.e., who
have no executive position in any of the firms in which they
are directors. Such big linkers are called network
specialists, even though they are often former presidents of
large firms. Of the 19 big linkers, 12 are network
specialists. Ten out of the 12, however, are outside chairmen
of the board of directors, a position which is often given to
the former president of the corporation.

Do the big linkers play an important role in linking firms of
different nationalities together? At first sight, it does not
particularly appear so. Of the 142 arcs carried by the big
linkers, 36 are international arcs (25.4 percent). In the
Western network as a whole the number of interlocks is 570,
of which 129 are between firms of different nationalities
(22.6 percent). The 19 big linkers induce a network between
50 firms in the sample. Forty-two form one component with 130
interlocks. (For the definitions of the graph-theoretical
concepts used here the reader is referred to Section 5.0.)
Two other components are 4-cliques (US General Electric –
Chrysler – Chemical Bank – Procter & Gamble and British
Insulated Callender's Cables – Mobil Oil – IBM – First
National City Bank). In the large component we find firms
from nine different countries. With the exception of Belgium-
Luxembourg all Western countries are represented. In other
words, less than 5 percent of all directors in the network
link 30 percent of the firms in the network in such a way
that firms from all Western countries are interlocked.
Conversely, if the big linkers are deleted, the remaining

directors carry a network that is much more fragmented along national lines. [7] The big linkers have indeed a high potential for international communication.

4.4 Types of interlocking directorates

4.4.0 Introduction

In the foregoing section we distinguished several types of interlocking directors. By doing so, we were able to trace some elementary characteristics of the structure of the international corporate elite. While it remained a personalistic approach, by the end of Section 4.3.2 it became clear that both the personal attribute of holding directorships and its distribution have a direct influence upon the structure of the network. In this section we will focus completely on the structural and institutional aspects of the study. The lines between firms will now be distinguished according to the types of interlocks that constitute these links. In Section 4.4.1 multiple interlocks will be considered and in Section 4.4.2 the interlocks will be distinguished according to the positions of the multiple director.

4.4.1 Multiple interlocks

A simple method of distinguishing between different types of interlocking directorates is to look at their multiplicity. The 'normal' interlocking directorate is carried by one person, who has a position in both corporations. There may, however, be more persons having positions in both corporations. If this is the case, we speak of a multiple

[7] The network without big linkers has been compared with the network as a whole (analyzed in Chapters 5 and 6). At multiplicity level ≥ 1 very little seems to have changed. Rather than the large component Morgan 127, we now find a large component Chemical Bank 119. At multiplicity level ≥ 2, however, an important change has taken place: the core component Dresdner Bank 58 has split into two components, Dresdner 15 (only German firms) and Morgan 33 (American, Canadian, Dutch and British firms) (compare Figure 5.7). And at multiplicity level ≥ 3 Morgan 33 has split into four strictly national components. Elimination of the big linkers does indeed cause a fragmentation of the network along national lines.

interlock or of a <u>line</u> <u>with</u> a <u>multiplicity</u> <u>equal</u> <u>to the</u>
<u>number</u> <u>of persons</u> <u>who</u> <u>have</u> <u>a</u> <u>position</u> <u>in</u> <u>both</u> <u>corporations</u>.
[8] This multiplicity is an indication of the intensity of
the line between two corporations. In Section 1.2 it was
assumed that two corporations are the more tightly linked,
the higher the multiplicity of the line between them. Thus,
by eliminating the lines with multiplicity one, one can
assume to have eliminated the less important interlocks from
the network. The first to do this were Sonquist and Koenig
(1975). We will use a more refined method than theirs of
stepwise elimination of multiple interlocks. This procedure,
which has been used by Stokman (1978), first eliminates the
lines with multiplicity one, then the lines with multiplicity
two, and so on. In this way we obtain a series of nested
networks, which we will analyzed in Chapter 6. In the
international network between 176 large firms in 1970 there
are 601 interlocks of which 281 are single. The multiplicity
of the lines is given in Table 4.4.

<u>Table</u> 4.4 Lines in the network according to their
          multiplicity

multiplicity	number of lines
1	281
2	78
3	26
4	12
5	4
6	3
total	404

4.4.2 <u>Weak</u>, <u>strong</u> <u>and</u> <u>tight</u> <u>ties</u>

As we suggested in Section 1.2 and elaborated in Section 4.1,
the positions held by a multiple director are of great
importance to the significance of the interlock that is
carried by this multiple director. From the different
positions discussed in Sections 1.1 and 1.2, five different
categories of positions have been constructed: three outside
positions (member of the advisory board, outside director and

[8] A line is defined as a direct relation between two firms
    regardless of how many interlocks exist between them. The
    multiplicity of a line is equal to the number of interlocks
    between two firms.

chairman of the board of directors) and two inside positions
(inside director and president).

Members of the supervisory board in a two-board corporation
have been placed in the category 'outside director'; members
of the executive board in a two-board corporation have been
placed in   the category 'inside director'. Non-director
executives have not been assigned a separate category since
only six of these carry an interlock. These six have been
lumped into the category 'inside director' (see Table 4.5).

<u>Table</u> 4.5 Interlocking directorates according to the position
          of the multiple directors

		outside			inside	
		AD	OD	CH	ID	TOP
outside	AD	3	43	7	11	12
	OD		273	75	73	74
	CH			7	6	2
inside	ID				10	4
	TOP					1

-----: weak ties
.....: strong ties (officer-interlocks)
,,,,,: tight ties

AD: Member of advisory board or committee
OD: Outside director in a one-board corporation; member of
     supervisory board in a two-board corporation
CH: Chairman of the board of directors in a one-board
     corporation; chairman of the supervisory board in a two-
     board corporation
ID: Inside director in a one-board corporation; member of
     the executive board in a two-board corporation
TOP: President or managing director in a one-board
     corporation; chairman of the executive board in a two-
     board corporation

Now the total number of interlocks is 601. Nearly half of these (273, or 45.4 percent) is carried by a person who is outside director in both firms. And if one looks at the interlocks carried by a person who has an outside <u>position</u> in both companies, the numbers rises to 408 (67.7 percent).

Furthermore, 93 interlocks (15 percent) are carried by the president of one of the companies, and if one adds those who are inside director in at least one of the interlocked companies, the number increases to 193 (32 percent). Of these 193 interlocks, 178 are carried by a person who is inside director or president in one company and outside director in the other. In 15 cases, however, the interlocking director has an executive position in both companies. Such an interlock is rare (2.5. percent of all interlocks) and indicates a concern relation between the interlocked corporations, although there is no <u>a priori</u> argument that the two corporations are hierarchically linked. Such interlocking directorates we will call <u>tight ties</u>. The remaining 178 interlocks carried by an inside director or a president do indeed indicate a dominance relation between the interlocked firms. If we assume the inside director or president to represent his 'own' firm A in the board of the firm B in which he has an outside position, the hierarchy line runs from A to B and the interlock between A and B can be given a direction. I will call such directed interlocks <u>strong ties</u>. Finally, the 408 interlocks carried by persons who have an outside position in both firms do not indicate a hierarchical line between the two interlocked companies, nor do they necessarily indicate a close relationship between the interlocked firms. I will call them <u>weak ties</u>. Two types of weak ties will be distinguished. The first is the secondary interlock, which is created when a person is an inside director in firm A and an outside director in firm B and firm C. Between B and C there exists a secondary interlock (see also Figure 4.1b). But not all weak ties are secondary interlocks. If a person has no inside position in any firm but is an outside director in more than one firm, he carries one or more weak ties that are not secondary interlocks.
It is possible to calculate the number of weak ties in the international network. As can be seen from Table 4.5, this number is 408, while the number of strong ties is 178. The proportion of weak ties in the network is roughly two-thirds, while the proportion of strong ties is roughly one-third. From Table 4.2 it is possible to calculate the maximum number of secondary interlocks in the network. To carry a secondary interlock a person must have in at least three firms a directorship. Fifty-three persons have directorships in three firms. These 53 persons carry a maximum of 53 secondary interlocks. The remaining 19 persons may carry more secondary

interlocks. Sixteen of them have directorships in 4 firms and thus carry a maximum of 48 secondary interlocks. One person has directorships in 5 firms, carrying a maximum of 6 secondary interlocks. Another has directorships in 6 firms, carrying a maximum of 10 secondary interlocks; and yet another has directorships in 7 firms, carrying a maximum of 15 secondary interlocks. The maximum number of secondary interlocks in the international network is 132. This means that at least 276 weak ties must be carried by persons who have no executive (inside) position in any of the firms in our sample. Such a person may either have an executive position in a firm outside the sample or no executive position at all. If the person has no executive position in a corporation, it is likely that he has been invited to sit on the boards of several corporations for specific expertise or contacts he has outside the business system. The weak ties he carries are then typically the unintended result of these independent corporation decisions. This may even be the case if the person is the president of a smaller firm and is invited for similar reasons to be on the board of several large ones. Although these weak ties generally do not indicate control or domination relations, they form an integral part of the business system and should not be neglected in the analysis.

If the network of strong ties is a network of control and domination, it can be assumed that the direction of control or domination is from the firm in which a executive position is held to the firm in which the outside position is held. If the network is regarded as an information network, then the information may go from the firm in which the outside position is held to the firm in which an executive position is held. [9] Warner and Unwalla (1967) called the strong ties officer-interlocks. Among the 1,131 United States firms they investigated, 1,552 officer-interlocks were found, 27.2 percent of the total number of interlocking directorates between these firms. This proportion is remarkably close to the proportion of strong ties in the international network (29 percent). The different types of interlocks (weak, strong, and tight ties) define different partial networks. The network containing only weak ties can be interpreted as a communication network, cementing the (international) business system. The network containing only strong ties (officer-interlocks) can be conceived as a dominance network, which,

[9] A control or dominance network is necessarily a network of information as well. But the reverse is not true.

at the higher levels of multiplicity, may indicate financial groups. Finally, the network containing only tight ties may indicate the existence of <u>concerns</u> formed by two or more firms. These partial networks will be analyzed in Chapter 6.

4.5 <u>Summary</u>

Although this book does not discuss the internal organization of corporations, it is necessary to compare the division of authority among the top committees of the corporations in different countries. In all corporations there exists a duality in the supervising function, associated with external control, and the executive function, associated with internal control. In the two-board corporations this duality has been 'solved' by the creation of a supervisory board and an executive board. This two-board system is dominant in continental Europe. Within the two-board system, there exist a 'German' and a 'Latin' variant. The one-board system is found in Anglo-Saxon countries. The duality of supervisory and executive functions is here reflected in the distinction between outside and inside directors.

The first important finding of this empirical study is that <u>executives</u> <u>who</u> <u>are</u> <u>not</u> <u>members</u> <u>of</u> <u>executive</u> <u>boards</u> <u>or</u> <u>boards</u> <u>of</u> <u>directors</u> <u>carry</u> <u>hardly</u> <u>any</u> <u>interlocks</u> <u>between</u> <u>the</u> <u>176</u> <u>firms</u> <u>of</u> <u>the</u> <u>sample</u>.

Of the 601 interlocks between these firms, 68 percent is carried by a person who has an outside function in both interlocked firms (<u>weak</u> <u>ties</u>), 29 percent is carried by a person who is an executive in one firm and outside director in the other (<u>strong</u> <u>ties</u> <u>or</u> <u>officer-interlocks</u>), while less than three percent is carried by an inside director in both companies (<u>tight</u> <u>ties</u>). In Section 4.4.2 we suggested a possible interpretation of these three types of interlocks, according to which the networks of weak, strong and tight ties can be fruitfully analyzed. Another difference between interlocks is based on the <u>network</u> characteristics of the carrier of the interlock. Thus a distinction was made between persons affiliated with at least one bank and persons affiliated only with industrial firms. The former we called <u>finance</u> <u>capitalists</u>. Interlocks carried by a finance capitalist have a different meaning from those carried by a non-finance capitalist. As expected from the theory of finance capital, the proportion of finance capitalists in the network is higher than that in the national networks in the Netherlands and the United States, where previous research has been done. Accordingly, it was found that the finance capitalists carry significantly more international interlocks.

A second relevant network characteristic is the amount of interlocks carried by one person. Those who carry six or more interlocks in the network are the <u>big linkers</u>. The number of big linkers in the network -nineteen- is much lower than the number of big linkers found in previous research on national networks. This can be explained by the fact that a restricted number of firms is included for each country in the sample. But even though the number of big linkers in our sample is relatively low compared to the number of big linkers in previous studies of interlocking directorates in the Netherlands and the United States, their role in the international network seems important. They link the different national (sub)networks together in an international network of communication.

Finally, a distinction was made according to the multiplicity of the lines in the network, defined as the number of interlocks between two firms. The higher the multiplicity of a line, the more intense the relation between the firms connected by that line. Based on this assumption, the networks nested according to the multiplicity of the lines will be analyzed in Chapter 6.

V NATIONAL AND INTERNATIONAL INTEGRATION

5.0 Introduction to some graph-theoretical concepts

In the next four chapters, we will analyze the network of
interlocking directorates according to the research design
presented in Section 3.3. A few introductory remarks will be
made here about the analytical tools to be used. Most of them
are based on graph theory, a special branch of mathematics,
the results of which are used in the social sciences for
quantitative structural analysis. Our presentation of some
graph-theoretical concepts will be very summary and non-
mathematical. For a more detailed and competent introduction,
the reader is referred to Harary (1972).
A graph is an object consisting of a non-empty collection of
points,P, and a collection of lines, R (relations). Each line
is incident with two points of the graph. A graph can be
considered as a representation of a structure. Consider, for
example, Figure 4.1a in Chapter 4. The structure of
interlocking directorates visualized in Figure 4.1a can be
represented by a graph consisting of the points a, b, c, d, e
and the lines (a,b), (a,c), (a,d), (a,e), (b,c), (b,d),
(b,e), (c,d), (c,e), (d,e), whose incidence relations can
also be presented in a matrix (Table 5.1).

Table 5.1 Adjacency matrix of a completely connected graph

	a	b	c	d	e
a	0	1	1	1	1
b	1	0	1	1	1
c	1	1	0	1	1
d	1	1	1	0	1
e	1	1	1	1	0

In the adjacency matrix the diagonal is empty, because lines
that are incident with only one point (loops) are not taken
into account.

To the points and lines of the graph information can be
added. To the points, for example, the names of firms can be
assigned. To the lines a direction can be assigned (as in
Figure 4.1b) or a multiplicity-number according to the number
of interlocks between two incident firms. A graph in which
information is added to the points and lines is called a
network.

One of the important general measures indicating the
compactness of a graph is the density. It is defined as the
actual number of lines (r) divided by the total number of
possible lines. If the number of points is P, then the total
number of possible lines is p(p-1)/2. In the adjacency matrix
of Table 5.1 the number of actual lines equals the total
number of possible lines: the density is 1. A graph with a
density of 1 is called a complete graph. In most cases,
however, the number of actual lines will be smaller than the
number of possible lines. Density varies between 0 (if no
lines between the points of a graph exist) and 1.

If two networks are compared in terms of density, it should
be remembered that the number of possible lines increases
with a quadratic factor when the number of firms (P)
increases. Strictly speaking, only networks with an equal
number of firms can be compared in this way. A graph is
bipartite if the collection of points can be divided into two
disjoint subcollections in such a way that within each
subcollection no incidence relations exist. In other words, a
bipartite graph consists of two disjoint sets of n points and
m points with k lines incident with the points that do not
belong to the same set. The density of such a bipartite graph
is k/(n*m).

Another general measure indicating compactness is the
connectivity of a graph. Two points are connected if there
exists a path between these two points. A path, connecting
two points u and v of a graph G, consists of the points u,
p(1), p(2), ...,p(1-1), v, such that u is adjacent to p(1),
p(1) is adjacent to p(2), and p(1-1) is adjacent to v. The
length of a path is given by the number of its lines. And the
distance between two points of a graph is given by the
shortest path between two points in that graph. From these
definitions a number of new concepts can be deduced. A graph
is connected if every pair of points is joined by a path. A
maximal connected subgraph of G is called a connected
component or simply a component of G. Thus, a disconnected
graph has at least two components. [1]

While density refers to the relative amount of lines in the
network, connectivity tells us something about the way in

[1] Strictly speaking an isolated point is also a component
    of graph G. Nevertheless, in the following chapters a
    distinction will be made between isolated points and
    components.

which the firms are linked together into components. The comparison of networks according to connectivity is also problematic since it is sensitive to the number of firms in the network as well.

There are several concepts of connectivity. In this book connectivity is defined as the fraction of pairs of points of a graph G joined by a path. [2] In his book, Graph Theory, Harary defines the connectivity of graph G as the minimum number of points whose removal results in a disconnected graph. Thus the connectivity of a disconnected graph is 0. If only one point c has to be removed to make G disconnected, the connectivity of G is one and the point c is called cutpoint. Analogously, line-connectivity of a graph G is the minimum number of lines whose removal results in a disconnected graph. If only one line y has to be removed to make G disconnected, the line-connectivity is one and the line y is called a bridge (Harary, 1972: 43). We have chosen another concept of connectivity, defined as the fraction of pairs of points of G joined by a path, because this concept can be used to compare disconnected graphs. To describe components of these disconnected graphs the concepts of cutpoint and bridge will be used.

In Section 4.4.1 we discussed a situation in which more than one person sit on the board of directors (or the executive board) of two companies, a and b. Between a and b then there exists a multiple line. Such a multiple line was defined - anticipating the exposition in this section - as a line with a multiplicity equal to the number of persons who have a position in both corporations. A high multiplicity indicates a thick tie between the two corporations, and the higher the multiplicity of the line, the thicker the tie. Thus, if the number of multiple lines in a graph G is high, the network is thick.

Apart from the analysis of the global structure of the network in terms of general network characteristics, emphasis will be placed on the position of singular firms in the

[2] The connectivity is calculated as

$$\frac{1}{n*(n-1)/2} \sum_{i=1}^{c} n[i] * (n[i] - 1)/2$$

where n is the number of firms, c is the number of components and n[i] is the number of firms in the component i.

network. To measure the centrality of firms, several graph-
theoretical concepts can be used.

Point centrality

As Freeman (1979) writes, the concept of centrality often is
used intuitively. The center of a star, for example, does
appear to be in some sort of special position with respect to
the overall structure (see Figure 5.1a). The center of a star
(s1) possesses two structural properties at the same time. It
has the maximum number of neighbors (adjacency-number or
simply adjacency) and it is maximally close to all other
points. These two aspects of centrality do not necessarily
coincide. In Figure 5.1b, b1 is maximally close to all other
points but has fewer neighbors than b2 and b5. Closeness can
be measured in terms of mean distance to all other points in
the graph. The measure is an inversion of the concept: the
lower the mean distance, the higher the closeness to all
other points. Furthermore, the measure can only be used in a
connected graph because the distance between two unconnected
points is not defined.

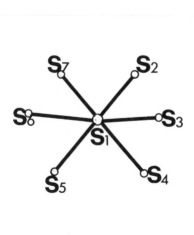

Figure 5.1a

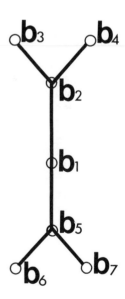

Figure 5.1b

In Figure 5.1a, s1 has an adjacency of 6 and a mean distance
of 1. All other points in Figure 5.1a have an adjacency of 1
and a mean distance of 1.8. In Figure 5.1b, b1 has an

adjacency of 2 and a mean distance of 1.7; b2 and b5 have an
adjacency of 3 and a mean distance of 1.8. All other points
in Figure 5.1b have an adjacency of 1 and a mean distance of
2.3.

We will call the adjacency local centrality, because it
measures the centrality of the firm in its direct
neighborhood. The mean distance will be interpreted as global
centrality, since it takes the distance to all other firms in
the component into account.

In Chapter 6 the Western network will be analyzed according
to the different levels of thickness as defined by the
multiplicity of the lines. The subsequent networks are nested
because from the thickest levels downwards each subsequent
network contains the same firms and lines plus the additional
lines with the multiplicity equal to the given multiplicity
level. This technique of nested network analysis is a first
approach to distinguishing clusters of heavily interlocked
firms.

5.1 General patterns in the international network

5.1.1 Compactness of the international network

The density of the international network of 176 firms is .03.
When comparing this density with the densities of several
national networks calculated in preceding studies, we should
remember that the density measure is sensitive to the number
of firms in the network (see Section 5.0). However, when a
network containing more than 176 firms has yet a higher
density, this can safely be regarded as an indication of that
network's greater compactness. Such is the case, for example,
with the network of 200 largest non-financial companies and
50 largest financial companies in the United States. In 1965
the density of the network of interlocks between these 250
firms was .08. [3] For the Netherlands the density of the
network of interlocks between the 86 largest firms in 1969
was .19. Although here the number of firms is much lower, the
density is so high that it would still be higher than the
density of the international network would be if 90 Dutch
firms would be added without any increase in the number of
lines in the network.

[3] Calculated from Dooley (1969: 317) who found 2480 lines
    between 250 firms in 1965.

The network of interlocks between 85 British firms in 1970 has a density of .05. When we add 91 British firms without adding any new lines, the hypothetical density of the resulting network is lower than the density of the international network. This is, of course, an extreme assumption. If one assumes that the number of lines increases proportionally with the number of firms, the density of the 'enlarged' British network would equal that of the international network. Since a comparison of the national subnetworks will show that the United Kingdom has the lowest density of all national subnetworks (see Section 5.1.2), it can be concluded that the international network has a lower density than most of the national networks.

But how are the firms in the international network connected? The connectivity of the network is .54, which is below the average connectivity of the national networks. The connectivity of the already-mentioned American network was .86: the Dutch network had a connectivity of .97; and the connectivity of the British network was .74. Taking into account the number of firms in the different networks, the connectivity of the American and Dutch networks is certainly higher than that of the international network, but this cannot be said a priori of the British network.
More important is the comparison of the component structure of the network. All national networks have one large component, plus a number of tiny ones and some isolated firms. In the international network there also exist one large component of 127 firms, a smaller one of 23 firms, two tiny components of 2 firms and 22 isolated firms. The correspondence of the component structure of the international network with that of the national networks becomes even more striking when the Japanese firms are set apart. The Japanese firms only interlock among themselves. One component of 23 firms consists solely of Japanese firms as does one of the tiny components as well. In the large component of 127 firms, on the other hand, no Japanese firms are found. Of the 30 Japanese firms included in the sample of 1970, 23 are connected (the second component), 2 are only connected with each other and 5 are isolated. The fact that none of the Japanese firms is interlocked with a non-Japanese firm indicates a reticent formation of the Japanese business system. Even though there was inadequate information concerning the composition of the boards of many Japanese firms (see Appendix A), it can be safely concluded that the Japanese corporate elite is not integrated into the international corporate elite. Whether this lack of integration has only 'economic' causes or may be induced by cultural barriers as well is hard to say here.

Because in the network of non—Japanese firms only the
Australian firms are completely isolated (see Table 5.2), we
will call this network the Western network. This Western
network has a connectivity of .76. The number of isolated
firms in the Western network is highest among the British and
French firms. The high number seems to reflect the low level
of compactness of the national network in these countries
rather than the lack of integration in the Western network.
We will come back to this in the following section.

Table 5.2 Distribution of isolated firms according to
          nationality

	Number of isolated firms	Total number of firms in the network
Australia	2	2
United Kingdom	8	30
France	4	17
Japan	5	30
Italy	1	9
Canada	1	11
United States	1	33
West Germany	0	19
Switzerland	0	10
Sweden	0	7
the Netherlands	0	6
Belgium/Luxembourg	0	3
South Africa	0	1

Some preliminary concluding remarks can be made about the
applicability of the two basic models deduced from the
economic theories of imperialism. Since the Japanese
corporate elite is completely cut off from the Western
network, the Japanese case follows the model deduced from the
theory of Bucharin. The corporate elites from all Western
countries are integrated into the Western network, in
conformity with the model derived from the Leninist and
Kautskian theories. In Section 5.2 the large component of
Western firms will be further analyzed to discover its
internal structure. Because the data on the composition of
the boards of Japanese firms are not complete (see Appendix
A), the Japanese network will not be analyzed in detail.

5.1.2 International integration of national networks

One way of estimating the amount of international integration
of the network is to compare the density of the national
subnetworks with that of the network as a whole. The national
densities are presented in the diagonal of Table 5.3. Even
though direct comparison is difficult because of the
different number of firms in the national networks and the
global network, the differences in density seem to be
considerable, also between the different national networks.
The density is particularly high for the Netherlands,
Switzerland, Sweden, Germany and the United States. Does this
mean that more lines exist between firms from the same
nationality than between firms from different nationalities?
The number of lines between firms from the same nationality
is 303 while the number of lines between firms from different
nationalities is 101. But this does not answer the question.
It is necessary to know the probability that a random
distribution of the total number of lines (404) among all
possible pairs of firms would result in a distribution in
which 303 or more lines are between firms from the same
nationality. According to a hypergeometrical distribution
this probability is less than 0.1 percent. There are more
lines between firms of the same nationality than between
firms of different nationalities. [4] To obtain an indication
of the integration of the national networks in the Western
network, we calculated the density of the bipartite network
between each national network and the rest of the Western
network. The results are presented in the last column of
Table 5.3. Because of the large denominator of these
bipartite densities, the fraction is given in three decimals
and the absolute number of international lines is added in
parentheses. Besides, the denominator increases with the
number of firms of the national networks, so that the
bipartite density contains a bias in favor of the countries
with a small number of firms in the sample.

Taking all this into account, we can draw some tentative
conclusions from the last column in Table 5.3. The
international integra¬ion of American and British firms seems
relatively high, given the fact that they are represented by
33 and 30 firms respectively. For the 'smaller countries',
Canada and the Netherlands, the international integration

[4] This result is even more convincing if one takes into
    account that of the 101 international lines 32 are carried
    by a person who is only a member of an advisory board of a
    foreign firm. For the national lines there are only 41
    advisory links out of 303.

seems also high. It may well be that the high amount of
international integration of Canadian, British and Dutch
firms is caused predominantly by their interlocks with
American firms. These results would thus indicate that
American domination is particularly strong in Canadian,
British and Dutch big business. To see whether this is true
we calculated the bipartite densities for each pair of
national sets of firms.

Table 5.3 Densities between the national networks and
bipartite densities between national networks and
the rest of the Western network (1970)

	USA	U.K.	BRD	Fr.	Can.	Swi.	It.	Swe.	Nl.	Nat.netw. versus rest of network
Number of firms:	33	30	19	17	11	10	9	7	6	
U.S.A.	.14	.02	.01	0	.04	.01	.02	.00	.04	.014 (54)
U.K.		.07	0	0	.02	0	.01	.00	.03*	.011 (38)
B.R.D.			.46	.01	0	.03	0	0	.08	.010 (25)
France				.13	0	.00	.00	0	0	.005 (12)
Canada					.22	0	0	.01	0	.015 (23)
Switz.						.60	.06	0	0	.011 (15)
Italy							.33	.03	.02	.012 (16)
Sweden								.48	.02	.007 (7)
Neth.									.67	.028 (24)

Legenda:
All densities except those in the diagonal are bipartite. The
densities of the network between countries cannot be compared
directly with the densities of the networks within countries
(in the diagonal). 0 in a cell indicates that no lines exist
between the national networks. .00 in a cell indicates that
the density of the bipartite network between two countries is
smaller than 0.005. Belgium and Luxembourg, Australia and
South Africa are not included in the table because the number
of firms from these countries is too small to allow any
interpretation of the measures given here. The firms from
Belgium/Luxembourg, Australia and South Africa are included,
however, in the category 'rest of the world' (last column).

[*] Since two firms in the sample are Dutch/British, the
bipartite density between the Netherlands and the United
Kingdom is not defined, because the sets of firms are not
disjoint; the figure is obtained by regarding Shell and
Unilever for a moment as separated into a Dutch and a British
firm, both of which are tightly interlocked. The figure 0.3
is certainly an underestimation.

The matrix of Table 5.3 shows that only in the case of Canada
is the international integration predominantly caused by
interlocks with American firms. The international integration
of British firms stems from interlocks with Dutch, Canadian
and American firms. The international integration of Dutch
firms stems from interlocks with German, British, American,
Italian and Swedish firms. This is clearly in accordance with
the model derived from the theory of Rowthorn as presented in
Section 3.2, in which British and Dutch firms have a strong
international orientation. The matrix of bipartite densities
also allows for a tentative falsification of the theory of
Mandel. According to the model derived from the theory of
Mandel, the continental EEC countries have an integrated
business system. Thus one would expect high bipartite
densities between these countries. As one can see in Table
5.3, this is not the case. Only West Germany and the
Netherlands have a high bipartite density, but between
German, French and Italian firms hardly any interlocks exist.
Finally, it is possible to say something about the theory of
super-imperialism. According to the model derived from this
theory, international integration is created predominantly
through interlocks that American firms maintain with firms
from other countries. Indeed, the United States has high
bipartite densities with four countries. However, it has been
shown already that the international integration of two of
these (the United Kingdom and the Netherlands) does not
exclusively stem from the interlocks with American firms.

Another way to see whether the international structure of
interlocking directorates is reflected in the theory of
super-imperialism is to delete the United States firms from
the network. According to the model derived from this theory,
one would expect the remaining network to break down into
national components, except for a few secondary interlocks
induced by an American executive who carries an interlocking
directorate with two foreign firms from different countries.
Deletion of the American firms, however, decreases the
connectivity of the Western network only slightly from .76 to
.62. Our first analysis of the structure of the Western
network, then, does not lend support to the model derived
from the theory of super-imperialism.

Mandel's theory, on the other hand, does not seem viable
either. Between the continental EEC countries there is not an
integrated structure of interlocking directorates and no
corresponding interrelation of the corporate elite from these
countries, apart from the integration of the Dutch and German
business system. This, however, can be far better explained
by the traditional ties between the Dutch and the German
economy, which antedate the Common Market. The position of

Canada in the Western network strongly resembles that of the Netherlands: its corporate elite is strongly interrelated with that of the large neighbor, i.e., the United States, while at the same time being related to the corporate elite in the United Kingdom. The specific position of the Dutch multinationals is that they connect the Anglo-Saxon network with the West German network.

5.2 The international network of Western firms

5.2.0 Introduction

If the Japanese firms are deleted, the general characteristics of the remaining network become more in line with the general characteristics of the different national networks. The density goes from .03 to .04, while the connectivity increases from .54 to .76. The connectivity of the non-Japanese network is now as high as the connectivity of the American network investigated by Dooley in 1965. The large component of 127 firms - which will be called Morgan 127 after the firm with the highest adjacency in the component - contains firms from 11 countries. Like the Japanese firms, the Australian firms are not in the component. It is indeed a component of Western firms. This large component will be analyzed by looking at the most central firms, according to local centrality and according to global centrality. The network of non-Japanese firms consists of 146 firms, 17 of which are completely isolated. The number of lines in the network is now 373.

5.2.1 Local centrality

Having sketched some general characteristics of the Western network as a whole, we turn now to the position of individual firms in this network. Using the concepts of point centrality presented in Section 5.0, we will first analyze the most central firms in the component Morgan 127 according to local centrality. Table 5.4 gives the top ten percent of most central firms according to adjacency. Morgan, Chemical Bank and Chase Manhattan have by far the highest adjacency-number, followed, after a gap of 5, by another New York bank, First National City, and the German BASF.

Table 5.4 Top ten percent in component <u>Morgan 127</u> according
         to local centrality

	Firm	Natio-nality	Product group	Adjacency number[*]
1	J.P. Morgan	U.S.A.	Banks	23
2	Chemical Bank	U.S.A.	Banks	22
3	Chase Manhattan	U.S.A.	Banks	20
4	First National City Bank	U.S.A.	Banks	15
5	BASF	W. Germany	Chemical	15
6	Royal Dutch/Shell	Neth./Brit.	Petrochemical	14
7	Daimler-Benz	W. Germany	Automobile	13
8	Deutsche Bank	W. Germany	Banks	13
9	Siemens	W. Germany	Electro-Tech.	13
10	Dresdner Bank	W. Germany	Banks	13
11	International Nickel Co.	Canada	Non-Ferrous	12
12	Metallgesellschaft	W. Germany	Non-Ferrous	12
13	AKZO	Netherlands	Chemical	12
14	Mannesmann [**]	W. Germany	Heavy Machin.	12
15	General Electric U.S.A.	U.S.A.	Electro-Tech.	12

[*] Number of adjacent firms in the component.

[**] Mannesmann and General Electric are included because
their adjacency-number is equal to that of International
Nickel Co. of Canada, Metallgesellschaft and AKZO.

German, United States and Dutch firms are overrepresented in
the top ten percent according to local centrality: they
constitute 47, 33, and 13 percent in the top 15 in local
centrality, while they constitute respectively only 23, 13
and 4 percent of all firms in the Western network (see also
Table 3.2). This is not surprising because the German,
American and Dutch networks have a relatively high density
(Table 5.3). A high local centrality does indicate a central
position in the respective national subnetworks. This
conclusion, however, leads to a warning about the
interpretation of the data. Firms of countries that are not
strongly represented in the sample will not score high on
local centrality even though their centrality position in the
national subnetwork is very high. Such is the case with the
Swiss firms. For this reason, the presence of the Dutch firms
in the top 15 in local centrality cannot be explained from
the density of the Dutch subnetwork, which contains only 6
firms.

According to the theory of bank control as well as to the
results of preceding studies, banks hold central positions in
the national networks. This alleged fact seems to be
supported by the position of the banks according to local
centrality. While the banks constitute 23 percent of the
firms in the sample, they constitute 40 percent of the top 15
in local centrality. A more detailed examination casts some
doubt upon a general conclusion. Indeed, the American banks
score very high, but the German banks do not score higher
than the German industrials and the Dutch banks are not
represented at all. Finally, the only Canadian firm
represented in the top 15 is the International Nickel Co. of
Canada. A further examination of the position of banks is
necessary.

5.2.2 Global centrality

The rank order according to mean distance does give a
slightly different composition of the top ten percent (Table
5.5). Morgan, Chemical Bank and Chase Manhattan are still the
most central firms, but Morgan has lost its lead to Chemical
Bank and Chase Manhattan. There is still a gap between these
three and the rest of the firms. Of the top 13 in global
centrality the German firms have lost their position to the
United States firms. While 7 German firms belonged to the top
15 in local centrality, only 2 belong to the top 13 in global
centrality. Now, the American and Dutch firms are still
(strongly) overrepresented, leading to the conclusion that
they owe their central position in the network to their
international contacts. Again, however, a warning is
necessary. First, a large number of adjacent firms has a
considerable impact upon the mean distance to all firms in
the sample. Secondly, the large number of American firms in
the sample may also depress the mean distance of American
firms in relation to other firms.

The banks are less central according to global centrality,
but they are still overrepresented in the top ten percent.
Part of their central position in mean distance can be
explained by the high number of adjacent firms, which eo ipso
influences the mean distance to all firms.

Table 5.5 Top ten percent in component Morgan 127 according
          to global centrality

	Firm	Nation-ality	Product group	Mean dist[*]
1	Chemical Bank	U.S.A.	Banks	2.25
2	Chase Manhattan	U.S.A.	Banks	2.26
3	J.P. Morgan	U.S.A.	Banks	2.34
4	Royal Dutch/Shell	Neth./Brit.	Petrochem.	2.49
5	General Electric U.S.A.	U.S.A.	Elect.-Tech.	2.52
6	Deutsche Bank	W. Germany	Banks	2.53
7	Bayer	W. Germany	Chemical	2.57
8	International Nickel Co.	Canada	Non-Ferrous	2.60
9	U.S. Steel	U.S.A.	Iron & Steel	2.61
10	Standard Oil (N.J.)	U.S.A.	Petrochem.	2.63
11	Procter & Gamble	U.S.A.	Food	2.69
12	AKZO	Netherlands	Chemical	2.70
13	Bethlehem Steel	U.S.A.	Iron & Steel	2.71

----

[*] Since global centrality is indicated by mean distance,
the relation between the concept and its operationalization
is inverse: the lower the mean distance, the higher the
global centrality.

5.2.3 Overall centrality

In Table 5.6 the overlap between the top ten percent in
global centrality (mean distance) and in local centrality
(number of adjacent firms) is given. Eight firms appear in
both: three New York banks, two Dutch firms, the Deutsche
Bank, International Nickel Co. of Canada, and General
Electric. The majority of the American industrials have a low
local centrality but a high global centrality, while the
majority of German industrials have it the other way around.
For all firms in Table 5.6 the percentage of foreign firms
among the adjacent firms is given. It appears that the firms
that score high both on local and global centrality are
adjacent to a large proportion of foreign firms, whereas the
firms that score high on only one of the centrality measures
are adjacent to a low proportion of foreign firms. Of the
seven firms, more than half of whose adjacent firms are
foreign, six are found in the overlap between high local
centrality and high global centrality, and one scores high
only on global centrality (United States Steel). The five
firms scoring high on global centrality have a line with at

least two of the three most central New York banks, while
those scoring high only on local centrality - with the
exception of Siemens and Dresdner Bank - do not. Since these
two firms are near to the top ten percent in global
centrality, we can assume that the high global centrality is
obtained through lines with the three most central banks. The
three banks in turn obtain a high global centrality through a
high adjacency and a strong international orientation.

Table 5.6 Global and local centrality in component <u>Morgan</u> <u>127</u>

GLOBAL CENTRALITY

	HIGH	Percentage of foreign firms among the adjacent firms	LOW	Percentage of foreign firms among the adjacent firms
HIGH	1 Morgan	57	1 Siemens	15
	2 Chemical Bank	54	2 Dresdner Bank	8
	3 Chase Manhattan	60	3 BASF	33.3
	4 Royal Dutch/Shell *	71	4 First Nat. City	20
	5 Deutsch Bank	23	5 Mannesmann	16
	6 Intern. Nickel Co.	75	6 Daimler-Benz	7
	7 AKZO	75	7 Metallgesellschaft	0
LOCAL CENTRAL-	8 General Electric	25		
ITY	1 Bayer	30		
	2 Procter & Gamble	0		
LOW	3 U.S. Steel	57	156	
	4 Standard Oil N.J.	17	FIRMS	
	5 Bethlehem Steel	20		

[*] Shell should be regarded as either Dutch or British if
one does not want to underestimate its international links.
Since it has lines with 4 Dutch firms and with 4 British
firms in the sample, it does not matter whether it is
regarded as Dutch or as British.

This may explain the high ranking of American firms in global
centrality, while at the same time explaining the high
ranking of the German firms in local centrality. Indeed, the
two German firms that score high on global centrality,
Deutsche Bank and Bayer, are also the only two German firms
that have direct links with two of the three most central New
York banks. The fourth New York bank, First National City,
does not score on the top ten percent global centrality for
the very reason that it maintains few direct links with
foreign firms. This finding is confirmed by the results of

Mintz and Schwartz (1979) who – using a centrality measure
that is some sort of combination of adjacency and mean
distance – found that in the network of United States firms
in 1969 First National City is less central than Chemical
Bank, but more central than Chase Manhattan and Morgan.

We may conclude from this first analysis that the cohesion in
the international network strongly depends on the
international orientation of the three most central New York
banks and on the international orientation of Shell, AKZO and
the International Nickel Co. of Canada.
The mean distance which we thought would indicate global
centrality appears to do so in combination with the adjacency
measure, which in itself indicates local, i.e., national,
centrality. Deutsche Bank, General Electric, Bayer, Procter &
Gamble, Standard Oil (N.J.) and Bethlehem Steel are
exceptions which have to be studied more in detail.

5.3 Economic centralization versus industrial concentration

As we saw in Chapter 1, the network of interlocking
directorates developed at the end of the nineteenth century,
especially in those countries which were at that time
industrially backward: Germany and the United States. At the
same time there was a rapid industrial and financial
concentration. This simultaneous development of industrial
concentration and economic centralization begs the question
of whether concentration and centralization are complementary
or supplementary phenomena. In other words, does a high ratio
of concentration go with a low measure of centralization or
is it the other way around. About industrial concentration in
different countries the following can be noted:
First, there is a large correspondence in rank-order of
concentration ratios for different industries in different
countries (George and Ward, 1975: 15: Nioche et Didier,
1969).
Secondly, there exist a hierarchy in the overall
concentration ratios for different countries, with the United
States, the Netherlands and Switzerland ranking highest (see
Table 5.7, second column). More detailed analysis shows that
Germany's concentration ratios increase drastically when the
number of large firms on which the ratio is based increases;
West Germany's concentration ratio is especially high in very
concentrated industries like the steel and chemical
industries. On the other hand, Great Britain's concentration
ratio decreases when more large firms are taken into
consideration (see Guibert et.al., 1975: 111). There is a
positive relation between the concentration ratio of a
country and its direct investment abroad. Countries with a

large share in total foreign investment also have a high concentration ratio.

Table 5.7 Relation between industrial concentration and internationalization of industry and banking

	Direct investment abroad in percentage of total amount of foreign investment in 1971 [*]	Importance of large enterprises in relation to manufacturing employment 1972 [**] (index Britain=100)
United States	52.2	124
United Kingdom	15.0	100
Switzerland	6.0	96
Benelux	4.0	95
France	4.6	56
Sweden	1.5	50
West Germany	4.6	44
Italy	2.0	32

[*] Source: Transnational corporations, 1978: 236. It would, of course, have been more accurate to relate these figures to the national 'industrial' product of each country.
[**] Source: Prais and Reid, 1976: 85.

There is a similar relation between sectoral concentration and internationalization. We find the largest amount of internationalization in those industries in concentration ratios are highest. This is true for both the United States (Vernon 1971a: 4) and continental Europe (Franko, 1976: 144). Besides, the great similarity in rank order of concentration per industry in the different countries has led some economists to conclude that growth of giant corporations in all countries is ultimately subject to rather similar factors and constraints (Prais and Reid, 1976:90). Such an observation could well be explained by the assumption that the factors and constraints that determine the behavior of these giant corporations stem from an international business system.

In Section 2.5.1 we argued that the network of interlocking directorates can be regarded as a form of economic centralization. A compact network of interlocking directorates thus indicates a high amount of centralization. In Table 5.3 it was shown that the density is relativily high in the national networks of the Netherlands, Switzerland,

Germany and the United States. If density is considered a
measure of compactness, economic centralization in these
countries is relatively high. If connectivity is taken as a
measure of compactness similar conclusions can be drawn. The
networks of West German, Swiss, Dutch and Swedish firms are
completely connected (connectivity 1), while the connectivity
of the United States network is .88. All other national
subnetworks are below .66. According to the concentration
ratios presented here, the United States, Switzerland and the
Netherlands also have a high industrial concentration (see
Table 5.7). In these countries, economic centralization is
supplementary, rather than complementary, to industrial
concentration. In Germany, the United Kingdom and Sweden,
however, this is not the case. [5] In Germany and Sweden a
relatively high amount of economic centralization goes with a
relatively low amount of industrial concentration. In the
United Kingdom it is just the other way around. As a result,
no general conclusion can be drawn here on the relation
between industrial concentration and economic centralization.
Given the fact, however, that the concentration ratio of
German industry is much higher in the industrial sectors
represented in the sample, the data support supplementarity
more than complementarity. This would also be in accordance
with Pennings' conclusion of a positive correlation between
concentration and centralization in American industries
(Pennings, 1980: 102).

Another finding from Table 5.7 is definitely supported by
analysis of the network of interlocking directorates. In
Table 5.7 a positive relation was established between
industrial concentration and share of total direct investment
abroad. The United States, the United Kingdom, Switzerland
and the Benelux ranked highest on both variables. From Table
5.3 we can conclude that the networks of these countries also
are relatively strongly integrated in the global network.

[5] In an elaborate study on the relation between frequency
of interlocking directorates and concentration ratio per
industry in the United States, Pennings (1980: 101) has
shown that such a positive relation between concentration
and centralization does indeed exist in the United States.
Our analysis shows that it is not easy to generalize from
analyses based on a national sample.

5.4 <u>Summary</u>

In this chapter we have analyzed some general characteristics
of the international network, focusing on the international
integration of the different national subnetworks. In Chapter
3 two models were constructed. In the first model an
integrated international business system was assumed; in the
second only nationally integrated business systems confronted
each other in the international 'space'. In the network of
interlocking directorates under survey there are
significantly more national than international lines.
Besides, the network of Japanese firms forms a highly
connected network which is completely cut off from the rest
of the network. These two facts clearly fit into the second
model corresponding to the theories of Bucharin, Mandel, and
Rowthorn. The network of Western firms, however, forms a
highly connected system of interlocking directorates. Further
analysis according to the rank-order of both local and global
centrality showed that the New York banks, Morgan, Chemical
Bank and Chase Manhattan, are by far the most central firms
in the network, followed by Royal Dutch/Shell, AKZO (Dutch)
and International Nickel and Co. of Canada. For all these
firms it was found that more than half of their neighbors are
foreign firms. The combination of local and global centrality
clearly indicates a high international orientation. Apart
from the firms mentioned above, the United States firms
scored very high on global centrality, whereas the German
firms scored high on local centrality. The German network is
not only dense, but also relatively self-contained. The
United States firms, on the other hand, clearly obtained a
high global centrality through their connections with the
three central New York banks.

In Section 5.3 the relation between industrial concentration
and economic centralization - expressed in the compactness of
the network of interlocking directorates - was investigated.
Existing data indicated a relation between industrial
concentration and internationalization of capital, both at
the level of the national economy and at the level of
industry. The question was raised of whether the <u>network</u> of
interlocking directorates has a high density in countries
with a high industrial concentration (in which case
interlocking directorates should be regarded as supplementary
to industrial concentration) or whether the opposite is true
(in which case interlocking directorates should be regarded
as complementary to industrial concentration). Conclusive
evidence to answer this question was not found. It seems that
the data available show some support for assuming
supplementarity rather than complementarity. Finally, a
positive relation between internationalization of capital and
integration of the national network into the global network
was established.

VI DOMINATION AND CONTROL

6.0. Introduction

In Chapter 5 we based our analysis on lines between firms
rather than on interlocks proper. In this chapter the
relation between two firms will be specified according to the
number of interlocks, which was defined in Section 4.4.1 as
the multiplicity of a line. Another typology defined in that
section was based on the function of the interlocking
director in each of two interlocked firms. Interlocks were
labeled as weak, strong or tight ties, depending on whether
the interlocking director had no inside position in either of
the firms, had an inside position in only one of the firms,
or had an inside position in both firms.
The multiplicity of lines typically indicates the intensity
of the relation between the interlocked firms as does the
distinction between weak ties and tight ties. Strong ties, on
the other hand, specify the direction of the relation, either
in terms of flow of information or in terms of control. Weak
and tight ties do not do this because in both cases the
interlocking director maintains the same type of position in
the two firms. In this chapter, we will measure the intensity
of the relation between firms primarily according to the
multiplicity of the lines. This will be done by eliminating
first the lines with a multiplicity of one (Section 6.1.1)
and second, the lines with a multiplicity of two (Section
6.1.2). In this way we successively eliminate the
interlocking directorates that indicate a relation with lower
intensity than the multiplicity investigated in a given step.
By the process of elimination, we obtain networks at
different levels of multiplicity. Each network contains the
same 146 firms, but the number of lines decreases with every
step. The network at multiplicity-level 3 is by definition
contained in the network at multiplicity-level 2. Therefore,
it can be said that the network at multiplicity-level 3 is
nested in the network at multiplicity-level 2. The higher the
multiplicity-level, the thicker the lines in the network, or
- in short - the thicker the network. The components in these
thick networks can be interpreted as clusters of heavily
interlocked firms, which form an integrated business system
with a high potential for communication, coordination and
control.

In Section 6.2 the network of officer-interlocks will be
analyzed, on the supposition that this network is more
purposive because the weak ties are eliminated. This may not
be immediately evident. The argument runs as follows. In
Section 4.4.2 we saw that weak ties can be divided into
secondary interlocks and other weak ties. A secondary

interlock is induced between firm A and firm B if an inside director of firm C sits on the boards of A and B. The strong ties between C and A and between C and B are assumed to be intended. But the secondary interlock between A and B may well be unintended. However, we saw also that at least 275 of the 407 weak ties are not secondary, because they are created by persons who have no inside position in any of the sample firms. Some of these persons may have been put on the boards of several firms because of their expertise or their contacts outside the business system; others are retired executives who have become network specialists. But some are executives of firms outside the sample. The person-cliques thus created (see Section 4.3.2) are typically the unintended result of decisions taken independently by these firms. Elimination of the weak ties, therefore, leaves the remaining network more purposive, since the creation of an officer-interlock generally requires a purposive decision by both firms. Clusters of heavily interlocked firms, therefore, indicate primarily a high potential for communication and a strong cohesion of the corporate elite. A high number of officer-interlocks indicates, apart from a high potential for communication, a high potential for control and domination.

6.1 Clusters of heavily interlocked firms

6.1.1 The network at multiplicity-level two

The partial network containing only lines with multiplicity two or more is, by definition, nested in the network analyzed in Section 5.2. It consists of the same 146 firms, but only 123 of the 373 lines still exist. In this network we find 12 components and 53 isolated firms. Each component is named after the firm with the highest local centrality. Thus, the large component analyzed in Section 5.2 is Morgan 127, Morgan being the firm with the highest adjacency, 127 being the number of the firms in the component. At multiplicity-level two, a score of 58 firms is still connected (Dresdner Bank 58). Furthermore, there is a Swiss component (Brown Boveri 8), an Italian component (Credito Italiano 4), a French component (Wendel-Sideror 3), a Swedish component (Ericsson 3), a British component (Westminster Bank 3), an American component (Standard Oil of California 3), and a French-Italian one (Citroen 3). Apart from these there exist four pairs of firms that are interlocked only with each other, as well as the 53 isolated firms [1] (see Figure 6.4). The small

[1] All Japanese firms are isolated at multiplicity-level two.

components are, with the exception of Citroen 3, national
components. Dresdner Bank 58, on the other hand, has an
international composition, although Swiss, French and Swedish
firms are not included. For Dresdner Bank 58, we have again
calculated the top ten percent according to local and global
centrality (see Tables 6.1 and 6.2).

Table 6.1 Top ten percent in component Dresdner Bank 58
          according to local centrality

	Firm	Nation-ality	Product group	Adjacency number[*]
1	Dresdner Bank	W. Germany	Banks	9
2	Deutsche Bank	W. Germany	Banks	8
3	J.P. Morgan	U.S.A.	Banks	7
4	Siemens	W. Germany	Electro-Tech.	7
5	Mannesmann	W. Germany	Heavy Machin.	6
6	AKZO	Netherlands	Chemical	5
7	Daimler-Benz [**]	W. Germany	Automobile	5
8	Metallgesellschaft	W. Germany	Non-Ferrous	5
9	First National City Bank	U.S.A.	Banks	5
10	Royal Dutch/Shell	Neth./Brit.	Petrochemical	5

[*] Number of adjacent firms in the component

[**] Daimler-Benz, Metallgesellschaft, First National City
Bank and Royal Dutch/Shell are included because they have the
same adjacency number as AKZO.

Table 6.2 Top ten percent in component Dresdner Bank 58
          according to global centrality

	Firm	Nation-ality	Product group	Mean dist[*]
1	Chase Manhattan	U.S.A.	Banks	4.05
2	Royal Dutch/Shell	Neth./Brit.	Petrochem.	4.05
3	Chrysler	U.S.A.	Automobiles	4.16
4	AKZO	Netherlands	Chemical	4.26
5	General Electric U.S.A.	U.S.A.	Elect.-Tech.	4.37
6	J.P. Morgan	U.S.A.	Banks	4.61

[*] Mean distance to firms in component

When we compare the component Dresdner Bank 58 with Morgan
127 in terms of local centrality, we see that the American
and German banks have changed place. Morgan still belongs to
the top three, but the Chemical Bank and Chase Manhattan do
not appear at all among the top ten percent. On the other
hand, Chase Manhattan now ranks highest in global centrality,
together with Chrysler and General Electric (U.S.). Morgan
and the two Dutch firms are the only firms still to score in
the top ten percent at both measures of centrality.
The overall picture is still the same. German firms score
highest on local centrality but not on global centrality;
American firms score highest on global centrality but not on
local centrality. Of the smaller components, Brown Boveri 8
contains eight out of ten Swiss firms in the network, the
other two now being isolated. The firms with the highest
local centrality, Brown Boveri and Sulzer (adjacency-number
6), are also the highest in global centrality (both have a
mean distance of 1.14). Exactly the same is true for the two
firms ranking second in local and global centrality. The fact
that these measures of centrality do not differentiate
indicates a network in which there are no regional
subnetworks. As will be shown later, the Swiss network has a
special shape (see Figure 6.3), indicating a high level of
national integration. On the other hand, a particularly low
level of national integration is found in the British
network, which at multiplicity-level two breaks down into
four separate components.

6.1.2 The network at multiplicity-level three

Elimination of the lines with multiplicity one and two
results in a partial network in which only those firms are
linked which have at least three directors in common. The
network at multiplicity-level three and more consists of 146
firms and 45 lines. The number of isolated firms is now 103.
The remaining 43 firms are divided over 7 components:
Dresdner Bank 17 contains 14 German and 3 Dutch firms; Morgan
10 contains 7 United States and 3 Canadian firms; Brown
Boveri 7 contains 7 Swiss firms; and Ferguson 3 contains 3
Canadian firms. Furthermore, Pechiney is linked to Rhone-
Poulenc (Pechiney 2), Commerz Bank is linked to Rheinstahl
(Commerz Bank 2) and Royal Dutch/Shell is linked to its
American daughter Shell Oil (Shell 2). All components are
visualized in Figure 6.4; the three largest components are
also drawn separately (Figures 6.1, 6.2, and 6.3). In Figure
6.1 the subnetwork of AEG, Dresdner Bank, Mannesmann, Siemens
and August Thyssen forms a block: it is not possible to
separate this subnetwork into two components by deleting one
of the firms. The subnetwork of AEG, Dresdner Bank and
Mannesmann is completely connected; it forms a clique. The
above-mentioned block is connected with the component through
lines with Siemens and Dresdner Bank. The line between

Siemens and Deutsche Bank is a bridge: elimination of this
line separates the component into two. The same is true for
the line between Deutsche Bank and AKZO. The density of
Dresdner Bank 17 is .13 at multiplicity-level three. The
density increases to .24 at multiplicity-level two, and to
.48 when all lines between the 17 firms are taken into
consideration. Dresdner Bank 17 grows rapidly denser at lower
levels of multiplicity. Nevertheless, AKZO and Deutsche Bank
remain cutpoints at multiplicity-level two, which indicates
that these two firms play a crucial role in connecting the
Dutch network with the German network. Deutsche Bank also
remains a cutpoint for a set of German firms.
The conclusion must be that the Dutch and the German networks
are heavily interlocked, the main cutpoint being the Deutsche
Bank whose elimination at multiplicity-level two separates
the German network into two components, one of which remains
interlocked with the Dutch network through AKZO. If such a
cutpoint would indicate the existence of two separate
business systems, their boundaries are not coincident with
the national boundaries.

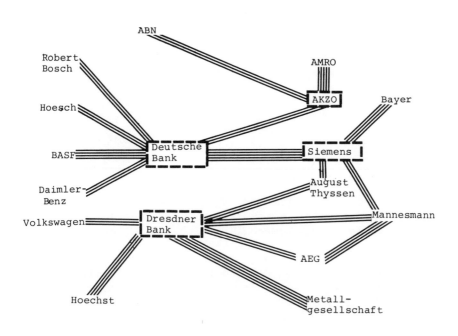

Figure 6.1 Component Dresdner Bank 17

A completely different structure is found in the United
States/Canadian component. Here all firms are cutpoints, thus
creating a tree (see Figure 6.2). Morgan is exceptionally
central, both in terms of local centrality and in terms of
global centrality. If Morgan is eliminated, the component
falls apart into two separate components and two isolated
firms. Here the two separate components divide the firms into
a United States group and a Canadian group.

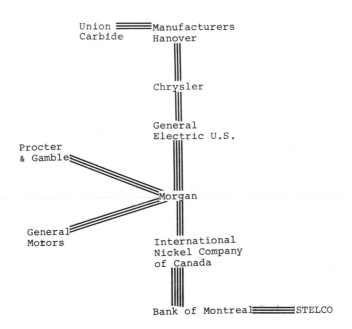

Figure 6.2 Component Morgan 10

The density of Morgan 10 is .20 at multiplicity-level three,
.27 at multiplicity-level two and .38 at multiplicity-level
one. The component Brown Boveri 7, on the other hand, is
itself a block: it is not possible to separate the component
by eliminating one of the points. Furthermore, within the
block the subnetwork formed by Brown Boveri, Gebr. Sulzer,
Ciba-Geigy and Schweizerische Kreditanstalt is completely
connected: it forms a clique. The density of Brown Bank 7 is
.62 at multiplicity-level three and increases only slightly
to .76 at multiplicity-level one. Compared with Dresdner Bank
17 and Morgan 10, Brown Boveri 7 loses very little of its

density at the higher levels of multiplicity. A network with
such an exceptional combination of density and thickness can
be called a _tenacious_ network, [2] indicating a strong
cohesion of the corporate elite.

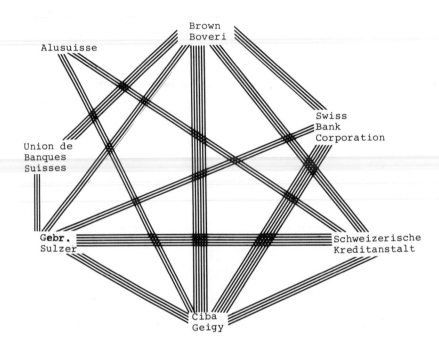

Figure 6.3 Component Brown Boveri 7

Here also we see that a relatively large block or even a
clique is often induced by big linkers: F.W. Schulthess, S.
Schweizer and A. Schaefer together carry 26 of the 70
interlocks   between   the   Swiss firms. When we neglect
multiplicity, the number of lines carried by the Swiss big

[2] A simple index of tenacity is the fraction of lines at
    multiplicity-level three and lines at multiplicity-level
    one. According to this index the tenacity of Brown Boveri 7
    is .81, that of Morgan 10 .52 and that of Dresdner Bank
    .27.

linkers is 20, while the total number of lines in the Swiss
network is 27. Besides, the big linkers connect the same
firms connected in <u>Brown Boveri</u> <u>7</u> (plus Nestlé). Although the
structure of the Swiss network is well established without
the big linkers, the above-mentioned persons are able to 'run
the system' all by themselves.

6.1.3 <u>Conclusions</u>

The component structure of the network at subsequent levels
of multiplicity has been visualized in Figure 6.4. The large
component <u>Morgan</u> <u>127</u> breaks down, when lines with
multiplicity one are eliminated, into one large and still
international component (<u>Dresdner Bank</u> <u>58</u>) and a number of
small, national ones. Of these small components <u>Brown Boveri</u>
<u>8</u> is the largest, and, together with <u>Pechiney</u> <u>2</u>, is also very
tenacious: at the higher levels of multiplicity they lose
little of their original density.
When the lines with multiplicity two are also deleted, the
large component <u>Dresdner Bank</u> <u>58</u> is separated into two major
components. These components, <u>Dresdner Bank</u> <u>17</u> and <u>Morgan</u> <u>10</u>,
are both binational: <u>Dresdner Bank</u> <u>17</u> contains only German
and Dutch firms; and <u>Morgan 10</u> contains only United States
and Canadian firms. And even these two highly interlocked
components break down into national components when the lines
with a multiplicity of three are also deleted.
We may also conclude that the countries with high density at
multiplicity-level one, <u>i.e.</u>, the Netherlands, West Germany,
Switzerland, and the United States (see Table 5.3), also
contain the highest amount of lines at multiplicity-level
three.

At this level, 16 out of 19 German firms, 7 out of 10 Swiss
firms, 4 out of 6 Dutch firms, 6 out of 11 Canadian firms, 8
out of 33 American firms, and 2 out of 17 French firms are
still part of the component. The German, Swiss and Dutch
firms are most heavily interlocked, more so than the United
States and Canadian firms, while the British, Belgian,
Italian, French and Swedish firms have few multiple lines.
For Belgian and Swedish firms this may be attributed to the
fact that no banks are included in the sample, but for the
other countries no such 'artifact' explanation is available.

Related to this conclusion is the discovery that 5 German
firms formed a block in <u>Dresdner Bank</u> <u>17</u> and all Swiss firms
formed a block in component <u>Brown Boveri</u> <u>7</u>, while United
States and Canadian components <u>Morgan 10</u> and <u>Ferguson</u> <u>3</u>
formed, at most, a <u>tree</u> structure.

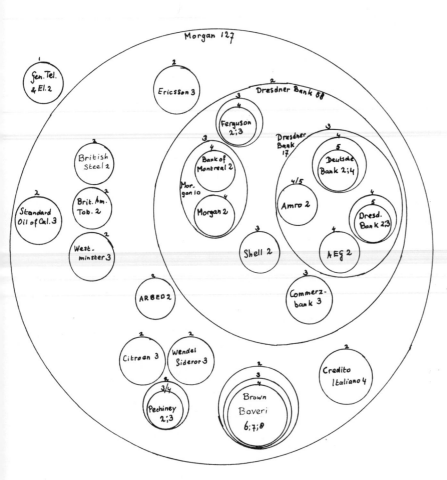

Figure 6.4 Nested components in the Western network of
interlocking directorates at multiplicity-level
one, two or more, and three or more

The continental European components have a relatively high
density at multiplicity-level one (.48 and .76), while Morgan
10 has a mere .38 at that level. The networks in the
Netherlands, Germany, and Switzerland have a compact core
comprising three-quarters of all firms in these countries.
The largest firms in these countries are part of an
integrated system of interlocking directorates indicating a
high potential for communication. Such an integrated circuit
may contribute to the cohesion of the corporate elite,
contain potential rifts and increase its strength as a
pressure group vis a vis the state.

6.2 The network of officer-interlocks

6.2.0 Introduction

In Section 4.4.2 a distinction was made between weak, strong
and tight interlocks, according to the position of the
interlocking director. Interlocks carried by a person who has
an outside position in both interlocked companies are weak
interlocks. Those carried by a person who is inside director
in one company and outside director in the other are strong
interlocks or officer-interlocks. These officer-interlocks
can be given a direction if one assumes that the officer
represents the interests of his 'own' company within the
company in which he is outside director. This implies an
influence from the former to the latter. Of course, this is
not always the case. It is often argued that an industrialist
is invited to be on the board of a bank to improve the bank's
relation with an important client. Such a relation, it is
said, does not influence or exercise control over the bank.

Although this may well be true, we will assume momentarily
that the majority of officer-interlocks indicates a dominance
relation, which can be expressed in the network by assigning
a direction to the interlock from the firm in which an inside
position is held to the firm in which an outside position is
held. In the network of officer-interlocks each interlock is
considered an arc, moving from the firm in which an inside
position is held towards the firm in which an outside
position is held. Each line, therefore, is directed; however,
depending on the multiplicity and the direction of the arcs,
there are several types of directed lines. The most simple
directed line is the one with multiplicity one. However, if
the multiplicity increases, the number of possibilities in
terms of composition of the line increases too.

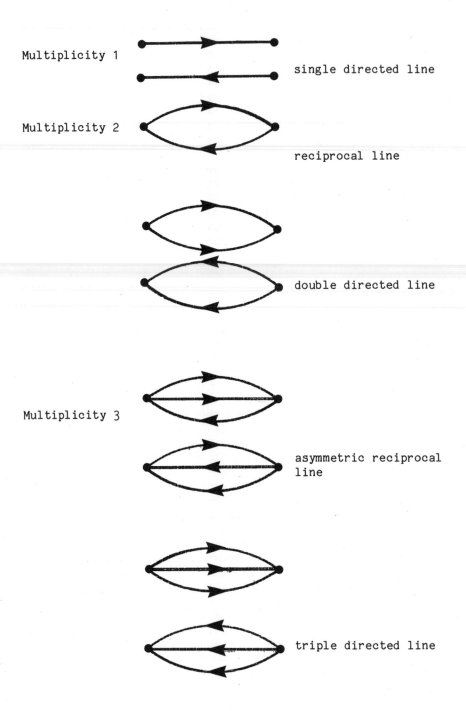

Multiplicity 1

single directed line

Multiplicity 2

reciprocal line

double directed line

Multiplicity 3

asymmetric reciprocal
line

triple directed line

Of course one could go on with such a taxonomy, but directed
lines with a multiplicity higher than three do not exist in
the network. To assign an empirical meaning to the above
types of lines is difficult enough as it is.

In a study on the automobile industry (Fennema, 1974) it was
found that all double and triple directed lines were
accompanied by a financial participation in the same
direction. The double and triple directed lines may therefore
be interpreted as control relations, even though there may
exist in some cases joint control by two or more
participating firms. Reciprocal lines, whether asymmetrical
or not, may accordingly be interpreted as mutual control
relations. The single directed lines, however, cannot be
interpreted as control relations without additional
information on financial and market relations between the two
firms. It is for this reason that the majority of officer-
interlocks indicate relations of dominance rather than
control. With this caveat in mind we will interpret the
network of officer-interlocks as a network of control and
domination.

6.2.1 Domination and control

6.2.1.1 The network of all officer-interlocks

The total number of officer-interlocks in the 1970 network
was 178 (see Table 4.5). In the Western network this number
is 163 or 29 percent of the total number of interlocks in
that network. These 163 officer-interlocks create 146 lines:
132 with a multiplicity of one, 11 with a multiplicity of two
and 3 with a multiplicity of three.
We will initially analyze the network of officer-interlocks,
neglecting the direction of the interlocks. In comparison
with the component structure of the network of all
interlocks, the large component Morgan 127 in the network of
all interlocks has broken down into Morgan 79, Lloyds Bank 6,
Italsider 4, National Westminster Bank 3, Bank of Nova Scotia
2, and Shell. Thirty-one firms are isolated. Although Morgan
79 is, like Morgan 127, an international component, the
British and Italian firms have become separated from the
large component and form separate national components.
British and Italian firms, therefore, do not participate in
the international network of control and domination which is
formed by the component Morgan 79. We will analyze this
component according to the local and global centrality of the
firms (Table 6.3 and 6.4) as we did for the large component
Morgan 127 (Table 5.4 and 5.5) and for the component Dresdner
Bank 58 at multiplicity-level two (Tables 6.1 and 6.2).

Table 6.3 Top ten percent in local centrality of the
         component Morgan 79 (officer-interlocks)

	Firm	Nation-ality	Product group	Adjacency number[*]
1	J.P. Morgan	U.S.A.	Banks	10
2	Dresdner Bank	W. Germany	Banks	8
3	Mannesmann	W. Germany	Heavy Machin.	8
4	Chase Manhattan	U.S.A.	Banks	7
5	Chemical Bank	U.S.A.	Banks	7
6	Deutsche Bank	W. Germany	Banks	7
7	Bayer	W. Germany	Chemical	7
8	Schweizer. Kreditanstalt	Switzerland	Banks	6
9	General Electric (U.S.)	U.S.A.	Electro-Tech.	6
10	AEG	W. Germany	Electro-Tech.	6
11	Robert Bosch	W. Germany	Electro-Tech.	6
12	Chrysler	U.S.A.	Automobiles	6

[*] Number of adjacent firms in the component

Table 6.4 Top ten percent in global centrality of the
         component Morgan 79 (officer-interlocks)

	Firm	Nation-ality	Product group	Mean dist[*]
1	Bayer	W. Germany	Chemical	3.01
2	Chemical Bank	U.S.A.	Banks	3.29
3	Deutsche Bank	W. Germany	Banks	3.29
4	J.P. Morgan	U.S.A.	Banks	3.30
5	Siemens	W. Germany	Elect.-Tech.	3.39
6	Schweizer. Kreditanstalt	Switzerland	Banks	3.51
7	Hoesch	W. Germany	Iron & Steel	3.54
8	Robert Bosch	W. Germany	Elect.-Tech.	3.64

[*] Mean distance to other firms in the component

A comparison of Tables 6.3 and 6.4 with 5.4 and 5.5 makes
clear that the most central firms in the network as a whole
are not the same as the most central firms in the network of
officer-interlocks. In the network of officer-interlocks the
New York banks are less central and the Dutch firms do not
even appear among the top ten percent in global or in local
centrality. On the other hand, a Swiss firm has entered the
top ten percent in both. The Dutch firms are less central in
the network of domination and control than in the network as
a whole. The same can be said for the New York banks. As we
have seen in Section 5.1.2, the Dutch firms and the New York
banks link the national networks into an international whole.
Their function is, in this respect, apparently one more of
international communication than of international domination
and control.

6.2.1.2 The network of control

Taking only multiple directed and reciprocal lines into
account, we find 10 components: Chrysler 13, Dresdner Bank 3,
and 8 pairs of firms (Shell ----> Shell Oil; Credito Italiano
----> Banco di Roma; Rhone-Poulenc ----> Pechiney; ARBED
----> Cockerill; AEG <----> Mannesmann; AKZO <----> AMRO;
Schweizerische Kreditanstalt <----> Alusuisse).

Although the lines between the German firms are generally
thicker than the lines between the American firms, the number
of multiple directed and reciprocal lines is higher in the
American network, which seems to contain more control lines.
Furthermore, there is a large similarity between the American
network at multiplicity-level three and more (undirected) and
the network of multiple directed lines. This becomes clear
when we compare Figure 6.2 and Figure 6.5.

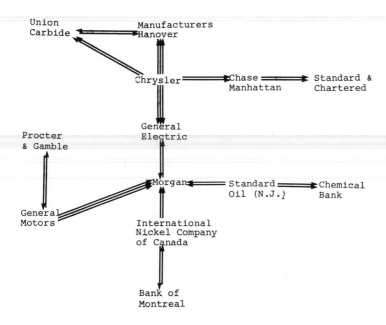

Figure 6.5 Component Chrysler 13

If we combine the firms and lines from Figures 6.2 and 6.5, adding the single directed lines and the double lines between these firms, we obtain a complete picture of the grouping around Chrysler and Morgan (Figure 6.6).

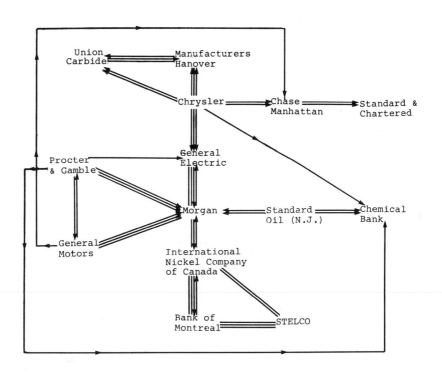

Figure 6.6 The grouping around Chrysler and Morgan

In Figure 6.6 four cliques can be distinguished: one
containing Chrysler, Manufacturers Hanover, and Union
Carbide; one containing General Motors, Morgan, and Procter&
Gamble; one containing International Nickel Co. of Canada,
Bank of Montreal, and STELCO; and one containing Morgan,
General Electric and Procter & Gamble. This last clique is
overlapping with the second, and is the only one that is not
persistent at multiplicity-level two and more. The cliques
are tied together with triple lines between Chrysler and
General Electric, between Morgan and International Nickel
Company of Canada, and between Manufacturers Hanover and
Union Carbide. As one can see from Figure 6.6, the structure

of the network is already complicated when all directed and multiple lines are taken into consideration. The complexity would be even higher if we were to draw the single undirected lines (weak ties) as well. The density of that network between the 14 firms would be .30, meaning that almost a third of the potential lines between these firms is actually realized.

There are few directed lines from banks to industrials. The only outgoing arcs from banks are those between Morgan and General Electric, between Morgan and International Nickel, between Manufacturers Hanover and Union Carbide and between Bank of Montreal and International Nickel. In all these cases there exists a reciprocal line between the firms. In fact, it is the industrials who have the majority of outgoing arcs, many of them to a bank. In this respect Chrysler is the most striking example with its multiple directed lines to Manufacturers Hanover, Chase Manhattan, General Electric and Union Carbide. This finding is very surprising in the light of the theory of bank control, and especially the idea of 'financial empires' with the banks in the center. Furthermore, it is not in line with empirical studies such as that done by Elsas and others on the Dutch network in 1976. They find that the largest commercial banks, ABN and AMRO, have together 67 outgoing arcs, 56 of which go to other financial institutions and 11 to industrial firms. These two banks have no incoming arcs from one and the same corporation, leading the authors to conclude that "no other corporation is permitted to coordinate the politics of these two banks" (Elsas, et.al., 1981: 30). Such a conclusion is certainly not warranted for the American network presented in Figure 6.6. Indeed, according to the interpretation of the Dutch research team, Chrysler is able to coordinate the politics of three large commercial banks (Manufacturers Hanover, Chase Manhattan and Chemical Bank). Such an interpretation makes it very hard to explain why Chrysler should have run into financial problems during the seventies.

To determine whether arcs from industrial firms to commercial banks really can be interpreted as dominance relations of the industrial firms over the banks we must look for the shareholding relationships between these firms. These are presented in Table 6.5.

Table 6.5 Percentage of the outstanding shares of the
company's stock held by the banks and the
corresponding interlocking directorates

	Percentage held by all banks [a]	Percentage held by	Latest year for data	Inter-locking direct-orates[b]
Chrysler	15	Manufacturers Hanover	0.4	1972 m/dir -->
		Chase Manhattan	4.0	m/dir -->
General Electric	20	Morgan Guaranty	0.6	1974 m/dir -->
		Citicorp	2.4	s/dir <--
General Motors	10	Morgan Guaranty	1.7	1974 m/dir -->
Procter & Gamble	10	Morgan Guaranty	5.1	1974 m/dir -->
Standard Oil N.J.	10	Chase Manhattan	2.7	? s
Union Carbide	10	Manufacturers Hanover	1.4	1975 m/reci.
IBM	15	Bankers Trust	2.5	1975 m/reci.
		Citicorp	2.3	1974 m/weak
Mobil Oil	15	Bankers Trust	7.2	1975 s/dir <--
		Chase Manhattan	2.2	1975 s/dir -->
RCA	10	Chase Manhattan	4.2	1972
Texaco	15	Manufacturers Hanover	0.9	1975
U.S. Steel	1	Morgan Guaranty	0.1	1974 m/dir <--
Metallgesellschaft		Dresdner Bank[c]	25.	1970 m/reci.
		Deutsche Bank	25.	1970 m/dir -->
Daimler Benz		Deutsche Bank	25.	1970 m/dir -->
Volkswagenwerke		Dresdner Bank		1970 m/dir -->
Thomson-Brandt		Banque Nationale de Paris [d]	3.2	1971 s/dir <--
		Credit Lyonnais	1.6	1971 ----

[a] Percentage of the shares of the company's stock held by
the trust departments of all commercial banks per 9/30/1969.
Source: Pastre, 1979.
[b] m: multiple line; s: single line; dir: directed line;
reci: reciprocal or two directed interlocks in opposite
directions.
[c] Source: Wer gehort zu Wem, 1971 (published by Commerz
Bank).
[d] Source: Morin, 1976.

There is no sign that large stockholdings are accompanied by outgoing officer-interlocks. On the contrary, although many of the large banks hold substantial blocks of shares of industrial companies in trust, the direction of the interlocking directorates between these banks and industrials is more often than not opposite to the shareholding relation. In nine out of twenty-one cases, the direction of the interlock is opposite to the shareholding, in three cases there exists a reciprocal relation, while in three other cases the direction of the interlock parallels the direction of the shareholding relation. These results are confirmed by the more extensive study of Mizruchi, comparing the stockholding of American banks with existing interlocks between those banks and industrial firms. He found that 46.2 percent of the large stockholdings was accompanied by an interlock, but less than half of these were carried by a banker (Mizruchi, 1980: 40).

Is it possible, then, that the industrial firms control the banks, rather than the other way around? There are two reasons not to accept such a conclusion.
First, there is very little evidence about the shareholding of industrial firms in the banks, due to the secrecy with which these shareholdings are kept. Second, it is often assumed that industrialists are invited to sit on the board of directors of a bank to strengthen the client relation with that bank rather than to exercise control. This was, for example, the position of Jeidels (1905: 151).

6.2.2 Financial groups

In the foregoing section we saw that the network of directed and multiple interlocks contains four cliques of completely connected firms, two of which (Procter & Gamble, Morgan and General Motors; and Procter & Gamble, Morgan and General Electric) overlap. In this section we raise the question of whether or not these cliques can be interpreted as the core of a financial group. The investigation of financial groups has a long tradition in which the work of Menshikov is an example. Menshikov distinguishes eight different New York groups, each of which he labels after the most important bank in it (Menshikov, 1969: 228 ff.). Of these the most important are Morgan Guaranty Trust Group, Chase Manhattan-Chemical Bank Group (Rockefeller group), Manufacturers Hanover Trust Group, and Le Sachs and Co./Lazard Freres. He further distinguishes the Ford group and a group of firms under joint control (Menshikov, 1969: 229). Chase Manhattan and Chemical Bank are the core banks of the Rockefeller financial group which through the Rockefeller Brothers Fund and Yale

University also hold at least $25 million common stock of
Chrysler (Schwartz, 1975: 35).

Table 6.6 Group affiliation according to Menshikov (1969)

		Number of adjacent firms in Figure 6.6	Menshikov [*]	[**]	[***]
1	Chrysler	5	D	25	A (20)/Humphrey – Hanna/ Mellon/B (2)
2	Morgan	5	A	100	
3	Procter & Gamble	4	A	60	E/Mellon
4	Chase Manhattan	3	B	100	
5	Chemical Bank	3	B	100	
6	General Electric	3	A	66	E/Boston/Humphrey – Hanna
7	General Motors	3	A	33	various
8	Manufacturers Hanover	2	D	100	
9	Union Carbide	2	D	50	Humphrey – Hanna
10	Standard Oil N.J.	2	B	75	A

[*] Financial group to which the firm belongs:
    A = Morgan Guaranty Trust group
    B = Chase Manhattan Chemical Bank/ N.Y Trust (Rockefeller
       Group)
    D = Manufacturers Hanover Trust Group
    E = Lehman Bros./ Goldman, Sachs and Co./ Lazard Frères
[**] Share of control in percentage
[***] Other controlling groups (share of control in
parentheses).

In Table 6.6 the affiliation of the ten United States firms
from Figure 6.6 is disclosed. The Menshikov data reveal a
group affiliation that conforms roughly to the pattern of
interlocking directorates presented in Figure 6.6. Indeed,
the main affiliation of both Union Carbide and Chrysler is
the Manufacturers Hanover Group, although Chrysler is partly
in the orbit of the Morgan Group (via General Electric in
Figure 6.6). Morgan, Procter & Gamble, General Electric and
General Motors belong to the Morgan Guaranty Trust Group,
although both General Electric and Procter and Gamble are
also under the influence of a group around Lehman
Bros./Goldman, Sachs and Co./ Lazard Frères. Lazard Frères
has, according to Menshikov (1969: 297), close connections
with the Rockefeller Group, which may explain the arc from
General Motors to Chase Manhattan, and the arc from Procter &
Gamble to Chemical Bank. Finally, Standard Oil is said to

belong to the Rockefeller Group, but is also under the
influence of the Morgan Group. This is reflected in multiple
directed lines to Chemical Bank and Morgan respectively. Our
data, therefore, seem to corroborate Menshikov's
interpretation of the structure of the United States big
business. Of course, it is possible that he also used the
network of interlocking directorates to arrive at his
interpretation, in which case this conclusion is rather
trivial. But, although Menshikov is vague about the
methodological aspects of his study, it is our impression -
and this is confirmed by Mizruchi (1980: 147) - that he
mainly used information on shareholding and other financial
relations. If so, the structure of directed double or triple
lines clearly indicates the existence of financial groups,
which, however, cannot be defined without reference to
shareholding and other financial relations. Chrysler, for
example, could easily be seen as the center of a financial
group including Union Carbide, Manufacturers Hanover, Chase
Manhattan, General Electric and even Morgan. Information on
shareholding and credit relations, however, reveals that,
rather than being the center of a financial group, Chrysler
is the meeting-point of at least three financial groups
(Manufacturers Hanover, Morgan and Rockefeller) and thus has
a very central position in the network of interlocking
directorates. This does not necessarily indicate a strong
financial position. On the contrary, Chrysler may well be a
constant source of anxiety for those financial institutions
that have stake in it. Through interlocks the banks maintain
close contact with the patient who needs permanent
(financial) care. At the same time, each bank is afraid that
if something happens to the patient, it may not have time to
save its investments. Rather than a sign of strength, a large
amount of interlocks with several banks may well be a sign of
weakness.
This argument underlines the fact that a firm can be central
in the network for different reasons. It can have a high
centrality because of its dominating position in a financial
group; it can also have a central position in the network as
a meeting-point for different financial groups. Mintz and
Schwartz (1981) distinguish these two positions as hubs and
bridges. [3]

[3] This concept of bridge is different from the concept used
    in this study and is similar to Harary's concept of
    cutpoint (1972: 26).

6.2.3 Constellations of interests

The component analysis of officer-interlocks so far does not
take the direction of the interlocks into account. The
direction of the interlocks is taken into account in the so
called strong component analysis (see Harary, 1972: 199 ff.).
A strong component in a directed graph (D) is a maximal
subgraph of D in which each point can reach the other points
in the subgraph through a directed path. A directed path
consists of a set of points and directed lines (arcs) between
these points in such a way that the starting point of the
directed path can reach its endpoint through a number of
points and consecutive arcs. The strong component cannot
contain a firm that can reach the other firms without being
reached by them in return. The idea of mutual control seems
immanent if the concept of strong component is applied to a
network of officer-interlocks. The concept of strong
component, therefore, seems an appropriate graph-theoretical
operationalization of the concept of constellation of
interests developed by Scott to define a financial group in
which no definite locus of control can be distinguished. [4]

In other words, there is no single company which is in a
control position vis a vis the other companies in the group.
Such is the typical structure of the strong component in
which reachability (and therefore dominance relations) are by
definition reciprocal, either directly or indirectly. The

[4] Using the graph-theoretical concept of strong component
    as an operationalization of Scott's concept of
    constellation of interests implies a more narrow and
    precise definition of the concept than his. Scott speaks of
    control by a constellation of interests if a corporation is
    controlled "by a loose grouping of major shareholders, who
    may nevertheless delegate some aspects of strategic control
    to professional managers or to the old controlling
    families" (Scott, 1979: 74). In a chapter on finance
    capital Scott maintains that "relations of effective
    possession and strategic control involving constellations
    of financial interests generate a structure of interlocks,
    the main significance of which is the communication of
    business information" (Scott, 1979: 103). In our definition
    of financial group the central element is the ability to
    raise funds autonomously for capital accumulation (see
    section 1.3). Control by a constellation of interests
    exists within a financial group where no fixed locus of
    control exists.

directed   graph defined by 146 firms and   the officer-
interlocks contains one strong component of 12 firms, one of
5 firms, one of 4 firms and three of 2 firms. A pair of firms
can only be a strong component if there exists a reciprocal
line between the two firms. Three such pairs form a component
in the   network: Manufacturers Hanover - Union Carbide;
Bankers Trust - IBM; and AMRO - AKZO. In such a component
each firm can reach all other firms in the component through
an uninterrupted series of arcs. We find a Swiss component
Alusuisse 4, a Canadian-United States component Morgan 5 and
a German component Volkswagen 12 (see Figures 6.7, 6.8 and
6.9).

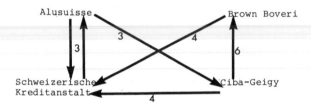

Figure 6.7 Strong component Alusuisse 4

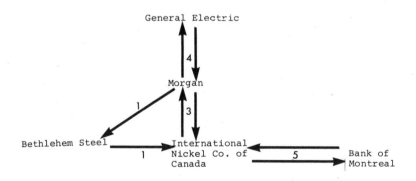

Figure 6.8 Strong component Morgan 5

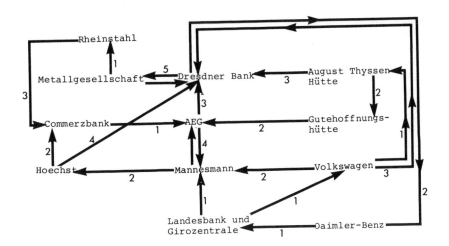

Figure 6.9 Strong component <u>Volkswagen</u> <u>12</u>

In Figures 6.7, 6.8 and 6.9, the numbers added to the arcs
indicate the multiplicity of the (undirected) line between
the connected firms. As to be expected, the strong components
in the officer-interlock network are relatively small, and
only one contains firms from more than one country. Two
strong components contain more than one bank, but only the
German component is a case in itself, since it contains no
less than twelve firms and has a very large diameter (8). As
we have already seen, the German business system is
characterized by a very strong integration and cohesion of
corporate elite. There are no clearly distinguished clusters
that can be interpreted as separate financial groups, as was
the case in the American network. Nevertheless, when we
compare the strong component <u>Volkswagen</u> <u>12</u> (Figure 6.9) with
the component <u>Dresdner</u> <u>Bank</u> <u>17</u> (Figure 6.1), it looks as if
there exist groupings around the large commercial banks:
Metallgesellschaft, Volkswagen, AEG and August Thyssen around
.Dresdner Bank; Hoesch, BASF, Siemens, Bosch and AKZO around
Deutsche Bank. There are many industrial firms in Germany
maintaining interlocks with several large banks.

There are two types of centrality in a strong component: the
first takes the outgoing arcs into account and the second

takes the incoming arcs into account. The adjacency can thus
be distinguished in the indegree (number of incoming lines)
and the outdegree (number of outgoing lines). In the Swiss
component the outdegree is highest for Alusuisse and Ciba-
Geigy, in the American component for Morgan, and in the
German component for Volkswagen. The indegree, on the other
hand, is in the Swiss component highest for the
Schweizerische Kreditanstalt, in the American component for
International Nickel, and in the German component for
Dresdner Bank. Again, the banks are not in all cases the most
central firms in the strong component, certainly not when one
looks at the outdegree. The conclusion from Section 6.2.2 is
confirmed in the analysis of the strong components: if these
strong components indicate constellations of interests, the
banks are not necessarily the central firms in such
constellations. Nevertheless, the fact that banks are central
in the network of interlocking directorates necessitates a
further analysis of their position.

6.3 Summary

In this chapter, the multiplicity and the direction of the
lines have been analyzed. The first analysis showed that the
international network breaks down into national components at
higher levels of multiplicity. This happens already at
multiplicity-level two with the Swiss, Swedish, French,
Italian and British networks. The French, Italian and British
networks fall immediately apart into separate components,
indicating a fragmentation of the national network itself.
The Swiss network, on the other hand, shows a remarkable
tenacity: its density decreases very little at the higher
levels of multiplicity. This is also the case, though to a
lesser extent, with the German/Dutch component and the United
States/Canadian component. At multiplicity-level four and
more, however, these tenacious binational networks also fall
apart into national components. The Swiss, German and Dutch
networks have a large and tenacious core, comprising roughly
three-quarters of the large firms. These integrated systems
of interlocking directorates provide a high potential for
communication, coordination and control. Furthermore they
indicate a strong cohesion of the corporate elite to the
containment of potential conflict and increase the strength
of the business community vis a vis the state. At higher
levels of multiplicity, the German firms increase their local
centrality but not their global centrality. For the United
States and Dutch firms the reverse is true, corroborating the
conclusion from Chapter 5 that they play a crucial role in
connecting the different national networks. The fact that the
Dutch firms and the New York banks are less central in the

network of officer-interlocks leads us to conclude that the
international network should be considered a network of
communication rather than a network of domination and
control.

Further analysis of the network of officer-interlocks reveals
that their number is larger in the United States network than
in the German network. While the German network is more
integrated and thicker, the American network seems more
purposive. At the higher levels of multiplicity the officer-
interlocks can be interpreted as control lines revealing the
cores of several financial groups. A detailed analysis of the
grouping around Morgan, Chrysler and Bank of Montreal,
however, reveals that for an accurate distinction of
financial groups additional information is necessary. A high
centrality in the network of domination and control does not
necessarily indicate a dominant position. If the centrality
is due to many interlocks with several banks, this may
indicate that the firm is dominated by several financial
groups. An unexpected finding was that there was no support
for the thesis of bank control, according to which bankers
dominate the boards of directors of large industrial firms.
Indeed it was found that more industrialists appear on the
boards of banks than vice versa, even in those cases where
the bank has a substantial shareholding in the industrial
firm. It seems that at least for the very large industrial
firms a bank tries to strengthen its relationship with them
by inviting the president of one or more of them to sit on
its board. This conclusion was strengthened by a strong
component analysis isolating clusters of firms with
reciprocal dominance relations. Three such components were
found. In only one was a bank found to have a central
position in terms of outgoing lines. In the other two the
banks were central in terms of incoming lines. In only one of
the three strong components were firms from different
countries found; this component consisted of three United
States and two Canadian firms. In the network of domination
and control, one may conclude, internationalization is only
visible between United States and Canadian firms. The
international aspect of the network of interlocking
directorates has to be found in the communication network in
the Atlantic business system. Since the banks are more
central in the network of communication than in the network
of control, one may assume that the banks play a significant
role in the international integration of the business system.
In the next chapter the focus will be on the international
structure of the banking system.

VII COMPETITION AND COOPERATION: the role of banks

7.0 Introduction

In the preceding chapters we considered whether, at the international level, there exists 'an integrated network of interlocking directorates, and we found that for the largest Western firms this is, indeed, the case. This network, however, seems to suggest a system of communication rather than a system of domination, one in which New York banks and Dutch multinationals play a significant role in cementing the national subnetworks into an international whole. Although these findings do not corroborate the predicted structure of the network derived from the theory of Bucharin, there is still a possibility that they concur with the expected structure derived from the Bucharinist-inspired theory developed by Rowthorn. According to him the (few) international interlocks are predominantly carried by American, British and Dutch multinationals (see Section 3.2). What has to be shown to discard all Bucharinist theories, including that of Rowthorn, is that the firms from the same nationality do not primarily cooperate at the national level to strengthen their position internationally, but that there exist international alliances between firms from different countries. The relation between competition and cooperation is fundamental for the choice between the different models presented in Chapter 3, and since it was demonstrated in Chapter 6 that the structure of interlocking directorates does not offer a rigorous test for identifying financial groups, an analysis of interlocking directorates cannot directly address the question of competition and cooperation. Furthermore, we have argued (in Chapter 2, Section 2.5) that there is a dialectical relationship between competition and cooperation involving different economic and institutional levels, e.g., regional, national and international, to name a few.

In this chapter we will analyze the international structure of cooperation and competition among banks by comparing interlocking directorates and international bank consortia. This emphasis on banks is guided by several theoretical and empirical arguments. The theoretical dimension has been elaborated in the theory of finance capital, presented in Chapter 1. Banks 'produce' a commodity (money) that is the most general and most 'abstract' of all. It can be transformed instantly - or nearly instantly - into any other commodity, be it means of production, labor power or consumer goods. Banks, therefore, play a central role in the allocation of capital and, thus, in the competition between firms and groups of firms. Close relations between

industrials and banks as, for instance, witnessed by interlocks between them are important mechanisms in obtaining money capital for productive investment. On this argument rests the concept of finance capital. [1]

Empirically, our earlier analyses have shown that banks maintain a central position in the network of interlocking directorates. Therefore, even though they may not be the centers of financial groups, we may temporarily assume that they have a large number of client-relations with industrial firms, relationships which we shall call spheres of interests. In Section 7.2 we will determine whether banks' spheres of interests are national or international in character. We will then analyze the overlap between financial spheres of interests as expressed in the number of meeting-points of each pair of banks. Such meeting-points — industrial firms that maintain interlocking directorates with at least two banks – are potential clients for each of the interlocked financial institutions and, therefore, are potential sources of conflict or competition among the banks. If there are many such meeting-points, this indicates a high potential for conflict (=competition); few or no meeting-points indicates the absence of direct competition. To investigate this interpretation, we will compare the structure of meeting-points between banks with the structure of international consortia, mechanisms which, we can more safely assume, indicate cooperation.
First, however, we will analyze in Section 7.1 the interlocking directorates between banks, since these are most likely to indicate the absence of conflict. In fact, the possibility of collusion was the main reason for the prohibition of interlocks among United States banks, specified in the Clayton Act of 1914 (see Section 1.2). However, since there are no international laws prohibiting

[1] Of course, banks are not the only firms engaged in the allocation of money-capital. In this sense Sweezy has correctly pointed out that "today's conglomerate-multinational corporations – and most of them have both characteristics – are essentially financial, not production units" (Sweezy, 1971: 31). However, this argument can only mean that finance capital is not restricted to bank capital invested in industrial firms, as Hilferding maintained. It does not contradict the assumption that banks, being predominantly engaged in allocating money-capital for productive investment, play a crucial role in the process of accumulation.

international interlocks among financial institutions and
since such legal prohibitions do not exist in all countries,
this is an appropriate starting point.

7.1 Interlocks among banks

If banks are as important in the interlock network as
suggested in Chapter 5, the network should break down when
banks are deleted. This is indeed the case: the number of
lines decreases from 404 to 170, and network density
decreases from 2.8 to 1.8 percent; the connectivity drops
from 54 to 30 percent. The compactness of the international
network is not due to the role of bankers, however. Only 29
out of 111 arcs between banks and industrial firms are
carried by bankers: industrialists sit on the boards of the
large banks, rather than bankers on the boards of the very
large industrial firms.

Between banks, on the other hand, there are relatively few
interlocks. In 1970 we find interlocks between the Japanese
banks, between three British banks and between two Italian
banks. All other interlocks are international interlocks,
most often carried by a European banker who sits on the
international advisory boards of Chase Manhattan, Morgan or
Chemical Bank (see Figure 7.1a).

The Japanese and the British networks are quite different
from those of the other countries. Six out of eight Japanese
banks in the sample form one component, which seems to be an
expression of the intricate financial structure of the
Japanese business system, the Zaikai, where cooperation
overrides competition (see Hadley, 1970). The Japanese
business system will not, for reasons explained in the
foregoing chapters, be analyzed here.

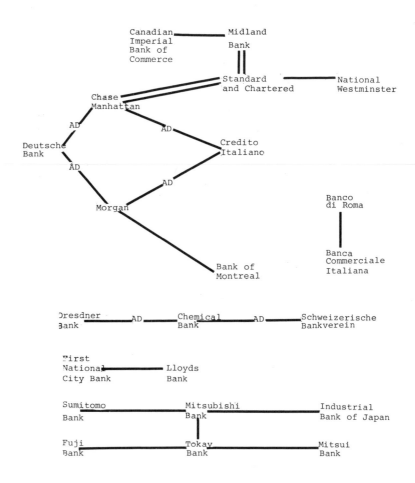

<u>Figure</u> 7.1a Interlocking directorates between the banks
           (1970)

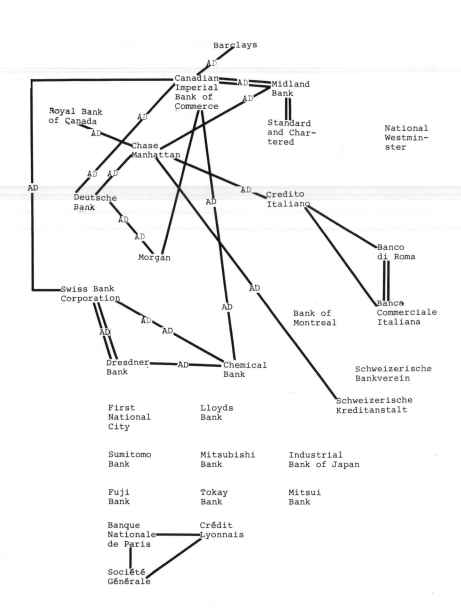

Figure 7.1b Interlocking   directorates   between   the   banks
            (1976)

For the British banks there is a different story. Although
only five British banks are included in the sample (smaller
British banks did not appear in the Fortune list (see
Appendix A)), these five banks controlled more than 90
percent of the commercial banking resources (see Table 7.1).
Such a high concentration was, apart from historical reasons,
due to three large mergers between 1968 and 1970. Barclays
DCO became a fully owned daughter of Barclays Bank and
changed its name to Barclays International. Standard Bank and
Chartered Bank formed the Standard and Chartered Banking
Group. National Provincial merged with Westminster into
National Westminster Bank. As a result of this merger boom
the total number of London clearing banks was reduced to
four, all of which are included in the sample. The remaining
Standard and Chartered is predominantly engaged in overseas
investment, taking advantage of the traditional position of
Standard Bank in South Africa and Chartered Bank in Asia. The
high concentration in the British banking system is, as
illustrated in Figure 7.1a, accompanied by economic
centralization in the form of interlocks between National
Westminster, Standard & Chartered and Midland. (For the
concept of centralization used here the reader is referred to
Section 2.5.1.)
How should this high rate of concentration and centralization
be explained? In his study on British finance capital
Overbeek (1980) refers to three factors. First of all,
finance capital was late to develop in Britain, because the
country's dominant position on the world market hampered the
formation of trusts and cartels flourishing in Germany and
the United States.

Table 7.1 Bank concentration in several European countries

	Share of total commercial banking resources of the 5 largest banks		
	1960	1970	1976
Netherlands	78	98	98
United Kingdom	77	93	95
Sweden	(80)[*]	80	87
France	61	65	63
BRD	(50)	50	(75)
Switzerland	(50)	50	46

[*] figures in parentheses are a rough estimation

Source: Thunholm, 1971: 104-106; personal communication with
Lars-Erik Thunholm.

Second, British banking was directed mainly at overseas
operations since the greatest profits could be obtained in
financing foreign trade and handling portfolio investment
abroad. Third, as a result of an early international
orientation, there existed important relations between
American and British capital. In fact a large part of
nineteenth century British export capital went to the United
States, and this portfolio investment in United States
railroads gave birth to some very powerful American
investment banks: for example, J.P.Morgan and Kidder, Peabody
& Co (Kotz, 1978: 26).

By 1970, some important financial relations between British
and American banks still remain. Chase Manhattan, for
instance, holds 13.8 percent of the shares of Standard and
Chartered Group, while National Westminster owns 9.2 percent
and Midland 4.6 percent, all of which are accompanied by
interlocking directorates (see Figure 7.1a). First National
City and Lloyds Bank jointly control Grindlays Bank, which is
reflected in an interlock between First National and Lloyds.

Although experts confirm a large amount of cooperation
between London clearing banks, Figure 7.1a shows that no
interlocking directorates exist among the four in our sample.
Interlocks are maintained between Standard & Chartered and
the two clearing banks - Midland and National Westminster -
which hold stock in the former. The structure of the British
banking system may, after all, be less exceptional than it
appears. Experts foresee growing competition among the
clearing banks. This is because the distinction between
deposit banks and merchant banks is, as in other countries,
vanishing, thus forcing both types to compete more
vigorously. This is also because of the Bank of England's
1971 attempt to break the cartel of London clearing banks
(Revell, 1973: 113; Spiegelberg, 1973: 119 ff).

To evaluate the extent to which this development has
influenced the network of interlocking directorates, Figure
7.1b gives a diagram of director exchanges among the sample
banks in 1976. By that year, the interlock between National
Westminster and Standard & Chartered had disappeared, because
National Westminster sold its holding to Midland Bank. The
number of interlocks among British banks thus had decreased.
This finding is consistent with Overbeek's conclusions.
Comparing the network of interlocking directorates among
twenty-six large industrial firms, four clearing banks, nine
of the large insurance companies and twelve of the most
important merchant banks for the years 1972 and 1976,
Overbeek finds that, although the total number of links
increased by almost 15 percent, the City as a subsystem had
not increased in density. He concluded that "to an increasing

extent the axis clearing banks - industrial companies is
becoming the most important one" (Overbeek, 1980: 117). The
year 1976 also witnessed a number of new interlocks among
French and Italian banks. In the French case interlocks were
established by J. de Larosiere de Champfeu who sat on the
boards of directors of the three French banks under
consideration. At the same time he was head of the Department
of Financial Activities, of the Ministere de l'Economie et
des Finance, and thus represented the French government in
these state-owned deposit banks. The interlocks among the
Italian banks were carried by U. Tabanelli who, in 1970, sat
on the boards of the Banco di Roma and the Banco Commerciale
Italiana. By 1976, he had added a directorship of Credito
Italiano. Tabanelli, who was at the time vice-president of
the Istituto Ricostruzione Industrial (IRI), represented the
IRI as the major shareholder in these three banks.

Both French and Italian deposit banks function more as a
para-state banking system than as a number of autonomously
competing institutions. Interlocks among these units should,
therefore, not surprise us nor should they be considered
indicative of the absence of competition. Both Tabanelli and
de Larosiere primarily serve an auditing function, because
both the Italian and French governments have refrained from
direct interference (Steuber, 1977: 78). Nevertheless, the
fact that this function is, by 1976, performed by only one
person in each country can indeed be regarded as a form of
centralization in the para-state banking system. According to
Morin, in his penetrating study of the structure of the
French banking system, the nationalized banks are
increasingly engaged in merchant banking and in the
internationalization of their activities. These new
developments increase competition among units and force their
association with financial groups based on private capital
(Morin, 1974: 173 ff). These private financial groups, like
the group Paribas, the group Empain and the group Suez, seem
to have a considerable impact on the strategy of the
nationalized and mixed-ownership financial institutions
(Morin, 1977: 72 ff).

It seems that in the United States, as well as in other
Western countries, the distinction between deposit or
clearing banks on the one hand and the merchant banks on the
other - institutionalized in the United States by force of
the Glass-Steagull Act in 1933, and in other countries
(except Germany and the United Kingdom) by similar legal
provisions forbidding deposit banks to engage in investment
activities - is fading away. This tendency will ceteris
paribus increase competition, especially among the large
commercial banks.

The number of international interlocks among banks increased
substantially between 1970 and 1976. In 1970, there were
eleven ties, six of which were carried by a European director
with a seat on the international advisory boards of Chase
Manhattan, Morgan or Chemical Bank. In 1976 there were
seventeen international interlocks, fifteen of which were
carried by a director who sat on the (international) advisory
board of at least one bank. In four cases, (Canadian Imperial
- Deutsche Bank, Canadian Imperial - Chemical Bank, Chemical
Bank - Schweizerische Bankverein and Morgan - Deutsche Bank)
the person was on the advisory boards of both banks.
The institution of advisory boards, established to provide
the banks with necessary international contacts, has spread
from the United States to other countries. The increase of
international advisory interlocks of the American banks may
well be related to the increasing importance of foreign
investment in relation to total earnings. While in 1970
foreign investment accounted for under 25 percent of total
earnings for all American banks in the sample except one, by
1976 this figure had risen to at least 40 percent (Table
7.2). Comparison of Figures 7.1a and 7.1b shows a
corresponding reshuffling of interlocking directorates. Only
eight interlocks were stable over the six-year period; six of
these were still carried by the same person. [2] The increase
in the number of interlocks among Western banks is a first
indication that, with the exception perhaps of the state-
owned or state-controlled financials, banks do not look for
national cooperation to strengthen their international
position vis-a-vis other 'national capitals', as the model
derived from the Bucharinist theories of imperialism implies.
On the contrary, there seems to be a tendency to increase
international consultation with foreign banks through a
network of advisory interlocks. According to the Leninist
theories of imperialism, the strategy of the banks would be
to strive for cooperation with those banks that can increase
their position at both a national and an international level.
Implicit here is that the banks are still competing with
their national rivals and have not merged into a 'state
capitalist trust'. The battlefield, however, is the
international rather than the national 'space'. This idea is

[2] Mokken and Stokman (1976b) use another definition of
    stability. They regard an interlock between two firms as
    stable if over the years the director creating the
    interlock disappears but the interlock remains. In our
    case, therefore, they would only consider two of the eight
    interlocks between banks as stable.

also expressed by the Swedish banker Lars-Erik Thunholm
(1971), who argued that the rapid internationalization of
banks stimulates and sharpens competition in the field of
international banking services, which "also tends to spill
over in the national areas." Moreover, he suggests that the
Euro-dollar market was the basis of this internationalization
at the end of the sixties, and is

> "the most perfect competitive money market in existence,
> untrammeled as it is by legal and institutional
> regulations. Access to this market increases the banks'
> efficiency to serve their customers both in the
> national and in the international field" (Thunholm,
> 171: 114).

The same argument is used by the Japanese Ministry of Finance
to restrict the expansion by Japanese banks of their foreign
branches. Such expansion would only lead to "needless"
competition among them (Schaft, 1980: 17, 18).

Table 7.2 American banks: share of foreign earnings in total
earnings (1970-1976)

	1970	1973	1976	Annual growth rate 1970-1975
First National City	40	60	72	33.2
J.P.Morgan	25	46	53	35.2
Chase Manhattan	22	39	78	26.9
Bank of America	15 [*]	24 [*]	40	37.7
Bankers Trust	14 [*]	40	64	38.4
Manufacturers Hanover	13	36	56	42.7
Chemical Bank	13	36	56	42.7
Western Bancorporation				

[*] estimation

Source: Transnational Corporations, 1978: 218

7.2 Overlapping spheres of interests

The tentative conclusion drawn from the analysis of
interlocking directorates among banks, that banks still
compete nationally and strive for international coalitions to
enhance their position nationally as well as internationally,
will be the starting point for an investigation of the
patterns of director overlaps between banks and industry. An
interlock between a bank and an industrial firm generally
indicates the existence of a client-relation between the bank
and the industrial firm. Here the set of client-relationships
between a bank and a number of industrial firms,
characterized by interlocks, is considered its sphere of
interests. We have emphatically discarded the idea that banks
somehow control the industrial firms through a set of
interlocks. Bank control is implausible if only because the
industrialists, and not the bankers, carry the interlocks
between banks and industrial firms.
In this section two questions will be addressed. The first is
whether the spheres of interests of banks overlap. An
indication of overlapping is the existence of large numbers
of meeting-points of banks through interlocks with the same
industrial firms. Such a meeting-point cannot be regarded
only as a board where two bankers meet. As we have seen,
meeting-points more often occur when executives of the same
industrial firm sit on the boards of two banks, both of which
have a financial stake in that firm. The second question is
whether the spheres of interests are national or
international. The analyses presented in Chapters 5 and 6
lead to the hypothesis that they are national.

To answer these questions, we will begin with an analysis of
the lines between banks and industrial firms in the 1970
sample. Of the 176 companies under investigation 41 are
banks; 221 lines connect the financials and industrials. But
does the patterning of these ties indicate a clustering of
meeting-points? Using a scaling-technique developed by Mokken
(1970) we can count the number of meeting-points of every
pair of banks and scale them according to the number of
points in common. For each group with a relatively high
number of meeting-points (a scale) a number of coefficients
are calculated to indicate the strength of the scale and the
contribution of each of the banks in the scale to that
strength. Hi is the relative number of meeting-points for
each bank with the other banks in the scale as compared with
the expected number in the case of statistical independence.
It evaluates whether a bank's total number of meeting-points
can be considered high. The difficulty is the number of lines
of a bank as a fraction of the total amount of possible lines
with that bank (in this case 135). [3] H is an overall

measure of the strength of a scale. If the banks in the
sample form scales, we may conclude that the banks of a
specific scale 'seek' meeting-points with each other, and
'avoid' meeting-points with banks belonging to other scales.
Strong scales indicate strong tendencies to do so.

Our use of such a scale-analysis assumes that the interlocks
between banks and industry are the result of strategic
decisions of the banks. A strong case for this is provided by
Pennings in his elaborate study of interlocking directorates
among American firms. He concluded that financial interlocks
   "are persuasive attempts by the financial firm to
   enhance its position with solvent firms that will be
   reliable customers for loans, bonds, and other forms of
   debt. Through these persuasive interlocks, the
   financial firms seek to secure good customers, and the
   nonfinancial firms benefit from the bank's commitment
   and access to information about the market" (Pennings,
   1980: 190).
The fact that the interlocks between banks and industrial

[3] This stochastic scale analysis was developed by Mokken
    (1970) and implemented in the program 'Mokken scale' (see
    also Stokman and Van Schuur, 1980 and Niemöller, Van Schuur
    and Stokman, 1981). Here the banks are conceived as the
    variables in the model, while a line between industrial I
    and bank X is seen as a positive score on the variable X.
    $\underline{H}i$ indicates the scalability of a bank in a certain scale.
    To be included in the scale requires $\underline{H}i$ >.30. For $\underline{H}$ it is
    assumed that
    .30 < H < .40 is a weak scale,
    .40 < H < .50 a moderate scale, and
    .50 < H a strong scale.
    For the relation between the scaling technique and the
    graph-theoretical approach see Stokman, 1977 and 1980.
    Application of the Mokken scale for the relations between
    banks and industry can meet two objections. First, the
    model on which the Mokken scale is based assumes that the
    variables (in our case the banks) are independent from each
    other. This condition is not fulfilled because there exist
    interlocking directorates among the banks (see Figure 7.1).
    Secondly, the model assumes a high number of positive
    scores (in our case interlocking directorates). Since the
    number of interlocking directorates between banks and
    industry is not very high (the density is only 4 percent),
    application of the Mokken scale takes on the character of a
    cluster technique rather than a scaling technique.

firms are carried preponderantly by industrialists who have
been _invited_ to be on the board of a bank supports the
postulate.

The Mokken scale-analysis of the 1970 data yields ten scales.
Three of these contain only two banks: Banque Nationale de
Paris/ Societe Generale; National Westminster Bank/ Lloyds
Bank; and Bank of America/ Manufacturers Hanover. All three
are _national_. Of the remaining seven, four are national and
three are binational (see Table 7.3). Ten banks cannot be
scaled: three Japanese, two British, two Canadian, one
French, one Italian and one American. These banks do not have
a significant overlapping sphere of influence with any of the
banks in the sample, nor do they significantly 'avoid' such
overlap. Two banks in the American scale would also fit into
another scale: Chemical Bank into the Dutch/American scale,
and Morgan into the Italian/American scale. The binational
scales are weaker than the national scales, while the number
of industrials connected to only one bank in these binational
scales is too high for definite conclusions. [4] The
British/Canadian scale is in fact solely based upon meeting-
points in International Nickel Company of Canada (2), Rio
Tinto Zinc and De Beers Consolidated; the Italian/American
scale is based on meeting-points in Italsider (4), Montedison
(2) and ENI; and the Dutch/American scale is based on
meeting-points in Shell (4), Unilever (2), and AKZO (2).
Without these international meeting-points between a total of
nine firms, there would be no binational scales at all. This
corroborates the conclusions suggested in Chapter 5, that the
majority of banks have overlapping spheres of interests at
the national level. Since we defined a sphere of interests as
the set of client- relations of banks, we may conclude that
rivalry exists significantly more between banks from the same
country than between banks from the different countries. Such
an interpretation is supported by Cohen's research on United
States banks. He concluded "that only six multinational banks
have built up a sizable clientele of MNCs from outside the
banks' home country" (Cohen, 1979: 37). If this is true for
the American banks, it must be even more true for the other
banks in the sample, which are in general less
internationally oriented.

[4] The total number of lines (221) between banks and
    industrial firms is very low for an application of the
    Mokken scale. In the case of the Japanese firms, the number
    of lines is so low that the scale has very little meaning.

Table 7.3 Scales of three or more banks based on meeting
          points in industrial firms (in 1970)

	Difficulty	H[i]
Japanese scale	H=.77 (strong scale)	
Sumitomo Bank	0.021	0.77
Fuji Bank	0.014	0.66
Mitsubishi Bank	0.014	0.66
Sanwa Bank	0.007	1.00
Industrial Bank of Japan	0.007	1.00
Swiss scale	H=.66 (strong scale)	
Schweizerische Kreditanstalt	0.062	0.67
Schweizerische Bankverein	0.048	0.59
Schweizerische Bankgesellschaft	0.041	0.74
German scale	H=.61 (strong scale)	
Dresdner Bank	0.083	0.65
Deutsche Bank	0.083	0.65
Commerz Bank	0.048	0.57
Landesbank und Girozentrale	0.041	0.52
American scale	H=.51 (strong scale)	
Chemical Bank	0.138	0.40
J.P. Morgan	0.138	0.50
First National City Bank	0.097	0.63
Bankers Trust	0.021	0.62
British/Canadian scale	H=.51 (strong scale)	
Canadian Imperial Bank of Commerce	0.055	0.47
Bank of Montreal	0.048	0.47
Barclays Bank	0.034	0.65
Dutch/American scale	H=.46 (moderate scale)	
Chemical Bank	0.138	0.36
Chase Manhattan	0.124	0.44
AMRO	0.034	0.60
ABN	0.028	0.54

Italian/American scale	H=.43 (moderate scale)	
J.P. Morgan	0.138	0.37
Credito Italiano	0.028	0.37
Banca Commerciale Italiana	0.028	0.41
Banco di Roma	0.021	0.41

Of course, if one assumes that meeting-points indicate cooperation rather than competition, then the Bucharin thesis would be supported: in that case banks are cooperating at the national level to strengthen their international position. But such a conclusion would make it difficult to explain the relatively small number of interlocks among banks from the same country. It would be even more difficult to explain why British bank do not tend to 'seek' each other out through meeting-points in industrial firms,even though they seem to cooperate more than banks from most other countries. The fact that even Chase Manhattan, Midland and Standard & Chartered, which are linked by multiple interlocks, do not 'seek' each other in meeting-points in industrial firms is convincing evidence against the interpretation of meeting-points as indicative of cooperation.

Only Japanese banks behaved, in 1970, according to a model in which meeting-points could be interpreted as cooperative: all Japanese banks that maintained interlocks with each other also 'sought' each other in meeting-points in Japanese industrials. This supports the conclusion from Chapter 5 that the Japanese business system is organized according to the model derived from the Bucharinist theories.

The general conclusion from this section is that Western banks tend to have overlapping spheres of interests at the national level. The largest potential for competition is to be found between banks from the same country. In the next section, cooperative behavior at the international level will be analyzed and juxtaposed with national patterns.

7.3 International bank consortia

In Section 7.2 we investigated overlapping spheres of bank
interests as a measure of competition. In this section we
analyze forms of cooperation among banks. On a national level
there are many cartels - and other agreements in which all
major banks participate. But what is the situation on the
international level? To answer this question we use data on
international bank consortia and joint-ventures. These forms
of international bank cooperation are the result of a process
of international expansion of trade and investment, which
accelerated rapidly during the sixties. Especially the
expansion of United States multinationals created a need for
international financial arrangements, resulting in the
development of the Euro-currency markets (see Junne, 1976).
Most international bank consortia and joint-ventures were
created to operate in these Euro-currency markets, which came
into existence during the sixties. The foundation of these
markets had been stimulated by four different events.

First, induced by the cold war, socialist countries began
transferring dollar deposits from America to Europe. The
Banque Commerciale pour l'Europe du Nord (Paris) and the
Moscow Narodny Bank (London) played an important role in
these transactions. Second, the elimination of sterling as an
international currency during and after the Suez crisis of
1957 caused the British banks to hold dollars, rather than
sterling, for international payments. Third, growth of Euro-
currency markets was stimulated by the Interest Equalization
Tax, created by the United States government in 1963 to
prevent American capital from profiting from differences in
interest rates between the United States and Europe. Rather
than limiting American capital investment in European bonds
and equity, it prevented American capital already invested in
Europe from returning home, thus creating a dollar market
outside the United States and mainly in London. Finally, the
post-1973 flow of 'petrodollars', which were 'recycled' into
the Western business system through the banks, had a
significant influence. Strictly speaking, Euro-currencies are
currencies held outside - and thus not under the jurisdiction
of - the country of origin. There came to exist a short-term
Euro-money market, which was initially a dollar market, but
later included German marks, Dutch guilders, etc. This Euro-
money market is dominated by the very large banks through
rather informal procedures. The long-term Euro-bond and
-equity market has developed alongside the Euro-money market.
The main actors in these exchanges are the international bank
consortia, which developed after 1963. More recently, a
medium-term Euro-currency market has emerged. Of course, the
oil-crisis of 1973 expanded the Euro-currency market

enormously by adding to the existing Euro-dollars the so-called petrodollars from the Arab countries, which saw their oil-revenues multiplied eight times between 1972 and 1974. Euro-currency loans more than doubled between 1973 and 1978 (Ruffini, 1979: 238) and the consortia founded after 1973 have been predominantly oriented to the Middle East, often with a dominant Arab participation (Schaft, 1980). For our purpose, however, only those consortia and joint-ventures that constituted a meeting-point between the 41 banks in the sample are of interest. In other words, only those containing at least two sample banks are considered. From different sources, 127 consortia were collected. [5] Meeting-points created by these consortia and joint-ventures can be interpreted as institutionalized forms of cooperation.

Again the question was raised of whether banks from the same country 'seek' such meeting-points, or whether they try to avoid them. The conclusions from Section 7.2 would lead us to expect that such meeting-points are systematically avoided by banks from Western countries. Using the Mokken scale analysis, we would expect to create scales that do not contain banks from the same country. The scale analysis creates nine scales. Five of these consist of two banks only: Chemical Bank/Schweizerische Kreditanstalt; First National City Bank/Fuji Bank; Morgan/The Industrial Bank of Japan; Lloyds Bank/ Standard and Chartered Banking Group; and Sanwa Bank/ Mitsui Bank. [6] The remaining four scales are presented in Table 7.4. The first two are very strong (H. 80 and H. 78). We call them Orion scale and EBIC scale after the international consortia that form the basis of each. Similarly, we call the third scale Europartners scale and the fourth SFE scale (Société Financière Européenne).

[5] Our main source was Steuber (1976), but additional information was obtained from experts from Dutch banks. Only those consortia and joint-ventures established before 1974 were taken into account.

[6] With the exception of the first, these five scales are strong.

Table 7.4 Scales   of   three   or   more   banks   based   on
          international bank consortia and joint ventures
          (1974)

	Difficulty	H[i]
Orion scale	H=.80 (strong scale)	
Landesbank und Girozentrale	0.063	0.71
Mitsubishi Bank	0.055	0.71
Chase Manhattan	0.055	0.71
Credito Italiano	0.047	0.71
National Westminster Bank	0.032	1.00
Royal Bank of Canada	0.032	1.00
Swiss Bank Corporation	0.008	1.00
Ebic scale	H=.78 (strong scale)	
Midland Bank	0.071	0.76
Deutsche Bank	0.071	0.76
Société Général (France)	0.071	0.80
AMRO	0.063	0.79
Western Bancorporation	0.008	1.00
Europartners scale	H=.61 (strong scale)	
Crédit Lyonnais	0.047	0.62
Commerz Bank	0.047	0.52
Banco di Roma	0.039	0.69
Societe Financiere Europeenne scale	H=.51 (strong scale)	
Bank of America	0.118	0.53
Barclays Bank	0.087	0.36
Dresdner Bank	0.063	0.59
Union de Banques Suisses	0.055	0.32
Sumitomo Bank	0.055	0.40
ABN	0.047	0.53
Banca Nazionale del Lavoro	0.039	0.59
Banque Nationale de Paris	0.032	0.69

This means that the banks in each scale show a common orientation toward international consortia. If, for instance, we find an international consortium in which Landesbank und Girozentrale participates, the probability is great that we find Mitsubishi Bank, Chase Manhattan, Credito Italiano and the other banks from the Orion scale in that consortium. The interesting feature of these results is not, of course, that the scales are international (which is just an artifact) but that they live up to our expectation: no one contains two banks from the same nationality, except Lloyds Bank/Standard & Chartered and Sanwa Bank/Mitsui Bank. As predicted, the Japanese banks display colluding behavior in the international capital market. The British banks, on the other hand, were not expected to seek cooperation in the international arena. However, this British scale is not based on an international consortium proper, but on the • Intercontinental Banking Service which contains two banks from New Zealand and Australia. Although formally it is international, it can more accurately be called a commonwealth consortium. Therefore, the cooperation should be regarded as a remnant of older forms of 'national' cooperation between the largest banks of the British Empire.

Not one of the scales - not even the Japanese or the British - contains banks with overlapping spheres of interests. This suggests that international cooperation is found among those banks which, competing at the national level, look for international support to strengthen their position both in the world market and at home. To give an example: Landesbank und Girozentrale forms a partnership with Chase Manhattan; subsequently the Deutsche Bank looks for cooperation with a competing American bank, i.e., Western Bancorporation. Dresdner Bank, in turn, looks for yet another American bank as its international partner, i.e., Bank of America, and so on.

The overall picture of the international banking system is one of competition among banks from the same country and cooperation among banks from different countries. Competition at the national level is transformed into cooperation at the international level, where each bank looks for a coalition with the 'enemies of its enemy's friends'. These coalitions, finding expression in international bank consortia, are not necessarily stable. The enemies of one's enemy's friends are not necessarily allies. And in a competitive international environment, they are even potential enemies. Arrangements within international consortia are, thus, subject to a prisoner's dilemma. They suit each partner, as long as the other partners stick to their commitments. But each participant is best off when all other partners fulfill their

obligations, while he does not. To preempt this potential, each member of the consortium tends to strengthen its position vis-a-vis its partners. So when, in 1973, the Europartners established a bank in the Netherlands, the German Commerzbank did not allow equal participation among all members, because this could have undermined its traditionally strong position in the Dutch business system (Steuber, 1977: 100). More recently, Commerzbank and Credit Lyonnais decided to establish separate branches in Paris and Frankfurt, contrary to the Europartners' expressed goal of integrating their network of foreign branches (Steuber, 1977: 104). Such a tendency is clearly self-inducing and it is no wonder that in recent years the major banks have been expanding their own network of foreign branches (Schaft, 1980; see also Channon, 1977: 148). [7]

Central to our conclusion is the fact that rapid change in international consortia, growth euphoria in the early seventies as well as stagnation after 1975, is a result of the interplay between competition and cooperation at the national and international levels. The expansion of international trade and investment during the sixties, and the subsequent developments of the Euro-currency markets, forced the banks to internationalize. And for the continental European banks, most of which lacked international experience and a network of branches and subsidiaries abroad, the most obvious strategy was to create international consortia with partners from the most important capitalist countries. These partners were chosen because they were the enemies of their enemy's friends.

This finding undermines the conclusions of the 1975 Dutch study by Helmers et.al. They concluded from the high network density, the central position of the banks, and the large number of meeting points between these banks, that there existed a unified center in the Dutch business system. They based their conclusion on the interpretation of meeting-points as indicative of cooperation and neglected the role

[7] The failure of the first consortium bank, the American Foreign Banking Corporation, incorporated in New York State in 1917 and liquidated in 1927, seems also due to such a prisoner's dilemma. According to a contemporary observer, "it soon appeared that the bank shareholders in such institutions were inclined to suspect one another, or to fear that through some lack of loyalty one or other of them would be disadvantaged (...)" (cited in Weston, 1980: 304).

played by international bank consortia. The interpretation
presented here does not imply an absence of cooperation among
banks at the national level. On the contrary, the number of
cartel-agreements, joint-ventures and consortia among banks
on the national plane is large (see for example Gans (1978:
569) for the Netherlands and Mintz and Schwartz (forthcoming)
for the United States). This fact does not contradict our
conclusions but can be explained within the model presented
here. The very fact that so many collusive arrangements exist
at the national level makes that competition takes on an
international form. The national financial markets are so
organized and divided among the major banks that the
possibilities for competition are very restricted. Indeed,
the international market is the only 'space' that has not
been subject to a rigid oligopolistic division. Read the
opinion of a leading banker on this topic:

"The trend towards internationalization has in it an
element of aggressiveness, of business-getting effort,
that cannot fail to increase the temperature of the
competitive atmosphere. Furthermore, the whole Euro-
dollar market, which is the basis of this
internationalisation, is a free-for-all market, and the
most perfect competitive money market in existence,
untrammeled as it is by legal and institutional
regulations" (Thunholm, 1971: 114).

The only country that does not fit nicely into this
interpretation is Japan, where existing forms of cooperation
(like the Federation of Economic Organizations) are so
strong, and the interpenetration of business and state so
firm, that it is possible to speak of a business system with
a unified center, the Zaikai, which has been succesful in
restricting entrance into international financial markets.
But even in this case, the situation is changing. By 1976
direct interlocks among Japanese banks disappeared (see
Figure 7.1b) while in 1979 the restrictions on international
expansion of banking were liberalized (Schaft, 1980: 18).

7.4 The American banks

The formation of international bank consortia is a fairly
recent phenomenon. Only 10 out of the 127 consortia in our
survey were established before 1969; the rest (117) were
established between 1969 and 1974. As suggested earlier, the
main cause of the sudden surge of international consortium
banks was the development of the Euro-equity and -bond
market, which was induced by the Interest Equalization Tax in
1963 and the various other programs for improving the United
States balance of payments.

From the point of view of American banks, the day-to-day
financial servicing of established customers could easily be
rendered through local branches abroad. Establishing such
branches in financial centers like London, Frankfurt or Paris
provided easy access to the short term Euro-currency market.
However, participation in the Euro-equity and -bond market
required detailed knowledge in which their European
competitors had an initial advantage. Thus, for American
banks, participation in a joint-venture with European banks
seemed to be a rational strategy. In addition, the huge
amount of capital demanded by large multinationals in the
equity- and bond market required international cooperation
between the banks. The total amount of international
emissions of bonds and equity grew from a mere 346 million in
1963 to 4,483 million in 1971 (Arnoult and Lemaire, 1972:
88).

The most important consortia with American participation are
the ORION group in which Chase Manhattan Bank, National
Westminster Bank, Royal Bank of Canada and Westdeutsche
Landesbank und Girozentrale are the main participants, and
the Societe Financiere Europeenne (SFE) in which the Bank of
America, Barclays Bank, Banca Nazionale del Lavoro, Banque
National de Paris, Dresdner Bank and Algemene Bank Nederland
(ABN) dominate (see Table 7.4). Many others - some as diverse
as Mandel (1970) and Thunholm (1971) - argue that the
foundation of international consortia should be regarded as a
defensive reaction against American penetration of European
banking. Although the Europartners may be regarded as an
example of a 'European' reaction (the participants of
Europartners are Credit Lyonnais, Commerz Bank and Banco di
Roma), the argument does not hold for international consortia
in general. American banks are to be found in six of the nine
scales and thus maintain an important position in the network
of international bank cooperation. There are, however,
important differences among United States banks. While in the
network of interlocking directorates the New York financials
- Chase Manhattan, Morgan and Chemical Bank - are central
(connected with 12.4 percent and 13.8 percent of all
industrials in the sample), in the network of international
bank consortia the West Coast banks - Bank of America and
Western Bancorporation - dominate (participating in 11.8
percent and 7.9 percent of all consortia and joint-ventures)
(see Table 7.5).

If participation in international consortia is a defensive
reaction, it is a defensive reaction of those American banks
that are marginal in the United States financial
establishment, and thus marginal in the network of
interlocking directorates. The New York banks Morgan,

Chemical Bank and Chase Manhattan, which are central in the network of interlocking directorates, are marginal in the network of international consortia. The only New York bank that is central in both of these networks is First National City, although it is more central in the United States network than in the global network of interlocking directorates (see Section 5.2). The other two New York banks are marginal in both the interlock system and the network of international consortia. Most interesting, however, is that the West Coast banks, Bank of America and Western Bancorporation, are both marginal in the network of interlocking directorates but central in the network of international consortia (see Table 7.5).

Table 7.5 American banks: interlocking directorates and international consortia

	Headquarters	1	2	
Chemical Bank	New York	13.8	0.8	
J.P. Morgan	New York	13.8	3.1	
Chase Manhattan	New York	12.4	5.5	
First National City	New York	9.7	7.9	
Manufacturers Hanover	New York	2.1	4.0	[*]
Bankers Trust	New York	2.1	-	[*]
Western Bancorporation	Los Angeles	2.1	7.9	
Bank of America	San Francisco	2.1	11.8	

1: Percentage of firms in the sample with which they interlock

2: Percentage of international consortia in which they participate

[*] not in scale

The assumption that participation in the network of international consortia is a defensive reaction now gains plausibility. The West Coast banks may well have sought to improve their international as well as their national position vis-a-vis the New York financial establishment through cooperation with European banks. [8] The sudden growth of international consortia can thus be considered as a reaction of European and West Coast banks against the dominance of the New York financial establishment. Our hypothesis that banks look for international cooperation with the enemies of their enemy's friends seems indeed more plausible than the model derived from the theory of Mandel in which American and European banks confront each other on the international market.

7.5 Summary

In this chapter the international organization of the banking system has been analyzed. Because banks play a crucial role in the process of allocation of capital, patterns of competition and cooperation in the banking system may indicate the structure of competition and cooperation in the international business system. In Section 7.1 we demonstrated that while few interlocks exist among banks from the same country, several cross-national (advisory) ties occur. The number of international advisory interlocks increased dramatically between 1970 and 1976, indicating an increasing need for international consultation. From the lack of direct links between banks from the same country (the exception being Japan), it was assumed that banks competed at the national level. This was supported by the analysis in Section 7.2 of meeting-points between banks maintaining director ties with the same industrial firm. Assuming that such meeting-points indicate overlapping spheres of interests, we found that, within countries, banks tend to share spheres of interests. This interpretation was strengthened when international consortia and joint-ventures were taken into account: meeting-points in international consortia were exclusively international (again, with the exception of

[8] The American banks in the sample have been arranged in Table 7.5 in order of centrality in the network of interlocking directorates (column 1). The rank order of the same banks according to the number of international consortia in which they participate is negatively correlated to the former rank order (T[a]= -.54).

Japan). Our analysis made clear that banks seek international
cooperation to strengthen their position, internationally and
nationally, vis-a-vis their national competitors. This
mechanism was described as a bank's search for the enemies of
its enemy's friends. Because of this mechanism, the
international consortia are inherently unstable. They suffer
from a prisoner's dilemma: being potential enemies, the
members of the consortia are permanently attracted to
parasitic behavior, hence the inclination of each participant
to undermine the consortium by developing an autonomous
international strategy. This explains the stagnation in
international consortia formation and the rapid increase in
the number of foreign branches of European banks (Section
7.3). In Section 7.4 we analyzed the role of the American
banks. It appears that the West Coast banks, which are
marginal in the United States financial establishment, try to
enhance their national position by active participation in
the network of international consortia. This supports the
hypothesis that banks seek cooperation with the enemies of
their enemy's friends and confronts the vision of Mandel who
explains international consortia in terms of an American
challenge. The model based on the Bucharinist theories of
imperialism can thus be discarded. The choice between the
Leninist- and Kautskian-inspired theories is still open. The
models of global structure of intercorporate relations
derived from them differ only insofar as the Kautskian-
inspired theories predict relatively stable relations whil
the Leninist-inspired theories assume that international
alliances are inherently unstable. Although the conclusion
from Section 7.3 that international consortia are inherently
unstable contradicts the basic assumption of the Kautskian
theories, the evidence presented for that conclusion is weak.
To investigate the stability of the structure of
intercorporate relations, it is necessary to compare the
network over time. This will be done in the next chapter.

VIII THE IMPACT OF WORLD CRISIS: changes in the network

8.0 Introduction

Up to this point our analysis has been predominantly static. Only in Chapter 7 did the longitudinal comparison of interlocks between banks allow for some tentative conclusions about developments in the international banking system. In this chapter the dynamic aspects of the models inspired by economic theories of imperialism are central.

In Section 3.2 we argued that the economic theories of imperialism, and especially the Bucharinist and Leninist variants, are theories of crisis. Therefore, economic world crisis should bring the international economic structure closer to the model derived from these theories. This means that, according to the Bucharinist theories, the international economic structure would become more nationalized, and according to the Leninist and Kautskian theories, it would become more internationalized. The difference between the two is that the Leninist theories assume an inherent instability of the structure, while the Kautskian theories emphasize permanency in the structure.

In terms of interlocking directorates this means that increased national densities together with a decreasing number of international lines would lend some support to the Bucharinist theories while an increase in the number of international interlocks would favor the Leninist and Kautskian theories. Large 'unexpected' changes in the network would support the Leninist as against the Kautskian theories.

The conclusion from Chapter 7 enabled us to construct a new model, which cannot be derived directly from any of the above mentioned theories. This model has been suggested by the empirical findings presented in this book and leans heavily on the interpretation of meeting-points of banks in industrial firms as overlapping spheres of interests. The spheres of interests overlap predominantly at the national level, indicating a high potential for conflict and competition between banks from the same country. The cartelization and regulation of financial markets make competition at the national level difficult and dangerous. Therefore, the banks look for markets that are not yet subject to a rigid oligopolistic division. The international financial market is just such a relatively free 'space', and that is the main reason why competition takes an international form. Accordingly, it can be assumed that increased competition will enhance the overlap between spheres of interests at the national level and at the same time create an increased need for international cooperation. For interlocking directorates this means that both national and international densities will increase simultaneously. And since competition increases in times of economic crisis, we

can assume that the economic world crisis that broke out in
1973 will have such an impact on the network of interlocking
directorates. Our choice of which year to investigate after
1973 was of course influenced by a practical consideration:
the availability of annual reports at the time we carried out
the investigation. Nevertheless, the choice of 1976 is
theoretically appropriate because it allows for a time lag
between the outbreak of the economic world crisis in 1973 and
the (possible) impact of this crisis on the structure of
interlocking directorates. Creating new interlocks and
destroying existing ones takes time. For one thing, a
strategic decision has to be made to do either one (or both).
For another, this decision has to be implemented. Very little
is known about these processes, which take place behind the
walls of a board room. In choosing 1976 we have assumed that
within a time span of three years some first results of these
decision-making processes will become visible in the
structure of the network of interlocking directorates.
The premise of the comparison of the networks in 1970 and
1976 is that in 1970 the coming economic world crisis was not
yet anticipated to the extent of influencing the structure of
interlocking directorates, while by 1976 the crisis had
already had a decided impact on it.
In the following section we will first sketch the economic
aspects of the crisis in terms of gross national product and
direct foreign investment of the advanced capitalist
countries, and second, relate these developments to the
expansion of international financial markets. Interlocking
directorates in 1976 will be analyzed according to our
research design and compared with the network in 1970.

8.1 A new economic world order?

The oil crisis in 1973 and the subsequent economic recession
undermined the assumption of the super-imperialist theories
that stable relations between capitalist countries and a
fixed order of imperialist powers - with the United States at
the top and the European powers and Japan at subordinate
levels - were typical for the post-war world. Much has been
said since about a new international economic order in which
the developing countries, and especially the oil-producing
ones, become increasingly important.

The focus of this study is upon the consequences of the
economic crisis for the structure of the international
business system of the advanced capitalist countries. Some
important changes in international investment have been
widely noticed. The recent influx of European multinationals
into the United States, for example, has received much
publicity.

Table 8.1 Gross national product and outflow of direct
          investment for developed market economies, 1971–
          1976

Year	Gross national product	Outflow of direct investment [*]	Outflow of direct investment as share of GNP (Percentage)
	(Billions of dollars)	(Billions of dollars)	
1971	2 181.2	12.8	0.59
1972	2 512.8	14.5	0.58
1973	3 061.2	22.7	0.74
1974	3 380.0	21.0	0.62
1975	3 757.1	25.0	0.67
1976	4 093.4	24.4	0.60

[*] including reinvested earnings

Source: Transnational corporations, 1978: 235

Table 8.2 Changes in the share of total foreign investment of
          the advanced capitalist countries, 1971–1976

	Share in total direct foreign investment of the developed countries (Percentage) [*]			Changes		Foreign investment received from developed countries (Perc) [**]		Changes
	1971	1973	1976	71–76	73–76	1973	1976	73–76
U.S.A.	54.0	52.6	50.7	−3.3	−1.9	18.9	19.9	+1.0
Un. Kingdom	15.5	14.0	11.9	−3.6	−2.1	16.0	13.7	−2.3
W. Germany	4.8	6.2	7.4	+2.6	+1.2	12.0	12.7	+0
Japan	2.9	5.4	7.2	+4.3	+1.8	1.1	1.1	−
Switzerland	6.2	5.8	6.9	+0.7	+1.1	2.4	3.1	+0.7
France	4.8	4.6	4.4	−0.4	−0.2	5.8	5.9	+0.1
Canada	4.2	4.1	4.1	−0.1	−	28.8	28.8	−
Netherlands	2.6	2.9	3.6	+1.0	+0.7	4.3	5.0	+0.7
Sweden	1.6	1.6	1.8	+0.2	+0.2	1.5	1.5	−
Belg./Lux.	1.6	1.4	1.3	−0.3	−0.1	3.0	4.4	+1.4
Italy	2.0	1.7	1.1	−0.9	−0.6	6.3	3.8	−2.5

[*] calculated from Transnational Corporations, 1978: 236

[**] calculated from Kragenau, 1979: 22

Table 8.1 gives an overall picture for the period 1971-1976 of the growth of international investment in relation to gross national product for the 'developed market economies', i.e., the advanced capitalist countries. It shows both a relative and an absolute increase in foreign investment until 1973, after which there is a stabilization.

From table 8.2 we see that between 1971 and 1976, the United Kingdom, the United States, Italy, France and Belgium/Luxembourg have suffered a relative decline in the share of direct investment abroad. Japan, West Germany, the Netherlands and Switzerland, on the other hand, have considerably strengthened their positions as capital exporters. Of the countries whose share in direct investment abroad has declined, Belgium/Luxembourg and the United States have received a larger part of the foreign investment. The United Kingdom and Italy, however, have lost heavily in the share of direct investment abroad and in foreign investment received. In this respect, they have become less integrated into the world economy.
In sharp contrast, there is an increasing integration of German and Dutch capital into the world economy. Both countries have increased their share in direct investment abroad, as well as in foreign investment received from other countries. Japan has received no additional foreign capital between 1973 and 1976, but it has increased its direct investment abroad. Between 1971 and 1976, West Germany has increased its share from 4.8 to 7.4 percent of the total foreign investment of the developed market economies. Another consequence of the economic world crisis is the enhanced position of the financial institutions. The financial sector has increased its international investment more rapidly than the industrial sector. In all countries, except the United Kingdom, the financial institutions have increased their share in foreign investment (Transnational corporations, 1978: 242, 243). As a result, the banks have come to depend for their profits more and more on foreign earnings. According to the figures from Table 7.2 forty percent or more of the earnings of all United States banks in the sample in 1976 were foreign earnings. In 1970 this was only the case for one (First National City). For non-United States banks the trend has been in a similar direction, although in most cases, as yet, less pronounced (Channon, 1977: 190).

Table 8.3 Euro-currency market size
based on foreign-currency liabilities and claims of
banks in major European countries, the Bahamas,
Bahrein, Cayman Islands, Panama, Canada, Japan,
Hong Kong, and Singapore.
Billions of dollars (rounded to the nearest 5
billion) at end of period.

	1970	1971	1972	1973	1974	1975	1976	1977	1978 *
Estimated size									
Gross	110	145	200	305	375	460	565	695	890
1	30	30	35	55	75	80	100	125	165
2	15	15	25	40	60	70	85	110	120
3	65	100	140	210	240	310	380	460	605
Net	65	85	110	160	215	250	310	380	475
4	25	35	45	65	100	115	145	190	235
5	30	35	45	75	95	115	140	160	195
6	10	15	20	20	20	20	25	30	45
7	81	76	78	73	77	78	79	76	74

[*] revised
1: Liabilities to non-banks
2: Liabilities to central banks
3: Liabilities to other banks (includes unallocated
   liabilities)
4: Claims on non-banks
5: Claims on central banks and on banks outside market area
   (includes unallocated claims)
6: Conversions of Euro-funds into domestic currencies by
   banks in market area (in European market area only)
7: Euro-dollars as percentage of gross liabilities in all
   Euro-currencies

We suggested in Chapter 7 that there is a relation between
the oil crisis and the international expansion of banks
because of the necessity for 'recycling' the so-called petrodollars. Indeed, it can be seen from Table 8.3 that the Euro-
currency market increased rapidly after 1972 and that the
share of dollars in this market increased with it, after a
decline from 1970 to 1973 (see Table 8.3, last row). (We will
not discuss the decline of the position of the dollar after
1976 because it falls outside the period under
consideration.) As a result of a manifold increase of the
Euro-currency market, foreign affiliates and branches
proliferated (see Table 8.4). Between 1971 and 1976 the 50
largest banks created 488 foreign establishments in developed
countries, an increase of nearly fifty percent. These

branches and affiliates were and remain predominantly
situated in the international financial centers (London,
Paris, New York, Luxembourg). The developing countries also
experienced an increase in foreign establishments of large
banks, also situated in financial centers (Hong Kong,
Singapore, Bahrein, the Bahamas, Cayman Islands) and operated
under minimal supervision from national or international
governmental agencies. International bank consortia and
joint-ventures have been and continue to be created
especially for these so-called 'off-shore' market places.

Table 8.4 World's largest 50 banks by country of origin, size
        of total assets and number of foreign affiliates,
        end 1971 and 1976 [a]

Country	Number of banks [b]		Assets (Billions of dollars)[c]		Foreign [d] affiliates developed market economies	
	1971	1976	1971	1976	1971	1976
United States	13	10	195	348	324	419
Japan	12	12	123	318	119	189
W. Germany	5	8	57	218	92	166
France	3	4	40	170	33	97
Un. Kingdom	4	4	58	102	77	169
Canada	4	4	40	93	80	99
Netherlands	–	3	–	64	–	65
Italy	5	2	54	53	76	67
Switzerland	3	2	27	43	42	44
Brazil	1	1	9	39	8	24
Total	50	50	603	1448	851	1339

[a]: Japanese bank figures reflect the status as of 30
     September; Canadian bank figures are for 31 October
[b]: Consolidated bank group
[c]: Excluding contra accounts. Currencies have been
     converted at the rates of exchange which were current at
     the time the accounts were made.
[d]: Includes subsidiaries, affiliates, foreign branches and
     representative offices. These data, the most reliable
     and comprehensive available, may not be complete or
     accurate in every case.

Source: Transnational Corporations, 1978: 215

Corresponding to the changing patterns of foreign investment
between 1970 and 1976 is a change in rank order of the
largest banks. Three German and three Dutch banks entered the
list of the world's fifty largest banks, while three United
States banks and three Italian banks dropped out (Table 8.4,
columns 1 and 2).

Although the relative importance of international investment
has declined in relation to the aggregated gross national
product of the advanced capitalist countries since 1973, this
has not led to a decline in internationalization of financial
institutions.
Furthermore, the relative decline in international investment
has not struck all countries equally. Traditionally
internationally-oriented corporations of the United Kingdom
and the United States have lost ground to the newcomers from
Japan and West Germany. The small but internationally-
oriented economies of Switzerland and the Netherlands have
also increased their relative share in international
investment. In other words, what we have here is a relative
stagnation of the Anglo-Saxon firms and an international
expansion of the continental and Japanese firms. Only the
Italian and French firms do not seem to follow this general
pattern. Accordingly, for the network of interlocking
directorates in 1976 we can expect that the continental
European firms have a more central position in the
international network at the expense of the Anglo-Saxon
firms, and that banks have a more central position as well.

8.2 Selection of the 1976 sample

To compare the network of interlocking directorates of 1970
with that of 1976, should we take the same firms that we
selected in 1970? This procedure has the advantage of keeping
the set of firms identical, so that only the interlocks
between them are subject to change. The disadvantage,
however, is that the changing structure of the world economy
is not taken into consideration because we have used
different selection criteria for the two samples. If, on the
other hand, we select the firms in 1976 by using the
selection criteria for 1970, we obtain a different set of
firms, which renders comparison of the networks more
difficult.

The first procedure is the one we will follow because it enables us to compare the years 1970 and 1976 in terms of the changing structure of interlocking directorates in the same set of firms. [1] In this set, three pairs of firms merged between 1970 and 1976 (Peugeot with Citroen; Pechiney with Ugine Kuhlmann; Dunlopp with Pirelli), reducing the total of 176 firms to 173. Apart from that, one firm (Consolidated Tin Smelters) was not included in 1976 because the annual report could not be obtained. The 1970 set thus contains 172 firms in 1976.

8.3 The international corporate elite

8.3.1 Finance capitalists

There is surprisingly little difference in the number of persons carrying the network in 1970 and in 1976. The number of persons who carried at least one interlock – defined as the international corporate elite in Section 4.2 – was 372 in 1970 and 369 in 1976.
All the same, the number of persons maintaining a position in at least one bank and at least one industrial firm – defined as finance capitalists in Sections 1.4 and 4.3.1 – increased considerably from 262 in 1970 to 301 in 1976. The financial aspect of the international network of interlocking directorates has become stronger between 1970 and 1976.
Has this tendency also enhanced the role of the bankers in the network? As we observed in Section 7.1, the role of the

[1] A new selection in 1976, based on the same criteria used for the 1970 set, would have contained many new firms, mainly from the petroleum and car industries, while some of the non-ferrous metal and iron & steel firms would have disappeared from the sample (see Fennema and Kleyn, 1979). Industries with a high profit rate are more represented in the new sample, while those with a low profit rate are less represented (see Fennema and De Jong, forthcoming). Such changes express the relative growth and concentration of the petroleum and automobile industries, which may influence the network even if these changes are not taken into account in the sampling. Since we concluded in Section 5.3 that industrial concentration and economic centralization are supplementary rather than complementary phenomena, we can expect oil and automobile firms to be more central in the 1976 network at the expense of the metal industries.

bankers was relatively small in 1970: of the 601 interlocks a
mere 41 were carried by a banker. In 1976 the number of
interlocks carried by a banker increased to 67. This increase
is not spectacular, however, since the total number of
interlocks also increased from 601 to 723 (see Table 8.5).
The bankers may have become more important in the network,
but they still carried less than 10 percent of all interlocks
in 1976.

In Section 4.3.1 it was argued and confirmed for 1970 that
finance capitalists carried significantly more international
interlocks. In 1976, 27.7 percent of the interlocks carried
by a finance capitalist were international, as against 18.8
percent of those carried by a non-finance capitalist. [2]

8.3.2 Big linkers

Between 1970 and 1976 the number of interlocks increased.
This is true when we look at the absolute number (from 601 to
723), at the number of interlocks per director (from 1.62 to
1.94) or at the number of interlocks per firm (from 3.42 to
4.19).
Furthermore, there was a marked centralization in terms of
personnel. This becomes clear when one looks at the number of
persons with a position in at least four firms. In 1970 there
were 19 such big linkers; in 1976 there were 32. In 1970 the
big linkers carried 24 percent of all interlocks; in 1976
they carried 37 percent of all interlocks. In fact, the
increase in the number of interlocks between 1970 and 1976
was exclusively caused by an increase in the number of big
linkers, since the number of multiple directors remained
stable (Section 8.3.1). Table 8.5 shows that the number of
interlocks carried by persons with a position in two or three
firms was 459 in 1970 and 451 in 1976. The big linkers, on
the other hand, carried 142 interlocks in 1970 and 272 in
1976.
The network created by the big linkers contains in 1976 a
large component of 61 firms from 11 countries in contrast to
one of only 42 firms from 9 countries in 1970. The big
linkers obviously play a more significant role in cementing
the different national networks into an international
network.

[2] The probability that in a random distribution of all
    interlocks at least 178 of the international interlocks are
    carried by a finance capitalist is less than 5 percent.

Table 8.5 Distribution of interlocking directorates (1970-
        1976)

n. of firms in which a a function is held (n)	n. of inter- locking directorates n(n-1)/2	n. of persons 1970	1976	n. of interlocks 1970	1976
7	21	1	4	21	84
6	15	1	-	15	-
5	10	1	5	10	50
4	6	16	23	96	138
3	3	53	57	159	171
2	1	300	280	300	280
Total:		372	369	601	723

We said in Section 4.3.2 that the big linkers have a high
potential for international communication. The considerable
increase in the number of big linkers and the fact that they
carried nearly two-fifths of all interlocks in 1976 as
against one-quarter in 1970 lead us to believe that
international communication and coordination in the network
have increased. This conclusion is underscored by the
increase in number of international interlocks. In 1970
eighteen percent of all interlocks were international
interlocks; in 1976 thus was 27 percent. In the next section
we will analyze this increase.

Apart from the increase in number, the change in position of
the big linkers is suprisingly large. Of the 19 big linkers
in 1970, only 9 retained a position in four or more firms in
1976. Of the remaining 10, three disappeared altogether and
thus no longer belonged to the international corporate elite.
In five years this seems to be a considerable reshuffle
although we have no comparable data on which to base such a
conclusion. It is impossible to say whether this sort of
reshuffle is an inherent characteristic of the international
corporate elite or induced by the economic world crisis.

8.4 International versus national integration

Up to this point we have confined our analysis to an analysis
of the international corporate elite and the overall number
of interlocks they carry. To compare the national and
international integration in 1970 and 1976, we calculated the
international as well as the national lines in the 1976
network. The total number of lines is 470 (see Table 8.7);
152 of these are international lines and 318 are national
lines. Although there are still significantly more national
lines [3] , the number of international lines has increased
absolutely as well as relatively when compared to 1970: 32.5
percent of all lines in 1976 were international as opposed to
25 percent in 1970. The international bipartite density has,
not surprisingly, increased for nearly all countries. Only in
the case of Italy and Sweden has there been no increase in
the international integration (see Table 8.6, column 4).
Although the total number of national lines has hardly
increased, the national densities of the different countries
have changed greatly. Of the nine countries with six or more
firms in the sample five have increased and four have
decreased in national density. The increase is most
spectacular for West Germany, France, Canada and Switzerland.
With the exception of Canada, these are also the countries in
which the international bipartite density has doubled.

The only country that has doubled in international bipartite
density and lost in national density is Holland. Here, the
addition in 1972 of a new binational firm (ESTEL) has
influenced the international density positively (through the
links of Hoesch as part of ESTEL) and the national density
negatively (through the addition of an extra firm in the
Dutch subset). However, since the absolute number of lines
has decreased from 10 to 9, the 'loosening' of the Dutch
network cannot be explained by this 'artifact' alone. Mokken
and Stokman (1979b) have analyzed the network of interlocking
directorates among about eigthy-five of the largest Dutch
firms. The density of this network declined considerably
between 1969 and 1972, and slightly between 1972 and 1976.
Between 1972 and 1976 the structure of the network changed
completely, as if to make up for the loss of communication
efficiency. This finding of Mokken and Stokman could be
extended to explain the position of the largest Dutch firms

[3] The probability that a random distribution of the total
    number of lines (470) among all possible pairs of firms
    would result in a distribution in which 318 or more lines
    are between firms from the same nationality is less than 1
    percent.

in the international network. Indeed, one could argue that
the enormous increase in international density was attained
at the expense of the national density, but that a drastic
restructuring of the national network compensated for the
drop in national density.

The other country where national density decreased while the
international (bipartite) density increased between 1970 and
1976 is Great Britain. Fortunately, an extensive study by
Overbeek provides us with a more detailed picture of the
development of the British network between 1970 and 1976.
Overbeek (1978) investigated the density of the network
between twenty-six large industrial corporations, four
clearing banks, nine large insurance companies and twelve of
the most important merchant banks. The density in the network
of interlocking directorates between these firms increased
from 9 percent in 1972 to 10 percent in 1976. This study
contradicts the findings for the British national network in
our sample but is in line with the expected correlation
between the increase in national and international densities.

Table 8.6 National and international densities (1970-1976)

| | 1970 | | | | |
| | 1 | 2 | 3 | 4 | 5 |
	n. of firms	n. of international lines	n. of national lines	international bipartite density %	national density %
United States	33	54	75	1.1	14.2
Un. Kingdom	30	38	29	0.9	6.7
W. Germany	19	25	78	0.8	45.0
France	17	12	18	0.4	13.2
Canada	11	23	12	1.3	21.8
Switzerland	10	15	27	0.9	60.0
Italy	9	16	12	1.1	33.3
Sweden	7	7	10	0.6	47.6
Netherlands	6	24	10	2.4	66.7
Belg./Lux.	3	3	1	0.6	33.3
Australia	2	0	0	0.0	0.0
South Africa	1	3	0	1.7	-
Japan	30	0	31	-	7.1
Total:		101	303		

	1	2	1 9 7 6 3	4	5
	n. of firms	n. of interna- tional lines	n. of nation- al lines	inter- nation- al bi- partite density %	nation- al den- sity %
United States	33	76	80	1.7	15.2
Un. Kingdom	29	44	24	1.1	5.9
W. Germany	19	65	95	2.1	55.6
France	15	22	26	0.9	24.8
Canada	11	26	18	1.5	32.7
Switzerland	10	27	32	1.6	71.1
Italy	9	17	10	1.1	27.8
Sweden	7	7	8	0.6	38.1
Netherlands	7	48	9	4.2	42.9
Belg./Lux.	3	10	1	2.0	33.3
Australia	2	3	0	0.9	0.0
South Africa	1	3	0	1.8	-
Japan	30	1	15	0	3.4
Total:		152	318		

If we explain the Dutch and British exceptions to the
expected correlations in this way, we may then conclude that
Table 8.6 suggests that international integration increased
in those countries where national integration also increased.
The finding corroborates the hypothesis formulated in Section
8.0 that in times of economic crisis the international
integration of the network of interlocking directorates
coincides with a national integration resulting from an
increased overlap between the spheres of interests of the
banks.

However, the density of a network is but one measure of its
compactness. The increase in the number of interlocking
directorates may have three different effects on the network.
First the connectivity of the network may increase, i.e., the
number of components may decrease. Second, the density may
increase, while the connectivity remains the same, i.e., the
paths within existing components become shorter. Third, the
multiplicity may increase, while the number of lines remains
the same, i.e., the lines between firms become thicker.
Of course in reality the three will appear simultaneously.

Indeed, between 1970 and 1976 the connectivity of the global network increased from 53.6 to 60.8 percent, due to the growth of the large component. [4] In contrast to the complete isolation of the Japanese component in 1970, in 1976 two Japanese firms became directly linked to the Atlantic component. Such an integration into the Atlantic network was predicted in Section 8.1 and has been mentioned by several authors. In reference to the automobile industry, Louis Wells, for example, notes:

"Although the president of one major European firm was still able to say in 1973 that he knew personally of all American and European automobile firms but had never met a top manager of a Japanese manufacturer, that situation was changing. The Japanese firms were beginning to develop ties with American firms through joint-ventures and they were establishing some loose ties with European manufacturers" (Wells, 1974: 251).

In addition to the growing number of connected firms, the increase in the number of lines led to an increasing density of the global network: from 2.6 to 3.2 percent. Finally, the multiplicity of the lines also increased. This growing thickness expresses itself by the growing number of lines at higher levels of multiplicity. For example, in 1970 the thickest line is between Deutsche Bank and Daimler-Benz with a multiplicity of 6. In 1976 the thickest line is still between Deutsche Bank and Daimler-Benz, but its multiplicity is now 9. In 1970 there are 19 lines with a multiplicity of 4 or more, while there are 31 such lines in 1976 (see Table 8.7).

The components of the network at different levels of tightness are shown in Figure 8.1.

To sum up, we find in 1976 a higher number of interlocking directorates, a higher average of interlocks per interlocking director and per firm, an increased density, an increased connectivity and an increased thickness of the network.

[4] Part of this increase in connectivity may also be due to the decreasing number of firms in the sample as a consequence of mergers between 1971 and 1976 (see Section 8.2). The increase in connectivity of the global network is predominantly caused by the increase in connectivity of the Western network from 75.6 in 1970 to 80.7 in 1976.

Table 8.7 Multiplicity of the lines in 1970 and 1976

Multiplicity	1970	1976
≥6	3	4
5	4	5
4	12	21
3	26	29
2	78	85
1	281	325
Total:	404	470

8.5 Centrality in the nested network (1976)

For 1976 we again analyzed the network of interlocking directorates at subsequent levels of thickness, starting at multiplicity-level one. We will compare this series of nested networks with that in 1970 (see Figure 8.1). In 1976 at multiplicity-level one there again exists one large component, Chase 134, which contains firms from all countries including Japan. The absolute separation between the Western business system and the Japanese business system has been broken by an interlocking directorate between the Canadian Imperial Bank of Commerce and Nippon Electric, which in turn brings the Sumitomo Bank into the Atlantic component. But rather than linking the former Japanese component to the former Morgan 127, these two Japanese firms, which are now part of the Atlantic component, are isolated from the other Japanese firms, which are now divided into four different components. There is an integration of some Japanese firms into the Atlantic business system and at the same time a fragmentation of the Japanese business system. The number of isolated Western firms has decreased, while the number of isolated Japanese firms has increased. [5]

The large component Chase 134 has a density of .05 and contains all interlocks between Western firms (457): this density is slightly higher than the density of Morgan 127 in 1970, which contained all but one of the lines between Western firms and had a density of 0.046. The overall density

[5] Because we could not obtain all annual reports for 1970, the results of the Japanese network are not very reliable.

of the Western network has increased. But what about the
internal structure of the large component? Has there been a
change in the rank order of most central firms? Table 8.8
gives the top ten percent most central firms according to
local centrality. When we compare this table with the same
table in 1970 (Table 5.4), we see that the adjacency-number
shows an overall increase. In 1970 the thirteen most central
firms average 15.2 neighbors; in 1976 this number has
increased to 20. In the period 1970-1976 the American banks
have lost their absolute top position in the rank order of
local centrality. Only Chase Manhattan has maintained its
position. J.P. Morgan, Chemical Bank and First National City
decreased not only relatively but in absolute number of
adjacent firms. That the restructuring of the international
network favored the continental European firms, as predicted
in Section 8.2, is apparent from the fact that Deutsche Bank,
Dresdner Bank and Schweizerische Bankgesellschaft increased
their local centrality. The position of the banks has not
been shaken. On the contrary, in 1976 seven rather than six
firms in the top ten percent in local centrality are banks.
This meets the expectation formulated in the introduction to
this chapter that during the economic crisis banks would
strengthen their central position in the network, both
through an increasing number of international advisory lines
with other banks (see Section 7.1) and through a higher
number of interlocks with industrial firms. Indeed the number
of lines between banks and industry increased from 221 in
1970 to 257 in 1976. Fifty percent of these are officer-
interlocks, as against 30 percent in the network as a whole
(see Section 8.6). This means that the interlocks between
banks and industry are in general more purposive.

Table 8.8 Top ten percent in component Chase 134 according to
         local centrality (1976)

	Firm	Natio-nality	Product group	Adjacency number[*]
1	Chase Manhattan	U.S.A.	Banks	27
2	Deutsche Bank	W. Germany	Banks	25
3	Can. Imperial Bank	Canada	Banks	22
4	Chemical Bank	U.S.A.	Banks	21
5	Dresdner Bank	W. Germany	Banks	21
6	Ford Motor Co.	U.S.A.	Automobiles	20
7	Mannesmann	W. Germany	Heavy Machin.	20
8	J.P. Morgan	U.S.A.	Banks	19
9	Schweizer. Bankgesell.	Switzerland	Banks	18
10	Volkswagen	W. Germany	Automobiles	18
11	Royal Dutch/Shell	Dutch/Brit.	Petrochem.	17
12	Daimler-Benz	W. Germany	Automobiles	16
13	Siemens	W. Germany	Elect.-tech	16

[*] Number of adjacent firms in the component.

Table 8.9 Top ten percent in component Chase 134 according to
         global centrality (1976)

	Firm	. Natio-nality	Product group	Mean dist[*]
1	Ford Motor Co	U.S.A.	Automobiles	2.11
2	Can. Imperial Bank	U.S.A.	Banks	2.18
3	Chase Manhattan	U.S.A.	Banks	2.20
4	Deutsche Bank	W. Germany	Banks	2.21
5	Chemical Bank	U.S.A.	Banks	2.23
6	Schweizer. Bankgesell.	Switzerland	Banks	2.29
7	Royal Dutch/Shell	Dutch/brit.	Petrochem.	2.35
8	J.P. Morgan	U.S.A.	Banks	2.36
9	Dresdner Bank	W. Germany	Banks	2.41
10	Bayer	W. Germany	Chemical	2.47
11	U.S. Steel	U.S.A.	Iron & Steel	2.47
12	Standard Oil N.J.	U.S.A.	Petrochem.	2.49
13	Volkswagen	W. Germany	Automobiles	2.50

[*] Mean distance to the other firms in the component

If we consider global centrality, it becomes even clearer
that the New York banks have lost their dominant position in
the network. Only Chase Manhattan remains among the top three
(see Table 8.9). Compared with the most central firms in
Morgan 127 the banks have become more strongly represented in
the top ten percent in global centrality, although Ford has
the highest global centrality in Chase 134. The Dutch firm
AKZO, the Canadian International Nickel and General Electric
(U.S.) have disappeared from both centrality scores, while
Schweizerische Bankgesellschaft, Ford, Volkswagen and
Canadian Imperial have entered both. In Chase 134 there is a
stronger overlap between local and global centrality than
there was in Morgan 127. This supports the conclusion that
there is more international integration in the network of
1976 than in the network of 1970.
The cohesion in the international network depends less on the
international orientation of the New York banks and the Dutch
multinationals. In 1976 the German firms are much more
pronounced, while the Canadian Imperial Bank of Commerce and
Schweizerische Bankgesellschaft also have a central position
in the international network. For details of the changes in
the component structure at multiplicity-levels two and three,
the reader is referred to Figure 8.1. In general there is a
stronger 'nationalization' at the higher levels of
multiplicity in 1976 than in 1970. There is even a
fragmentation in the Dutch, Italian and Japanese networks.
The main changes, however, occur in the French network where
mergers in the automobile and iron and steel industries have
induced a thickening of the network (see Figure 8.1: Pechiney
7 at multiplicity-level two and Pechiney 4 at multiplicity-
level three). In the American network at multiplicity-level
three, the 1970 component Morgan 10 has broken down into a
Canadian component Ferguson 6 and United States component
Morgan 6. In Europe things are more complicated. On the one
hand, there are two separate Dutch components (AMRO 2 and ABN
2) at multiplicity-level three; on the other hand, Shell is
part of the German component Dresdner Bank 19, while in 1970
Shell formed a separate component with its American
subsidiary Shell Oil. This exception to the tendency towards
'nationalization' in 1976 may possibly be explained by the
problems confronting German industry during the oil crisis
because of the lack of an independent German oil industry.
This enabled Shell to penetrate the German chemical market
and subsequently to become heavily interlocked with German
industrials.

So far, the analysis of the network of 1976 supports the
model summarized in the introduction to this chapter. The
economic world crisis did lead to an increased competition
between the banks, expressed in a higher overlap of spheres

of interests at the national level; hence, we see the
increased density of most national networks and a tendency
towards 'nationalization' of the international network at the
higher levels of multiplicity. Such an interpretation is
further supported by the analysis of the lines between banks
and industry. Application of the Mokken scale analysis to the
lines between banks and industry in 1976 yields eleven
scales, most of which bear no resemblance to the scales in
1970 (see Table 7.3). Only the United States, German and
Swiss scales still exist in 1976. The number of binational
scales has decreased from three to one, while there now exist
two Italian and two United States scales, the latter two
being formed by the West Coast banks and the New York banks
respectively. Only First National City fits into both scales
and can therefore be regarded as a sort of junction between
the West Coast and the New York interests. The specific
position of First National City was already apparent in Table
7.5 where it scored equally high on adjacency in the network
of interlocking directorates and on participation in
international bank consortia. The overlapping spheres of
interests have become more national in the period 1970-1976
and in the case of the American banks, even more
regionalized. [6]

8.6 Domination and control in the 1976 network

In Chapter 6 the network of officer-interlocks in 1970 was
analyzed and interpreted as a network of domination and
control. It was shown that the international interlocks were
predominantly weak ties, based on an outside position in the
interlocked firms. Such weak ties were interpreted as
channels of communication rather than of domination and
control. Tight ties, based on an inside position in both
interlocked firms, were interpreted as concern relations.
Such tight ties appeared to be rare. Table 8.10 gives the
distribution of these different types of interlocks for the
1976 network.

[6] The Italian banks form two separate scales (Credito
    Italiano/Banco di Roma and Banca Nationale del Lavoro/Banca
    Commerciale Italiana); however, since the two scales are
    based on one meeting-point in each case, this is not very
    meaningful.

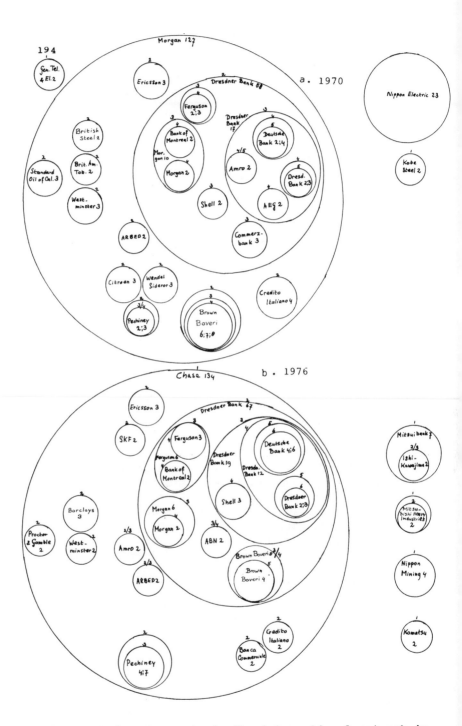

Figure 8.1 Nested components in the international network in 1970 and 1976

Table 8.10 Interlocking directorates according to the
position of the interlocking director in both
firms (1976)

		outside			inside	
		AD	OD	CH	ID	TOP
	AD	12	76	15	. 10	20 .
outside	OD		293	97	. 87	85 .
	CH			8	. 7	4 .
inside	ID				, 6	3 ,
	TOP				,	0 ,

-----: weak ties
.....: strong ties (officer-interlocks)
,,,,,: tight ties

AD: Member of advisory board or committee
OD: Outside director in a one-board corporation; member of
     supervisory board in a two-board corporation
CH: Chairman of the board of directors in a one-board
     corporation; chairman of the supervisory board in a two-
     board corporation
ID: Inside director in a one-board corporation; member of
     the executive board in a two-board corporation
TOP: President or managing director in a one-board
     corporation; chairman of the executive board in a two-
     board corporation

Compared to 1970 (see Table 4.5) the number of weak ties
(outside – outside) has increased from 408 (68 percent) to
501 (69 percent); the number of officer-interlocks has
increased from 178 (30 percent) to 213 (30 percent) and the
number of tight ties has decreased from 15 (2.5 percent) to 9
(1.3 percent).
Thus, although the absolute number of weak ties and officer-
interlocks has increased, the relative number of weak ties in
relation to the officer-interlocks has remained remarkably

stable. In 1970 as well as in 1976 nearly one-third of all
interlocks are officer-interlocks, while two-thirds are weak
ties.

The network as a whole has become more dense between 1970 and
1976. This is not attributable to either a spectacular
increase in the density of the network of control and
coordination or an increase in the network of communication.
In other words, the functions performed by the international
network of interlocking directorates do not seem to have
changed between 1970 and 1976.
The structure of the network of officer-interlocks has,
nevertheless, changed considerably. A component-analysis of
this network in 1976, neglecting the direction of the
officer-interlocks, shows that the national fragmentation in
1976 is not as strong as it was in 1970 but moves in the same
direction: the British and Italian firms form separate
components, while the majority of firms forms a large
component Chase 99 (comparable to Morgan 78, see Section
6.2.1.1). In terms of both local and global centrality the
German banks have become more central while the United States
banks have become less central: only Chemical Bank has
retained its 1970 position. Furthermore, the Canadian
Imperial Bank of Commerce belongs in 1976 to the top ten
percent most central firms in component Chase 99. In the
network of officer-interlocks, the German, Canadian and Swiss
banks have strengthened their positions at the expense of the
American firms.

In Section 6.2.0 it was argued that the network of multiple
directed and reciprocal lines (the network of officer-
interlocks at a higher multiplicity-level) can be interpreted
as a network of control. A complete rearrangement of the
components has taken place. All American firms are now
isolated, while the German and Swiss firms form the bulk of
the still interlocked firms. Only Shell 2 and Pechiney 2 form
stable components over the years. New components in 1976 are
Brown Boveri 6, August Thyssen 3 and Deutsche Bank 2. The
network of control has become looser in America and thicker
in West Germany and Switzerland.

So far, the direction of the officer-interlocks has been
neglected. The strong component analysis takes the direction
of these officer-interlocks into account. A strong component
is defined as a direct subnetwork in which all firms can
reach each other through a consecutive series of arcs. There
exists in a strong component a mutual reachability of the
firms; this compelled us in Chapter 6 to consider the strong
component as an operationalization of the concept
constellation of interests (see Section 6.2.). The German and

Swiss strong components from 1970 (see Figures 6.7 and 6.9) still exist in 1976, although in the German strong component the number of arcs has tripled, and the most central firm (Deutsche Bank) did not even belong to the strong component in 1970. The United States/Canadian strong component in 1970 (<u>Morgan</u> 5, see Figure 6.8) has disappeared completely. The enormous reshuffle of strong ties and the instability of the strong components make it difficult to believe that strong components do indicate constellations of interests, unless one assumes that the constellations of interests are in themselves very unstable structures.

Rather, it seems plausible that clusters in the network of control stem from temporary alliances and client-relationships between banks and industry. Compared to 1970, banks have become more central in the strong components; however, since they have in 1976 as many incoming as outgoing arcs, there is still no reason to assume them to be in a controlling position <u>vis-a-vis</u> industrial corporations.

8.7 <u>Summary</u>

Until 1973 international direct investment increased in absolute terms as well as in relation to gross national product. After 1973 there was a relative decline of international direct investment. During the economic crisis, Japan, West Germany, the Netherlands and Switzerland increased their share in foreign investment, while the United Kingdom, United States, Italy, France and Belgium/ Luxembourg suffered a relative decline. Taking capital imports into account as well, there was a marked integration into the world economy of West Germany, Japan and the Netherlands, and a marked disintegration of the United Kingdom and Italy. In all countries, except the United Kingdom, the banks increased their relative share in capital export and, notwithstanding the contraction of international investment after 1973, spectacularly enhanced their international position.

On the basis of the findings in Chapters 6 and 7, we predicted a stronger overlap of the spheres of interests of the banks at the national level and at the same time an increasing international integration of the network, especially through the Japanese, German and Dutch national subnetworks. Both tendencies were indeed found to exist. The number of big linkers increased over time and with them the international centralization in the network of communication. The international network also become <u>thicker</u> between 1970 and 1976, but in the opposite direction: at the higher levels of multiplicity the components have become more national. The analysis allows for the conclusion that competition between

banks at the national level has increased, leading to a
stronger overlap in spheres of interests between banks from
the same nationality.
Although a certain national integration has taken place in
many Western countries, international integration in the
network of interlocking directorates has been much stronger.
Except for the Netherlands, the strongest international
integration was found for those countries who also
experienced an increase in the density of their national
networks.
These findings are contradictory if they have to be explained
according to the two models derived from the Bucharinist
theories on the one hand, and the Leninist and Kautskian
theories on the other hand. But they can be explained in our
own model, summarized in Section 8.0. This model is based on
an interpretation of meeting-points between banks in
industrial firms as overlapping spheres of interests, and on
the dialectical relation between the national and the
international business system. International interlocks are
primarily an expression of coordinating activities with the
enemies of the enemy's friends. This mechanism, explained in
Chapter 7, produces uneasy alliances, due to the prisoner's
dilemma that the allies are potential enemies for one
another. The oil crisis has induced a further
internationalization of the banking system expressed in many
international advisory interlocks between banks. At the same
time, and due to increasing competition, banks from the same
nationality have tried to strengthen their relations with
industrial firms through more interlocks, forcing each other
to follow suit. This has led to a higher density of most of
the national networks, while at the same time fragmentation
has increased at the higher levels of multiplicity (see
Figure 8.1). For this reason increasing density at the
national level goes with increasing integration in the
international network.

> Men see little, presume a great
> deal, and so jump to the
> conclusion.

John Locke

IX SUMMARY AND CONCLUSIONS

9.1 Introduction

In this final chapter, we will discuss some of the important findings of our investigation and take the liberty of formulating a few conclusions that are not, as yet, based on hard empirical evidence, but may nonetheless stimulate further research.

In the first chapter, we argued that the development of interlocking directorates among large business corporations at the end of the nineteenth century can be explained by Hilferding's theory of finance capital. In Chapter 2 we showed that the same phenomenon can also be explained by the neo-classically inspired theory of the 'new economists'. We found that both theoretical approaches provide similar and, for the explanation of networks of interlocking directorates, compatible conclusions. We chose the theory of finance capital as the framework for this study, because it provides a better explanation for the internationalization of capital.

The international network of interlocking directorates can be regarded as an indication of the internationalization of finance capital. The existence of such a network, demonstrated in Chapter 5, supports the notion of international finance capital, especially because banks are the most central firms in this international network. The strengthening of the international network and the increased centrality of banks between 1970 and 1976 are only further evidence. In times of crisis, banks will more central because:

> "capital accumulation on a given technical basis has to
> be abandoned, and capital has to be amassed in money
> form to enable its organized reinsertion into at least
> partially renewed production processes. The mobility of
> banking capital (...) entitles it to prominence in
> periods of restructuration of capital" (Van der Pijl,
> forthcoming).

This interpretation needs, of course, other evidence than the banks' position in the network of interlocking directorates. In his thesis, Van de Pijl shows that banks increased their

Furthermore, international restructuration of capital has
been evidenced by the relative increase of German, Dutch and
Swiss international investment and the corresponding
ascendance of these countries' firms in the network of
interlocking directorates. A further analysis of this
phenomenon would require comparison of the position of
different industries over time, both in terms of profit rate
and in terms of network centrality. Such an analysis has not
been undertaken in the present study because the size of our
sample is too small to have sufficiently large product groups
to compare. It will be attempted, however, in a transnational
study of intercorporate structures to be edited by Stokman,
Ziegler and Scott. [1]

9.2 The structure of the international corporate elite

Because the concept of international finance capital is a
very general one, it helps little in explaining the specific
structure of the international network. We therefore examined
the economic theories of imperialism (Chapter 3) and from
them derived two basic models from which we were a to predict
a certain structure of the network of corporate interlocks.
From the theories of Bucharin and those who follow his basic
tenets, we deduced that there exists a cohesive network of
corporate interlocks at the national level cementing the
unity of the business system and expressed in the concept of
state capitalist trust. Since competition takes the form of
international rivalry between these state capitalist trusts,
few international interlocks exist and international cohesion
is weak. The model derived from the Bucharinist theories of
Mandel and Rowthorn deviate only slightly from this model.
According to Mandel, there exists a growing network of
corporate interlocks among firms from EEC countries,
indicating the integration of the Common Market. The model
derived from Mandel's theory would have cohesive national
networks and few international interlocks, except for the
continental Common Market countries, where international
interlocks would abound. Rowthorn's theory would also lead us
to believe that there are few international interlocks,

[1] This project, sponsored by the European Consortium for
    Political Research, will analyze the network of
    interlocking directorates among the 250 largest
    corporations in 9 countries. These countries are Austria,
    Belgium, West Germany, Finland, France, Italy, the
    Netherlands, United Kingdom, United States, and
    Switzerland.

except for the Dutch and British multinationals, which, for
the lack of a strong nation state, tend to accommodate the
policies and structures of business systems other than their
own.

The second basic model we derived from the theories of
Kautsky and Lenin. According to both theories one would
expect a cohesive network of interlocking directorates
between firms from different countries. From the Kautskian
theory of super-imperialism and the Leninist theory of
Poulantzas, we deduced that this international network is
dominated by American firms. Such dominance may find
expression in the direction of the interlocks between United
States and non-United States corporations. Since the theories
of imperialism are typically theories of crisis, one would
expect the actual structures of interlocking directorates to
come closer to the respective models during economic crisis.
Thus, we assumed that if the structure of interlocking
directorates between 1970 and 1976 were to come closer to one
of the two basic models, this would support the theories on
which that model was derived.

The results of our investigation definitely contradict the
model derived from Bucharinist theories. There exists a
cohesive international network of interlocking directorates.
Because the international interlocks are predominantly weak
ties, the network should be considered primarily a
communication network rather than a network of domination and
control. The network has increased in density between 1970
and 1976 mainly through an increase of international
interlocks from 25 percent in 1970 to 32.5 percent in 1976.
The need for international consultation clearly has grown,
and, as a result, the international corporate system has
become more integrated, largely as a result of an increase in
the number of big linkers in the network.

Only the 1970 Japanese network conforms to the model derived
from the Bucharinist theories. There are in 1970 no
interlocks between Japanese firms and firms from other
countries. Moreover, there are many direct interlocks among
Japanese banks. The Zaikai, an informal organization of
Japanese big business, in which the state plays an important
part, can indeed be regarded as a sort of state capitalist
trust. By 1976, however, the complete isolation of the
Japanese network had been lifted: two Japanese firms were
related to a Canadian bank, the remaining Japanese network
had become fragmented, and the interlocks among the banks had
disappeared. Because of incomplete data on the Japanese
corporate directors we did not analyze the Japanese network,
emphasizing instead the network of non-Japanese firms. In

this network the Australian firms were also isolated, so it could be properly called a Western or Atlantic network, consisting of one very large component and a few isolated firms.

Between 1970 and 1976 the Western network had become denser and more connected. We found as well a higher average of interlocks per multiple director and an increased thickness of the Western network. Such developments could have been explained by the theories of Kautsky and Lenin or one of their successors if the national networks had not become denser at the same time, especially in those countries which had also become more integrated in the international network. Because this combination of trends is difficult to explain by any of the economic theories of imperialism presented in Chapter 3, it encouraged us to take up the conclusions from the analysis of international bank cooperation from Chapter 7 and present our own model. According to this model, banks have overlapping spheres of interests at the national level, indicated by meeting-points through industrial firms. These overlapping spheres of interests induce them to compete. Competition at the national level, however, is hampered by a rigid oligopolistic division of the national financial markets. Therefore, banks look for international expansion and international alliances to strengthen their position at home and abroad. In the seventies, these alliances took the form of international bank consortia in which banks seek cooperation with the enemies of their enemies' friends. These consortia operate in international financial markets, which are contrary to the national financial markets, "free for all" because they are untrammeled "by legal and institutional regulations" as the Swedish banker Lars-Erik Thunholm noted in 1971. This argument is very similar to that of Hilferding for the explanation of international investment but has been specified here to explain the international strategy of banks. Moreover, we have shown with a stochastic scale analysis that the structure of interlocking directorates between banks and industry and the structure of international bank consortia correspond with this model.

The banks that have joined an international consortium are, however, confronted with a prisoner's dilemma because the enemies of their enemies' friends are not necessarily allies. On the contrary, they are potential competitors. Hence there is the inclination of each participant to undermine the consortium by developing an autonomous international strategy alongside the strategy of the consortium. This makes international consortia inherently unstable and explains why the consortium boom from the beginning of the seventies suddenly stagnated after 1975.

The model presented in Chapters 7 and 8 sheds a new light on the relation between international strategy and international structure. It shows that the structure of the international corporate interlocks depends on the strategy of these corporations. But it also shows that, once the structure has come into existence, the strategic freedom of the individual firms is severely restricted. If the majority of banks participate in international consortia, those remaining have no choice but to form an international consortium as well. And vice versa, once a number of banks in a consortium start to undermine it with a separate international strategy, the 'loyal' banks can not do otherwise than develop an autonomous strategy as well. Two important theoretical conclusions can be drawn fro this finding. The first is that the structure of corporate interlocks is relatively independent from the strategy of each of the corporations; it is the unintended result of a multitude of separate strategies. The second is that the structure itself constrains the strategic options of each individual firm. This underlines the theoretical propositions put forward by Norbert Elias in terms of 'gamemodels':

   "(...) the course of the game cannot be determined by
   any of the players. One can express this also
   positively by saying: the course of the game has in its
   turn power over the behaviour and the thinking of each
   of the individual players" (Elias, 1971: 104).

The emphasis on the relation between strategy and structure is the quintessence of the network approach. We found, for example, that the West Coast banks, which were marginal in the network of interlocking directorates, were very central in the network of international bank consortia. This was interpreted as a defensive strategy. Being marginal in the United States financial establishment, these banks looked for international alliances to strengthen their position both at home and abroad.

9.3 Conflict or cooperation?

The conclusion that banks seek international alliances with the enemies of their enemies' friends leans heavily on the interpretation of meeting-points between banks as overlapping spheres of interests. However, the term meeting-point is somewhat misleading here because far more industrialists are found on the boards of banks than bankers on the boards of industrial firms. In the majority of cases, the term refers to a situation where two banks have executives of the same industrial firm on their boards. This finding is consistent

with the result of Mizruchi's study of interlocking
directorates among 167 American corporations in 1974. Of the
officer-interlocks between banks and industry 40 percent was
carried by bankers, while the remaining 60 percent was
carried by industrialists. The Dutch network, on the other
hand, showed an inverse relation. Of the officer-interlocks
between the two largest commercial banks, AMRO and ABN, and
the 200 largest industrials 72.5 percent was carried by an
executive of one of the banks, while 27.5 percent was carried
by an industrialist (Elsas et.al., 1981: 21).

This inconsistency may be explained by the fact that the
Dutch sample is relatively large and therefore included much
smaller industrial firms than Mizruchi's sample or our own
sample. If banks send executives to small industrials and
receive executives from large ones, this would account for
the small number of banker-interlocks in our sample, which
contains only very large corporations. If this is true, the
thesis of bank control will have to be rejected, or at least
restricted to the smaller industrial firms. The notion of
power balance, again put forward by Elias, is a useful
concept to characterize the relation between banks and
industry, because the weaker of the two has nevertheless
power over the stronger. Control or domination stems from an
asymmetrical power balance, in which power relations are
always reciprocal.
But power relations are not only reciprocal, they are also
multipolar, because they depend not on dyadic relations but
on the specific position of each of the two firms in the
network of corporate interlocks. The power relation between
one bank and one industrial firm cannot be studied in
isolation from the network of which both firms are a part.

Furthermore, according to Elias, the term power balance also
points to the process aspect of power. And indeed, although
it is difficult to determine the precise position of the
power balance between banks and industry, comparison of the
network of 1970 with that of 1976 has shown that banks have
become more central. From this we may conclude that the power
balance has changed in favor of the banks. This does not, in
our opinion, support the theory of bank control because the
number of banker-interlocks is still small. Control is much
too strong a concept to describe the asymmetry in the power
balance between banks and very large industrial corporations.

Furthermore, our use of the concept of sphere of interests
should not be mistaken for the concept of sphere of influence
used by Hilferding and other authors at the beginning of this
century. Implicit in the concept of sphere of influence is

the notion of bank control, which may have been correct at
that time but has since become untenable. [2] The concept of
overlapping spheres of interests is based on the assumption
that meeting-points between banks indicate potential conflict
rather than cooperation. It is, however, difficult to
distinguish corporate relations according to conflict and
cooperation on the basis of interlocking directorates alone,
just as it proved difficult to determine financial groups on
the basis of interlocking directorates. Even though it has
been demonstrated that multiple directed interlocks indicate
control relations, the analysis of the network of officer-
interlocks in Chapter 6 showed that clusters of heavily
interlocked firms do not unequivocally indicate financial
groups. In the component of heavily interlocked American
firms, for instance, Chrysler was the most central firm in
1970, but further evidence suggested that the ailing
automobile firm was a junction of three financial groups, if
indeed such groups existed at all. This finding underlines
the suggestion of Mintz and Schwartz (1981) that high
centrality in the network may indicate hubs or bridges. It
was also shown in Chapter 6 that arcs between banks and
industry most often run from industry to banks, and even
where banks hold substantial blocks of shares of industrial
corporations, the majority of accompanying interlocks are in
the opposite direction.
These findings seem to support the cooptation theory, that
corporations invite representatives of organizations to sit
on their boards in an attempt "to anticipate environmental
contingencies and to control their relations with other
companies" (Allen, 1974: 393, 394). Here the coopting
corporation is implicitly regarded as the more powerful one.
Although cooptation is generally attributed to Selznick
(1949) and subsequently to such American sociologists as
Thompson (1967) and Aldrich (1979), the argument was
developed as early as 1905 by Otto Jeidels to explain
interlocks between German banks and the iron and steel
industry. Jeidels also noted, however, that bankers often had
a large number of directorships in industrial firms, giving
them a very influential position in these firms. Whether the

[2] According to Mizruchi's study there has been a decline in
    the proportion of bankers carrying interlocks with
    industrial firms. In 1912 this proportion was 58 percent;
    it remained constant until 1935, but had declined to 40
    percent by 1974. This and a decline of bank centrality in
    the American network suggest a decline in the amount of
    bank control (Mizruchi, 1980: Table 5-17).

interlock is a cooptation- or a control relation seems to depend on the power balance between the interlocked industrial and financial firms. <u>Size</u> is definitely an important variable in determining the relative power position of industrials <u>vis-a-vis</u> the banks, and this may well explain why the very large corporations often have a representative on the boards of the interlocked banks, while the smaller ones tend to have bankers on their own boards. From the network perspective, the industrial's position in the network may also partly determine its power position <u>vis-a-vis</u> the banks. A suggestion for further research, therefore, is to investigate the relation between network position and type of financial interlocks of the industrial firms in the network.

9.4 The meaning of interlocking directorates

Although our analysis has not focused on the dyadic relations created by each interlock, we have made a typology of interlocks and defined different networks accordingly. Strong ties are based on inside-outside relations whereas weak ties are based on outside-outside relations. The weak tie network has been interpreted as a communication network, whereas the strong tie network has been interpreted as a potential control and domination network. In Chapter 6 we saw that the international interlocks are predominantly weak ties, indicating that the international network is a network of communication rather than control. In this international network of communication the New York banks and the Dutch multinationals play a prominent role. Morgan, Chase Manhattan and First National City in particular scored very high on local as well as global centrality. The binational character of Shell and Unilever contributes, of course, to their central position in the international network. Most firms that scored high on local as well as global centrality had neighbors more than half of which were foreign.

By 1976, the dominant position of the New York banks had declined somewhat, although they were still very central in the international network. The analysis of the 1976 network in Chapter 8 supports the assumption that centrality in the network indicates a dominant position in the international business system. First, it was found that the increased internationalization of banking between 1970 and 1976 corresponded with a more central position of the banks in the international network. Second, countries that had increased their share in international investment between 1970 and 1976 - West Germany, the Netherlands and Switzerland - also spectacularly increased their integration in the international network. For German, Dutch and Swiss firms in

the sample, international density doubled between 1970 and
1976. Multiplicity-analysis in Chapter 6 showed that the
firms from these countries are also heavily interlocked
nationally; roughly three-quarters of them form a compact and
tenacious network. These integrated systems of interlocking
directorates provide a high potential for communication,
domination and control. They also indicate a strong cohesion
of the corporate elite in these countries, which may
contribute to the containment of potential conflict and
increase the strength of the business community vis-a-vis the
state. The network in Canada and the United States, on the
other hand, is less heavily interlocked. Fewer firms remain
connected at higher levels of multiplicity, and the United
States/Canadian component has a tree structure, rather than a
block form, at multiplicity-level three and more. Analysis of
the network of strong ties or officer-interlocks showed that
there are proportionally more officer-interlocks in the
American network than in the German, Swiss and Dutch
networks. This suggests that, although the American
corporations are less heavily interlocked, the American
network is more purposive from an institutionalist
perspective: in the American network more interlocks result
from a explicit decision of two firms to create a director
tie.

9.5 The international corporate elite

From a personalistic point of view, the weak ties, abundant
in West Germany, the Netherlands and Switzerland, may also be
purposive. Collecting directorships may be a very purposive
activity indeed, and the persons whom we called 'big linkers'
may contribute greatly to a strong cohesion of international
elite. As we noted in Chapter 1, this book is a study of the
international elite of corporations rather than of the
international corporate elite. Nevertheless, we have made
some observations on the international corporate elite by
singling out two categories of multiple directors. First, we
defined those multiple directors holding a position in at
least one financial firm as finance capitalists. In general,
these finance capitalists connect financial corporations with
production corporations and thus create the institutional
links that are typical of finance capital. Since our sample
consisted only of the very large corporations in different
countries, it was in line with the theory of finance capital
to find a higher proportion of finance capitalists in this
international network than in the national networks studied
previously. Furthermore, the proportion of finance
capitalists among multiple directors increased from 70
percent in 1970 to 82 percent in 1976. From this we were able

to conclude that the financial aspect of the international
network had become more important. Nevertheless, the role of
the bankers in the network between banks and industry is
relatively modest. In 1970 26 percent of the directed
interlocks between banks and industrial firms was carried by
a banker, while in 1976 it was 18 percent. The explanation
for this apparent contradiction should be sought in the size
of the corporations included in the sample. As we suggested
in Section 9.3, the cooptation principle dominates the
interlocking behavior of banks vis-a-vis very large
corporations with the result that finance capitalists are
here predominantly industrialists. They carried in 1970
significantly more international interlocks. Although they
carried even more in 1976, the difference is not significant.

Second, we defined as big linkers those multiple directors
holding a position in at least four firms in the sample. If
none of the positions were executive, the big linkers were
called network specialists, e.g., retired presidents of large
corporations. Big linkers, and especially network
specialists, generally perform a communication function
rather than a function of dominance and control. They are
often engaged in formulating broad business strategies for
handling economic and political problems. Rather than
representing specific business interests, such as those of a
corporation or a financial group, they are the promotors of
sections of the business community, or even the business
community as a whole (Mills, 1956: 121). It is the big
linkers, in our opinion, who tackle such problems as how to
handle the oil crisis, how to influence governments, how to
enhance or to oppose trilateralism, and the like. The big
linkers, therefore, are the most political of the corporate
elite. They are, in fact, the informal opinion leaders in the
top echelons of corporate power, without actually
participating in the corporate organization. Koenig has shown
that in the United States, big linkers were more likely than
other corporate directors to contribute to Richard Nixon's
1972 reelection campaign (Useem, 1980: 63). Useem calls the
big linkers in American business the "inner group", who
    "constitute a distinctive segment of the capitalist
    class, and (...) in the social organization of the
    class (...) are likely to take a particularly active
    role in the institutional governance" (Useem, 1979:
    558).
Strangely enough, the authors of Graven naar Macht derive
from the Dutch data a completely different conclusion. There
exists, according to their findings, a division of labor
between those directors who specialize in interlocking with
other corporations and those who specialize in interlocking
with governmental agencies (Helmers et.al., 1975: 341). The

Dutch team, however, does not consider single directors, which may explain part of the difference with the results of Useem.

More important, there is reason to assume that both may be right. There may exist a division of labor between the directors of one firm in the sense that some are supposed to exercise influence over other firms, while others are specialized in influencing specific policy areas of government. The network specialists, however, are not specialized in a specific policy area; rather, they are engaged in formulating general and broad business strategies. Nor are they engaged in exercising influence on behalf of a particular corporation; they are opinion leaders who shape the policy outlook of large segments of the business community. The big linkers, therefore, combine 'business' and 'governmental' positions; those who carry less than four positions may well be divided into 'financial and commercial specialists' and 'policy specialists'. Too little systematic investigation of the structure of the corporate elite and its relation to the state apparatus in different countries has been done to draw any conclusions. [3]

The international corporate elite, however, has hardly been investigated at all. In our 1970 sample of 176 corporations 19 big linkers were found, but the number had increased to 32 in 1976. More than half were network specialists, i.e., they had no executive position in any of the sample firms. The increasing importance of the big linkers is, as was shown in Chapter 8, related to the integration of the international networks. In 1970 the big linkers carried 24 percent of all interlocks; in 1976 they carried 37 percent. By 1976 the big linkers played a significant role in cementing the national networks into an international whole. One could say that the international network has shown a considerable degree of centralization in terms of personnel. Further analysis of the international corporate elite, and especially of the big linkers, may shed light on the international class formation in the Atlantic area. Such research is necessary to determine whether the 'model' of the structure and development of corporate interlocks presented in the last chapters of this book corresponds with a specific structure of the international corporate elite. Only if it does can one

[3] The argument developed here will be tested in a forthcoming study of multiple directors among Dutch colonial enterprises and their participation in shaping colonial policy between 1945 and 1962.

attempt to develop an 'alternative' and empirically founded economic theory of imperialism. As we argued in Chapter 3, a theory of imperialism is essentially a theory about the relationship between the economic and the political international structure. The international corporate elite plays in that respect a crucial role, because it forms the link between the two.

REFERENCES

Aaronovitch, S., 1961,
   The Ruling Class. A study of British Finance Capital.
   Lawrence & Wishart, London.

Agersnap, Fleming, 1980,
   Analysis of interorganizational relations. Paper
   prepared for the workshop Markets, Hierarchies and
   Politics, ECPR conference, 24 - 30 March 1980, Florence.

Aglietta, M., 1978,
   Internationalisation des relations financières et de la
   production. In: Weiller, Jean et Jean Coussy (eds.),
   Economie Internationale (II) Mouton, Paris/Den Haag.

Alba, Richard D., 1973,
   A graph-theoretic definition of a sociometric clique.
   The Journal of Mathematical Sociology, Vol 3: 113-126.

Alchian, Armen A. and Harold Demsetz, 1972,
   Production, Information Costs and Economic Organization.
   American Economic Review, Vol 62: 777-795.

Aldrich, Howard E., 1979,
   Organizations and Environments. Prentice-Hall, Englewood
   Cliffs, N.J.

Allard, Patrick, et.al., 1978,
   Dictionnaire des groupes Industriels et Financiers en
   France. Editions du Seuil, Paris.

Allen, Michael Patrick, 1974,
   The structure of interorganizational elite cooptation:
   interlocking corporate directorates. American
   Sociological Review, Vol 39: 393-406.

Allen, Michael Patrick, 1978,
   Economic interest groups and the corporate elite
   structure. Social Sience Quarterly, Vol 58, 4: 597-614.

Andreff, Wladimir, 1976,
   Profits et Structures du Capitalism Mondial. Calmann-
   Levy, Paris.

Andreff, Wladimir, 1982,
   Firme et système economique: la nonlieu de la théorie
   des droits de propriété Critiques des nouveaux
   economistes. Maspéro, Paris (à paraitre).

Andreff,Wladimir et Olivier Pastrè, 1979,
    La genèse de banques multinationales et expansion du
    capital financier international. Communication présentée
    au colloque Sur les Banques et Groupes Financiers
    (C.E.R.E.M.,   Université   de   Paris-X-Nanterre)   9-10
    novembre.

Anthonisse, J.M., 1971,
    The rush in a directed graph. Mathematisch Centrum,
    Amsterdam.

Antitrust subcommittee, 1965,
    Interlocks   in   Corporate   Management.   Antitrust
    subcommittee of the Committee on the Judiciary, House of
    Representatives,   89th   Congress,   1st   Session,   U.S.
    Government Printing Office, Washinton D. C.

Arndt, Helmut, 1974,
    Wirtschaftliche   Macht.   Tatsachen   und   Theorieen.
    C.H.Becke, München.

Arrighi, Giovanni, 1978,
    The Geometry of Imperialism, The Limits of Hobson's
    Paradigm. NLB, London.

Bain, J.S., 1956,
    Barriers to new competition. Harvard University Press,
    Cambridge.

Baran, Paul A. and Paul M. Sweezy, (1966)1968
    Monopoly Capital. An essay on American Economic and
    Social Order. Penguin Books, Harmondsworth, Middlesex.

Barrat Brown, Michael, 1973,
    The Controllers of British Industry. In: Urry, John and
    John Wakeford (eds.), Power in Britain. Heinemann
    Educational Books, London.

Baruch, F., 1962,
    Grote   macht   in   klein   land.   Een   beeld   van   het
    monopoliekapitaal en zijn invloed in Nederland. (2
    delen) Pegasus, Amsterdam.

Baudhuin, 1946,
    Histoire economique de la Belgique 1919-1939 (tome II).
    E. Bruijlant, Brussel.

Bearden, James et.al., 1975,
    The nature and extent of bank centrality in corporate
    networks. Paper delivered at the Annual Meeting of the
    American Sociological Association.

Bendix, R., 1956,
    Work and Authority in Industry. Harper & Row, New York
    and Evanston.

Berle A.A., 1954,
    The 20th Century Capitalist Revolution. Harcourt Brace,
    New York.

Berle, A.A. and G.C. Means, 1932,
    The modern corporation and private property. Macmillan,
    New York.

Böhm-Bawerk, Eugen Von, 1914,
    Macht oder Ökonomischer Gesetz? Zeitschrift fur
    Volkswirtschaft, Sozial-Politik und Verwaltung, Vol 23:
    206-71.

Bonacich, Phillip, 1972,
    Technique for analyzing overlapping memberships. In:
    Costner Herbert (ed.), Sociological Methodology, Jossey-
    Bass, San Francisco.

Bourdieu, Pierre et Monique de Saint Martin, 1978,
    Le patronat. Actes de la Recherche en Sciences Sociales,
    no. 20-21 (Mars/Avril): 3-82.

Bouvier, Jean, 1967,
    Les Rothschild. Fayard, Paris.

Bouvier, Jean, 1973,
    Un siecle de banque francaise. Hachette Litterature,
    Paris.

Brady, R.A., 1943,
    Business as a System of Power. Columbia University
    Press, New York. (with a foreword by Robert Lynd).

Bucharin, Nicolai, (1918) 1972,
    Imperialism and World Economy. The Merlin Press, London.

Bunting, David, 1976,
    Corporate Interlocking, Part I- The Money Trust.
    Directors and Boards, Spring 1976: 6-15.

Bunting, David, 1979,
     Efficiency, Equity, and the Evolution of Big Business.
     Paper read at the Annual Meeting of the Western Economic
     Association, Las Vegas.

Bunting, David and Jeffrey Barbour, 1971,
     Interlocking   Directorates   in   Large   American
     Corporations, 1896-1964. Business History Review, Vol
     45, 3: 317-335.

Burch, Philip H., 1972,
     The managerial revolution reasessed. Family control in
     America's large corporations. Lexington Books, Lexington
     (Mass).

Burnham, James, (1941) 1960,
     The managerial revolution. Indiana University Press,
     Bloomington.

Camps, Miriam, 1974,
     The Management of Interdependence: A preliminary view.
     New York.

Capital I,
     Marx, Karl, Capital, A critique of Political Economy.
     Vol I. Lawrence and Wishart, London, 1970.

Capital III,
     Marx, Karl, Capital. A critique of Political Economy.
     Vol III. Progress Publishers, Moscow, 1959.

Chandler Jr., Alfred D. and Fritz Redlich, 1961,
     Recent Developments in American Business Administration
     and their Conceptualization. Business History Review,
     Spring 1961: 1-27.

Channon, Derek F., 1977,
     British Banking Strategy and the International
     Challenge. MacMillan, London and Basingstoke.

Chevalier, J.M., 1970,
     La structure financiere de l'industrie americaine et le
     probleme du controle dans les grandes societes
     americaines. Edition Cujas, Paris.

Citoleux, et.al., 1977,
     Les groupes de sociétés en 1974: une méthode d'analyse.
     Y.Citoleux, D.Encaoua, B. Franck et M.Héon. Economie et
     Statistique 87 (Mars, 1977): 53-63.

Clement, Wallace, 1977,
    Continental Corporate Power. Economic linkages between
    Canada and the United States. Mc Clelland and Stewart
    Limited, Toronto.

Coase, R., 1937,
    The nature of the firm. Economica, no. 4.

Cohen, Robert B., 1979,
    Structural change in international banking and its
    implications for the U.S. economy. Submitted to Special
    Study on Economic Change of the Joint Economic Committee
    U.S. Congress (preliminary draft).

Cypher, James M. 1979,
    The Transnational Challenge to the Corporate State.
    Journal of Economic Issues, Vol 13, 2: 513-542.

Daems, Herman, 1978,
    The Holding Company and Corporate Control. Nijhoff,
    Leiden/Boston.

Dahrendorf, Ralf, 1959,
    Class and Class Conflict in Industrial Society.
    Routledge & Kegan, Paul, London.

De Boer, H., 1957,
    De commissarisfunctie. De Bussy, Amsterdam.

De Brunhoff, Suzanne, 1976,
    Etat et Capital. Recherches sur la politique economique.
    Presses Universitaires de Grenoble/ Francois Maspèro,
    Paris.

De Jong, H.W., 1979,
    Paradoxale economie. Spruijt, van Mantgem & De Does,
    Leiden.

De Vroey, Michel, 1973,
    Propriete et pouvoir dans les grandes entreprises.
    C.R.I.S.P., Bruxelles.

De Vroey, Michel, 1975,
    The owners' interventions in decision-making in large
    corporations. A new Approach. European Economic Review,
    Vol 6: 1-15.

Dixon, Frank Haigh, 1914,
    The significance of interlocking directorates in railway
    finance. Journal of Political Economy, Vol 22 : 937-954.

Domhoff, G. William, 1970,
    The Higher Circles. The Governing class in America.
    Random House, New York.

Domhoff, G. William, (ed), 1980,
    Power Structure Research. Sage Publications, Beverly
    Hills, London.

Dooley, Peter C., 1969,
    The interlocking directorate. American Economic Review,
    Vol 59: 314-323.

Elias, Norbert, 1971,
    Wat is sociologie? Het Spectrum, Utrecht/Antwerpen.

Elsas, Donald A., Frans N.Stokman and Frans W.Wasseur, 1981,
    The Dutch network of interlocking directorates in 1976.
    Its overall structure and different types of interlocks.
    Paper presented at the meeting of the E.C.P.R. Research
    Group on Intercorporate Structure, Bad Hamburg, Germany,
    April, 27-10, 1981,

European Financial Almanac, 1974,
    European Financial Almanak, 1974-1975. (Gower Press),
    Deventer, Kluwer.

Fennema, Meindert, 1974,
    Car firms in the European Communities. A study on
    personal linkages, joint-ventures and financial
    participations. Paper prepared for the ECPR Workshop on
    Internationalization of Capital, Strasbourg, March,
    1974.

Fennema, Meindert, 1975,
    De multinationale onderneming en de nationale staat.
    SUA, Amsterdam.

Fennema, Meindert, 1976,
    Graven naar macht. Enkele opmerkingen bij de theorie en
    praktijk van het onderzoek naar de machtspositie van de
    economische en politieke elite in Nederland. De Gids,
    Vol 139: 96-106.

Fennema, Meindert and Peter de Jong, 1978,
    Internationale vervlechting van industrie en bankwezen.
    In: A.W.M. Teulings (ed.), Herstructurering van de
    industrie. Samsom, Alphen a/d Rijn: 137-164.

Fennema, Meindert and Huibert Schijf, 1979,
    Analysing interlocking directorates: theory and methods.
    Social Networks, Vol 1, 4: 1-36.

Fennema, M. and W. Kleyn, 1979,
    Interlocking directorates at the international level:
    1970-1976. (in collaboration with P. de Jong and H.
    Schijf). Paper prepared for the workshop on
    Interorganizational Networks between Large Corporations
    and Governments". ECPR Joint Sessions of Workshops
    ,Brussels, April 1979.

Fennema, Meindert et Peter de Jong, forthcoming.
    Profits et Structures du Capitalisme Mondial: Une
    critique. Critiques de l'economie politique.

Franko, L.G., 1976,
    The European multinationals. A renewed Challenge to
    American and British Big Business. Harper & Row, London,
    New York etc.

Freeman, Linton C., 1979,
    Centrality in Social Networks. Conceptual Clarification.
    Social Networks, Vol 1, 3: 215-239.

FTC - Report, 1951,
    Report on interlocking Directorates. Federal Trade
    Commission, U.S. Government Printing Office, Washington
    D.C.

Frommel, S.N. and J.H. Thompson, 1975,
    Company Law in Europe. Kluwer, Deventer.

Galbraith, J.K., (1967) 1968,
    The New Industrial State. Signet Books, New York.

Gans, M.P., 1978,
    Bankconcentratie, concurrentie en het emissiebedrijf.
    Economisch-Statische Berichten, no 3157: 568-570.

George, Kenneth D. and T.S.Ward, 1975,
    The structure of industry in the EEG. An International
    Comparison. Cambridge University Press, Cambridge.

Giddens, Anthony, 1973,
    The class structure of the advanced societies.
    Hutchinson, London.

Gille, B., 1967,
     Histoire de la maison Rothschild. Tome 2. Droz, Paris.

Gordon, R.A., (1945) 1966,
     Business Leadership in the large corporation. University
     of California Press, Berkeley.

GRADAP, 1980,
     Gradap User's Manual (eds. F.N. Stokman and F.J.A.M. van
     Veen) Publication 3 of the inter-university project
     group G R A D A P (University of Amsterdam, University
     of Groningen, University of Nijmegen).

Gramsci, Antonio, 1971,
     Selections from the prison notebooks. Edited and
     translated by Quintin Hoare and Geoffrey Nowell Smith.
     Lawrence and Wishart, London.

Guibert, Bernard, et.al., 1975,
     La mutation industrielle de la France. Du traite de Rome
     a la crise petroliere. Les collections de l'INSEE,
     Paris. (2 tomes).

Hadley, Eleanor M., 1970,
     Antitrust in Japan. Princeton University Press,
     Princeton (N.J.).

Hagemann, Wilhelm, 1931,
     Das verhaltnis der deutschen Grossbanken zur Industrie.
     Wilhelm Christians Verlag, Berlin.

Harary, F., 1972,
     Graph Theory. Addison-Wesley, Reading (Mass.).

Helmers, H.M., et.al., 1975,
     Graven naar Macht. Op zoek naar de kern van de
     Nederlandse ekonomie. Van Gennep, Amsterdam.

Herman, Edward S., 1972,
     The Greening of the Board of Directors? The Quarterly
     Review of Economics and Business: 87-95.

Hermansson, C-H., 1971,
     Monopol och Storfinanz- de 15 familjerna Raben &
     Sjogren, Stockholm.

Hilferding, Rudolf, (1910) 1968,
     Das Finanzkapital. Eine Studie uber die jungste
     Entwicklung des Kapitalismus. Europaische
     Verlagsanstalt, Frankfurt am Main.

Hilferding, Rudolf, 1914,
     Organisationsmacht und Staatsgewalt. Neue Zeit, Vol 32,
     2: 140-?

Hilferding, Rudolf, 1927,
     Organisierter Kapitalismus. Referat Sozialdemokratischer
     Parteitag, 1927, Kiel.

Hobson, J.A., (1902)1968,
     Imperialism: A study. London.

Hobson, J.A., 1906,
     Evolution of modern capitalism. A study of machine
     production. (New and Revised Edition). The Walter Scott
     Publishing Co. , London.

Hoivik, T and N.P. Gleditsch, 1970,
     Structural parameters of graphs: A theoretical
     investigation. Quality and Quantity Vol 4: 193-209.

Houssiaux, J., 1958,
     Le pouvoir de monopole. Sirey, Paris.

Hughes, Michael, John Scott and John Mackenzie, 1977,
     Trends in Interlocking Directorships: An international
     comparison. Acta Sociologica, Vol 20, no 3: 287-292.

Invloedsstructuren, 1971,
     Invloedsstructuren van politieke en ekonomische elites.
     IWP, Amsterdam.

The international petroleum cartel, 1952,
     The international petroleum cartel. Staff report to the
     Federal Trade Commission submitted to the subcommittee
     on monopoly of the select committee on small business,
     United States Senate. Government Printing Office,
     Washington D.C. (reprint, 1975).

Israelewicz, E. et D. Kessler, 1979,
     Elements d'interpretation de l'internationalisation du
     systeme de credit.Communication presentée au colloque
     sur les Banques et Groupes Financiers (CEREM, Université
     de Paris-X-Nanterre) 9-10 novembre.

Jacquemin, Alexis P., 1967,
     L'entreprise et son pouvoir de marche. P.U.F., Paris.

Jacquemin, A.P. and H.W. De Jong, 1977,
     European Industrial Organization. MacMillan, London.

Jalée, Pierre, 1970,
    L'imperialisme en 1970. Maspéro, Paris.

Jeidels, O., 1905,
    Das Verhaltnis der deutschen Grossbanken zur Industrie
    mit besondere berucksichtigung der Eisenindustrie.
    Verlag Duncker & Humbolt, Leipzig.

Junne, Gerd, 1976,
    Der Eurogeldmarkt. Seine Bedeutung fur Inflation und
    Inflationsbekampfung. Campus Verlag, Frankfurt/New York.

Kautsky, Karl, (1914) 1970,
    Ultra Imperialism. New Left Review, Vol 59 :   40-48
    (original in Die Neue Zeit, Vol 11, 9 (1914)).

Keynes, John Maynard, (1926) 1972,
    The End of Laiser-faire. Collected Writings, Vol IX,
    MacMillan, London and Basingstoke: 272-294.

Knowles, James L., 1973,
    The Rockefeller Financial Group, In: Ralph L. Andreano,
    Superconcentration/ Supercorporation: A collage of
    opinion on the Concentration of Economic Power. Warner
    Modular Publications, Book I.

Koenig, Thomas, Robert Gogel and John Sonquist, 1979,
    Models of the Significance of Interlocking Corporate
    Directors. American Journal of Economics and Sociology,
    Vol 38, 2: 173-186.

Koenig, Thomas and Robert Gogel, 1981,
    Interlocking Corporate Directorships as a Social
    Network. American Journal of Economics and Sociology,
    Vol 40, 1: 37-49.

Kotz, David M., 1978,
    Bank Control of Large Corporations in the United States.
    University of California Press, Berkeley, etc.

Kragenau, H., 1979,
    Internationale   Direktinvestionen.   Ergänzungsband
    1978/1979, Hamburg.

Lampman, 1959,
    Changes in the Wealth held by Top Wealth Holders 1922-
    1956. Review of Economics and Statistics, (November,
    1959).

Larner, R.J., 1966,
    Ownership and control in the 200 largest non-financial
    corporations, 1929 and 1963. The American Economic
    Review, Vol 51 : 777-787.

Lenin, V.I., (1916) 1964,
    Imperialism, the highest stage of capitalism. Collected
    Works Vol 22. Progress Publishers, Moscow.

Levine, J.H., 1972,
    The sphere of Influence. American Sociological Review,
    Vol 37: 14-27.

Levine, Joel H. and William S. Roy, 1979,
    A study of Interlocking Directorates: vital concepts of
    organization In: Holland, Paul W. and Samuel Leinhardt
    (eds.), Perspectives in Social Network Research.
    Academic Press, New York etc.:349-378.

Lhomme, Jean, 1966,
    Pouvoir et société économique. Editions Cujas, Paris.

Lintner, John, 1972,
    The financing of corporations. In: Edward S. Mason
    (ed.), The corporation in modern society. Atheneum, New
    York.

Llewellen, 1971,
    The ownership income of management. New York.

Lundberg, Ferdinand, 1937,
    America's Sixty Families. New York.

Lupton, Tom and C. Shirley Wilson, (1959) 1973,
    The social background and connections of 'Top decision-
    makers' in: Urry, John & John Wakeford (eds.), Power in
    Britain. Heinemann Educational Books, London: 185-204.

Mace, Jules L., 1971,
    Directors: Myth and Reality. Harvard Graduate School of
    Business Administration, Boston.

Machlup, F., 1952,
    The political economy of monopoly. J. Hopkins Press, New
    York.

Magdoff, Harry, 1969,
    The age of Imperialism. MR Books, New York.

Mandel, Ernest, 1970,
    Europe versus America. Contradictions of imperialism.
    NLB, London.

Marglin, Stephen A., (1971) 1976,
    What do bosses do? The origins and functions of
    Hierarchy in Capitalist Production. In: A. Gorz (ed.),
    The devision of Labour. Harvester Press, Hassock.

Mariolis, Peter, 1975,
    Interlocking Directorates and Control of Corporations.
    Social Science Quarterly, Vol 56: 424-439.

Mariolis, Peter, 1977,
    Interlocking directorates and finance control: a peak
    analysis. Paper presented at the 1977 meeting of the
    A.S.A.

Martinelli, Alberto, Antonio M. Chiesi, Nando Dalla Chiesa,
    1981,
    I grandi imprenditori italiani. Profilo sociale della
    classe dirigente economica. Fentrinelli, Milano.

Means, G.C., 1932,
    Interlocking directorates. Encyclopaedia of the Social
    Sciences, Vol 8, MacMillan , New York.

Medvin, Norman, 1974,
    The energy cartel. Who runs the American oil industry.
    Vintage Books, New York.

Menshikov, S., 1969,
    Millionaires and managers. Progress Publishers, Moscow.

Metcalf Committee, 1978,
    Interlocking Directorates among major U.S. Corporations.
    U.S. Senate 95 th. Cong, second session, Subcommittee on
    Reports, Accounting and Management of the Committee on
    Governmental Affairs. Senate Document 95- 107, April
    1978.

Michalet, Charles-Albert et Catherine Sauviat, 1979,
    L'internationationalisation bancaire. Le cas Francais.
    Communication presentée au colloque sur les Banques et
    Groupes Financiers (C.E.R.E.M., Universite de Paris-X-
    Nanterre) 9-10 novembre 1979.

Mills, C. Wright, (1956) 1959,
    The Power Elite. Oxford University Press, London/New
    York/Oxford.

Mintz, Beth and Michael Schwartz, forthcoming,
    The Structure of Power in the American Corporate System.

Mintz, Beth and Michael Schwartz, 1981,
    The structure of intercorporate unity in American
    Business. Social Problems (dec.1981).

Mizruchi, Mark S. and David Bunting, 1979,
    The structure of the American corporate network: 1904-
    1919. Paper presented at the Interorganizational
    Relations Session of the A.S.A. Annual Meeting at
    Boston, september 1979.

Mizruchi, Mark, 1980,
    The structure of the American corporate network: 1904-
    1974. (Ph. D. Dissertation) Department of Sociology,
    State University of New York at Stony Brook (to be
    published by Sage Publications).

Mokken, Robert J.,1979,
    Cliques, clubs and clans. Quality and Quantity, Vol 13 :
    161-173.

Mokken, R.J. and F.N.Stokman, 1974,
    Traces of Power II. Interlocking directorates between
    large corporations, banks and other financial companies
    and institutions in the Netherlands in 1969. Paper
    presented at the Joint Sessions of Workshops of the
    European Consortium for Political Research. Strasbourg,
    March-April, 1974.

Mokken, R.J. and F.N. Stokman, 1976,
    Power and influence as political phenomena. in Brian
    Berry (ed.), Power and Political theory: some European
    perspectives. Wiley, New York: 33-53.

Mokken, R.J. and F.N. Stokman, 1978,
    Traces of Power IV. The 1972 Intercorporate Network in
    the Netherlands. Department of Sociology, University of
    Groningen.

Mokken, R.J., and Stokman, F.N., 1979a,
    Corporate-governmental networks in the Netherlands.
    Social Networks, Vol 1, 4: 333-358.

Mokken, Robert J. and Frans N. Stokman, 1979b,
    Traces of Power V. Information and cooptation.
    Comparitive analysis of two intercorporate networks in
    the Netherlands. Paper prepared for the Workshop on
    Interorganizational Networks between large corporations
    and government. E.C.P.R. Joint Sessions of workshops ,
    Brussels , april 17-21, 1979.

Morin, Francois, 1974,
    La structure financiere du capitalisme francais.
    Calmann-Levy, Paris.

Morin, Francois, 1977,
    La banque et les groupes industriels a l'heure de
    nationalisations. Calmann-Levy, Paris.

Niemöller, B., W.H. van Schuur and F.N. Stokman, 1980,
    Stochastic cumulative scaling. STAP User's Guide, vol 4,
    part 1. University of Amsterdam, Amsterdam

Niemöller, Kees and Bert Schijf, 1980,
    Applied network analysis. Quality and Quantity, Vol 14 :
    101-116.

Nioche, J.P. et M.Didier, 1969,
    Deux etudes sur la dimension des entreprises
    industrielles. Collections de l'INSEE- Serie
    "Entreprises" (E 1).

Norich, Samuel, 1980,
    Interlocking Directorates, the Control of large
    Corporations and Patterns of Accumulation in the
    Capitalist Class in: M.Zeitlin (ed.), Classes, Class
    conflict and the State. Winthrop Publishers, Cambridge
    (Mass.).

N.R.C.- Report, 1939,
    The structure of the American Economy. U.S. National
    Resources Committee, U.S. Government Printing Office,
    Washington D.C.

Ornstein, Michael D.,1980,
    Assessing the Meaning of Corporate Interlocks: Canadian
    Evidence. Social Science Research, 9: 187-306

Overbeek, Henk, 1978,
    Finance capital and crisis in Britain. Paper presented
    for the CSE Annual Conference, Bradford, July 14-16,
    1978.

Overbeek, Henk, 1980,
    Finance Capital and Crisis in Britain. Capital & Class
    11 : 99-120.

Palloix, Christian, 1973,
    Les   firmes   multinationales   et   le   proces   d'
    internationalisation. Maspéro, Paris.

Palloix, Christian, 1975,
    L'internationalisation du capital. Elements critiques.
    Maspéro, Paris.

Palmer, John P., 1972,
    The Separation of Ownership from Control in Large
    Industrial Corporations. Quarterly Review of Economics
    and Business, Vol 3: 55-61.

Pastré, Olivier, 1979,
    La   strategie internationale des groupes financiers
    Americains. Economica, Paris.

Patman Committee, 1968,
    Commercial Banks and their Trust Aktivities: Emerging
    Influence on the American Economy. Staff report for the
    Domestic Finance Subcommittee of the House Committee on
    Banking and Currency, 90 th Congress, second session.
    U.S. Government Printing Office, Washington D.C.

Payne, P.L., 1967,
    The Emergence of Large Scale Companies in Great Britain,
    1870-1914. Economic History Review, Vol 10: 518-542.

Pennings, Johannes M., 1980,
    Interlocking Directorates. Origins and Consequences of
    Connections Among Organizations' Board of Directors.
    Jossey-Bass, San Francisco/London.

Perlo, Victor, 1957,
    The Empire of High Finance. International Publishers,
    New York.

Perroux, F., 1962,
    L'economie du XX siecle, Presses Universitaires de
    France, Paris.

Pfeffer, Jeffrey, 1972,
    Size and Composition of Corporate Boards of Directors:
    The Organization and its Environment. Administrative
    Science Quarterly, Vol 16: 218-228

Van der Pijl, Kees, forthcoming.
     Imperialism and Class Formation in the North Atlantic
     Area. (Diss.).

Poensgen, Otto H., 1980,
     Between Market and Hierarchy - The role of Interlocking
     Directorates. Zeitschrift fur die gesamte
     Staatswisschenschaft, Vol 136: 209-225

Poulantzas, Nicos, 1974,
     Les classes sociales dans le capitalisme aujourd'hui.
     Editions du Seuil, Paris.

Pujo Committee, 1913,
     U.S. Congress House Banking and Currency Committee,
     Report of the Committee Appointed Pursuant to H.R. 429
     and 504 to Investigate the concentration of Control of
     Money and Credit, 62 nd Cong., second sess. (Washington
     D.C. : U.S. Government Printing Office, 1913).

Prais, S.J. and Caroline Reid, 1976,
     Large and small manufacturing entreprises in Europe and
     America. In: Jacquemin, A.P. and H.W. De Jong (eds.),
     Markets, corporate behavior and the state. Martinus
     Nijhoff, The Hague.

Radice, Hugo, 1975(ed.),
     International Firms and Modern Imperialism. Selected
     Readings. Penguin Books, Harmondsworth, Middlesex.

Revell, Jack, 1973,
     The British Financial System. MacMillan, London and
     Basingstoke.

Riesser, J., (1906) 1910,
     Die deutschen Grossbanken und ihre Konzentration im
     zusammenhang mit der Entwicklung der Gesamtwirtschaft in
     Deutschland. Gustav Fisher, Jena.

Rochester, Anna, 1936,
     The Rulers of America. International Publishers, New
     York.

Rowthorn, Bob, 1971,
     Imperialism in the seventies. Unity or Rivalry? New Left
     Review, Vol 69: 31-59.

Ruffini, P.B., 1979,
    Banques   multinationales   et   système   bancaire
    transnational. These pour le Doctorat d'Etat de Sciences
    Economiques, Paris X.

Salvadori, Massimo, 1979,
    Karl Kautsky and the Socialist Revolution 1880 - 1938.
    New Left Books, London.

Schaft, Wolfgang, 1980,
    International Banks. A documentation of their foreign
    establishments. Verlag Weltarchiv GMBH, Hamburg.

Schijf, Huibert, 1980,
    The Bussiness Elite; a note on top functionaries in the
    networks of interlocking directorates at the turn of the
    century. Paper prepared for the Researchgroup on
    Intercorporate Structures, E.C.P.R. Joint Sessions of
    Workshops, Florence, March 1980.

Schonwitz, Dietrich, und Hans-Jürgen Weber, 1980,
    Personelle Verflechtungen zwischen Unternehmen: Eine
    wettbewerbspolitische Analyse. Zeitschrift fur die
    gesamte Staatswisschenschaft, Vol 136: 98-112.

Scott, John, 1978,
    The   intercorporate   configuration: substructure and
    superstructure. Paper prepared for the Workshop on
    Interorganizational Networks between Large Corporations
    and the State, E.C.P.R. Joint Sessions of Workshops,
    Grenoble, April 1978.

Scott, John, 1979,
    Corporations,   classes   and   capitalism. Hutchinson,
    London.

Selznick, Philip, 1949,
    TVA and the Grass Roots. Harper, New York.

Shepherd, William G, 1970,
    Market Power & Economic Welfare. Random House, New York.

Shoup, Laurence H. and William Minter, 1977,
    Imperial Brain Trust. The Council on Foreign Relations
    and the United States Foreign Policy. Monthly Review
    Press, New York and London.

Sonquist, John A. and Thomas Koenig, 1975,
    Interlocking directorates in the top U.S. corporations.
    A graph theory approach. In: New Directions in Power
    Structure Research (ed. by G. Williams Domhoff). The
    Insurgent Sociologist, Vol 5, 3: 196-229.

Soref, Michael, 1980,
    The finance capitalists. In: M. Zeitlin (ed.), Classes
    Class Conflict and the State. Winthrop Publishers,
    Cambridge (Mass.).

Spiegelberg, Richard, 1973,
    The City. Power without accountability. Quartet Books,
    London.

Stanworth, Philip en Anthony Giddens, 1975,
    The modern corporate economy: interlocking directorships
    in Britain, 1906-1970. Sociological Review, Vol 23, 1:
    5-28. 5-28

Steuber, Ursel, 1976,
    International Banking. The foreign activities of banks
    of principle industrial countries. Sijthoff, Leiden.

Steuber, Ursel, 1977,
    Internationale Bankkooperation. Deutsche Banken in
    internationalen Gruppen. Fritz Knapp Verlag, Frankfurt
    am Main.

Stokman, F.N., 1977,
    Roll calls and sponsorship. A methodological analysis of
    Third World group formation in the United Nations.
    Sijthoff, Leiden.

Stokman, Frans N. and Wijbrandt H. van Schuur, 1980,
    Basic scaling. Quality and Quantity, Vol 14: 5-30.

Stuurman, Siep, 1978,
    Kapitalisme en burgelijke staat. SUA, Amsterdam.

Sweezy, Paul M., 1953,
    Interest Groups in the American Economy. In: The Present
    as History. Essays and Reviews on Capitalism and
    Socialism. Monthly Review Press, New York/London.

Sweezy, Paul M., (1942) 1956,
    The theory of capitalist development. Monthly Review
    Press, New York.

Sweezy, Paul and Harry Magdoff, 1969,
    The Multinational Corporation. Monthly Review (Oct. and
    Nov. 1969).

Thompson, James D., 1967,
    Organizations in Action. McGraw-Hill, New York.

Thunholm, Lars-Erik, 1971,
    Banking structure and bank competition. In: Banking in a
    changing world. Associazione Bancaria Italiana, Roma:
    99-120.

TNEC-report, 1940,
    Investigation of concentration of economic power.
    Monograph No 29. The distribution of ownership in the
    200 largest non-financial corporations. U.S. Government
    Printing Office, Washington D.C.

Transnational Corporations, 1978,
    Transnational Corporations in World development: a
    reexamination. Commission on Transnational corporations,
    United Nations, New York.

Useem, Michael, 1978,
    The inner group of the American capitalist class. Social
    Problems, Vol 25: 225-240.

Useem, Michael, 1979,
    The social organization of the American business elite
    and participation of corporation directors in the
    governance of American institutions. American
    Sociological Review, Vol 44: 553-572.

Useem, Michael, 1980,
    Corporations and the corporate elite. Ann. Rev. Sociol.,
    Vol 6: 41-77.

Valkhoff, J., 1941,
    De eigendom in de moderne maatschappij. Handelingen van
    de Nederlandsche Sociologische Vereeniging. No.9 (maart
    1941): 21-41.

Van der Pijl, K., 1979,
    Classformation at the international level. Capital and
    class, 9: 1-22.

Van der Pijl, Kees, forthcoming,
    Class formation in the North Atlantic Area, 1941- 1974.
    Dissertation.

Varga, Y., 1968,
      The problems of Inter-Imperialist Contradictions and
      War. Politico-Economic Problems of Capitalism, Moscow.

Verloren van Themaat, P., 1963,
      The Antitrust policy of the European Economic Community.
      In: Comparative aspects of antitrust law in the United
      States, the United Kingdom and the European Economic
      Community. London.

Vernon, Raymond, 1971,
      Multinational Enterprise and National Security. Adelphi
      paper 74, Institute for Strategic Studies, London.

Vernon, Raymond, (1971) 1973,
      Sovereignty at Bay. The Multinational Spread of U.S.
      Enterprises. Penguin Books, Harmondsworth, Middlesex.

Vessière, M., 1978,
      La structure des cumuls dans le champ politique et dans
      le champ économique en Belgique. Paper prepared for the
      Workshop on Interorganizational Networks between Large
      Corporations and Government, E.C.P.R. Joint Sessions of
      Workshops, Grenoble, April 1978.

Villarejo, D., 1961/1962,
      Stock ownership and the control of corporations I, II
      and III. New University Thought, Vol 2, 1: 33-77 and Vol
      2, 2: 47-65.

Warner, W. Lloyd and Darab B. Unwalla, 1967,
      The system of Interlocking Directorates. The emergent
      American society, Vol 1, Large scale organizations.
      (eds. W. Lloyd Warner, Darab B. Unwalla, John H. Trimm)
      Yale University Press, New Haven/London.

Weber, Max, (1922) 1925,
      Grundriss der Sozialokonomik, III Abteilung, Wirtschaft
      und Geschellschaft. Zweite, vermehrte Auflage. Verlag
      von J.C.B. Mohr (Paul Siebeck), Tübingen.

Weiss, Rainer, 1978,
      Internationale Zentralisation des Kapitals. IWP-
      Berichte, Vol 12: 66-69.

Wells, Louis T., 1974,
      National Policies in an international industry: The
      Europeans and the automobile. In: R.Vernon (ed.), Big
      Business and the State: changing relations in Western
      Europe. MacMillan, London etc.

Westerman, W.M., 1920,
     De concentratie in het bankwezen. (Tweede bijgewerkte
     druk) Martinus Nijhoff, 's Gravenhage.

Weston, Rae, 1980,
     Domestic and Multinatinal Banking. The Effects of
     Monetary Policy. Croom Helm, London.

Whitley, Richard, 1974,
     The city and Industry: the directors of the large
     companies, their charcteristics and connections. In:
     Stanworth, P. and A. Giddens (eds.), Elites and Power in
     British Society. Cambridge University Press, London.

Wibaut, F.M., 1903,
     Trusts en Kartellen. A.B.Soep, Amsterdam.

Wibaut, F.M., 1913,
     De nieuwste ontwikkeling van het kapitalisme. De nieuwe
     Tijd, Vol 18: 284-339.

Wilcox, Clair and William G. Shepherd, 1975,
     Public Policies toward Business. Richard Irwin,
     Homewood, Illinois.

Zeitlin, Maurice, 1974,
     Corporate Ownership and Control: The Large Corporations
     and the Capitalist Class. American Journal of Sociology,
     Vol 79, 5: 1073-119.

Zeitlin, Maurice, 1976,
     On class theory of the large corporation: response to
     Allen. American Journal of Sociology, Vol 81: 894-903.

Zschocke, Helmut, 1970,
     Siemens Konzern- Electroimperium in der Expansion. DWI-
     Berichte, Vol 21, 7: 33-36.

Zijlstra, Gerrit Jan, 1979a,
     Networks in public policy: Nuclear Energy in the
     Netherlands. Social Networks, Vol 1, 4: 359-389.

Zijlstra, Gerrit Jan, 1979b,
     The organization of organizations; interlocking
     directorates and their analysis . Paper prepared for the
     Workshop on Interorganizational Networks between Large
     Corporations and Governments. ECPR, Brussels, April,
     1979.

page

page

APPENDIX A: SELECTION OF THE FIRMS

1. INDUSTRIAL FIRMS

1.1. Selection of the industrial firms.

To operationalize the concept 'large firm' is not easy. Most common indices
are sales, assets and number of employees. This last index has the disadvantage
that it contains a bias in favour of the socalled 'labour intensive industry'.
Chosing the amount of assets as an indicator for the bigness of a firm has the
disadvantage that the value of the assets is often manipulated in the accounts
of the firm, mainly for tax reasons.
Although to some extend the same can be said for sales, we think that the
compilers of the Fortune directories made the right choice in taking sales
as an indicator for size and ranking the firms accordingly in the 'Fortune
lists'.
In order to select the industrial firms we used the Fortune directories of 1971.
Our aim was to select about 150 firms. If we had taken only the largest firms,
92 of the 150 firms in the sample would have been American. This would make
international comparison very difficult.
We therefore constructed five categories:

A. Firms, located in one of the EC countries[1] in 1970;

B. British firms;

C. American firms;

D. Japanese firms;

E. Firms, located in other countries

From each category the 26 largest firms were selected, except for category A, from
which we selected 41 firms. This was done because our study concentrates upon
the European Communities. Had we restricted our sample to 26 firms from EC-
countries, there would have been no Belgian and Luxembourgian[2] firms in the
sample, and only very few French firms.
For A, B, D and E we used "The 200 largest industrials outside the U.S.", Fortune,
August 1971.
For C we used "The 500 largest industrial corporations in the U.S.", Fortune,
May, 1971.
We selected 145 firms from 14 countries. For 8 of these 145 no information about
the Board of Directors could be found.

They were deleted. Royal Dutch/Shell and Unilever appeared twice in the
sample. Due to their binationality they were both in category A and B.
Thus we were left with 135 industrial firms, which appear in table II to VI
Table I shows the number of firms per country.

Table I

Number of industrial firms per country in the sample	
United States	25
United Kingdom	25
Japan	22
Federal Republic	15
France	14
Canada	7
Switzerland	7
Sweden	7
Italy	5
Netherlands	4
Belgium/Luxembourg	3
Australia	2
South Africa	1

1.2. Internationality of the firms

As a criterium for internationality we decided to use the Judge-list of
multinational business enterprises in the Yearbook of International Organizations
1970/1971 (13th ed.) edited bu the Union of International Associations, Brussels
1971. This list includes only those companies which have an affiliate in at
least 10 foreign countries.
A.J.N. Judge started to compile such a list in the Yearbook of International
Organization 1968, in which he writes:

> "A certain amount of inconsistency over the definitions of
> subsidiary and associate is to be expected. The definitions
> used by the editors of "Who Owns Whom" are:
> 'A subsidiary is defined as a company more than 50 percent
> of the share capital of which is owned by another company
> which in the directory is therefore defined as parent company.
> A company is classified as an associate when it is so
> described by itself or where it has announced that it has
> acquired a substantial interest in another company or where
> published information is available that it owns not less than

10 percent of the share capital of the other company. Members
of industrial consortia are listed as associates. Any company
of which another company is the associate as already defined
is regarded as being in association with that other company'." [3]

The definitions used by the editors of "Directory of American Firms Operating
in Foreign Countries" are:

"This Directory includes only those firms in which American
firms or individuals have a substantial direct capital investment in the form of stock, as sole owner, or as a partner in
the enterprise.
'Branches' and 'subsidiaries' are included but not distinguished
or defined." [3]

It is clear that there is a definitional muddle. Judge goes on by saying:

"The lack of adequate distinction between branches and subsidiaries or associates in the source on US corporations makes
it difficult to compare details on European and American organizations in the tables. Due to inclusion of more information
on branches in the American source the figures for American
organizations are all scaled upwards."
(The source in question was not "Who Owns Whom", M.F.) [3]

This muddle is caused by the fact that Judge depended for his information on
the existing directories. [4]
In the introduction of the 'revised Judge-list' it is said that

"this time all figures are derived from "Who Owns Whom" which
will account for the unexpected result of a comparison of the
two sets of figures for the USA (12th edition) and this may
also permit comparison of European and American organizations." [5]

For reasons explained above and for apparent inaccuracies -Philips was not
included in the Judge-list 1970/71 to give but one example- we did not trust
the Judge-list 1970/1971 completely. We therefore decided to collect
additional information on those firms which owned or partly owned production-
plants in 10 or more countries according to the Judge-list 1968 or according
to its annual report. This is indicated in the tables I to V with one (x)
or two (x x) asterisks respectively.
In addition we counted the number of EC-countries in which a subsidiary or
affiliate was held. This information is also included in table II to VI.
It was taken from the Annual Reports of 1970.

Table II

41 largest companies of EC-countries in 1970

	Nationality	Rank Fortune	Number of countries in which subsidiaries and affiliates [7]	Number of EC-countries in which subsidiaries and affiliates [2]
1. Royal Dutch/Shell	Dutch/British	1	61	5
2. Unilever	Dutch/British	2	31	5
3. Volkswagenwerk A.G.	German	3	12	3
4. Philips' Gloei-lampenfabriek N.V.	Dutch	4	29[*]	5
5. Siemens A.G.	German	10	13	4
6. Farbwerke Hoechst	German	11	43	4
7. Daimler-Benz A.G.	German	12	12	3
8. August Thyssen-Hütte	German	13	17	4
9. Badische Anilin-und Sodafabrik A.G.	German	14	22	4
10. Montecatini Edison (Montedison)	Italian	15	14	3⁻
11. Fiat SpA	Italian	16	25[*]	4
12. Renault [8]	French	20	23	5
13. Farbenfabrik Bayer A.G.	German	21	39	3⁻
14. AEG-Telefunken	German	24	16[*]	5
15. AKZO	Dutch	28	18[* *]	5
16. Rhône-Poulenc S.A.	French	29	27	5
17. Cie Française des Petroles	French	30	28	5
18. Ente Nazionale Idrocarburi [8]	Italian	34	39	3
19. Mannesmann A.G.	German	36	14	4
20. Fried.Krupp Hütten Werke A.G.	German	37	2[* *]	2
21. Saint-Gobain/Pont-à-Mousson	French	38	16[* *]	5
22. Pechiney	French	42	29	3

Table II (continued)

	Nationality	Rank Fortune	Number of countries in which subsidiaries and affiliates [7]	Number of EC-countries in which subsidiaries and affiliates [2]
23. Cie Générale d'Electricité S.A.	French	43	14	x
24. Robert Bosch GmbH	German	44	19	4
25. ELF (ERAP) [8] [9]	French	45	26 (11 **)	5
26. Hoesch A.G.	German	47	14	5
27. Citroën S.A.	French	48	13	2
28. Peugeot	French	49	5 **	2
29. Metallgesell-schaft A.G.	German	50	17	2
30. ARBED	Luxembourg	52	5 **	2
31. Rheinstahl A.G.	German	54	1 **	1
32. Gutehoffnungs-hütte A.G.	German	56	19(1 **) [11]	1
33. Petrofina	Belgian	58	21	5
34. Pirelli	Italian	60	18 **	3
35. Michelin [9]	French	62	11 **	5
36. Ugine Kuhlmann	French	65	10 **	3
37. Wendel Sideror [9]	French	72	1 **	1
38. Italsider [8]	Italian	75	x	x
39. Thomson Brandt [10]	French	76	9 **	3
40. Usinor [10]	French	80	1 **	1
41. Cockerill	Belgian	94	3 **	2

  x   Figures from the Judge-list 1968
x x   Figures from the annual report
  -     The annual report did not give exact information on foreign subsidiaries. The number given is a conservative estimate.
  x   No information available from any sources.
 --   No annual report available; firm not included in our sample

TABLE III

26 largest companies of the United Kingdom in 1970

	Rank Fortune	Number of countries in which subsidiaries and affiliates [7]	Number of EC-countries in which subsidiaries and affiliates [2]
1. Royal Dutch/Shell	1	85	5
2. Unilever	2	27	5 (14)
3. The British Petroleum Company Ltd.	5	52	5
4. Imperial Chemical Industries Ltd.	7	46	4
5. British Steel Corporation [8]	8	19	1
6. British Leyland Motor Corporation Ltd	22	33	3
7. General Electric (English)	27	36	5
8. British-American Tobacco Company Ltd.	32	19	5
9. National Coal Board [8] [12]	33	1	0
10. Courtaulds Ltd.	40	31	2
11. The Dunlop Company Ltd.	55	29	3
12. Associated British Foods	57	--	--
13. Reed International Ltd.	59	16	4
14. Guest, Keen & Nettlefolds Ltd.	61	27	3
15. British Insulated Callender's Cables Ltd.	68	17 *	2
16. Imperial Tobacco Group Ltd.	69	13	2
17. Hawker Siddeley Group Ltd.	70	20	2
18. Rio Tinto Zinc Corporation Ltd. [9]	74	20	5[+]
19. Consolidated Tin Smelters [9]	83	18 * *	3
20. Ranks Hovis McDougall Ltd.	85	14	3
21. Tube Investment Ltd.	91	20 (12 * *)	2
22. Unigate Ltd.	100	10	1
23. The Union International Co. Ltd. [9]	102	18	5
24. Coats Paton Ltd.	103	22	4
25. The Bowater Paper Corporation Ltd.	107	14	3
26. Thorn Electrical Industries Ltd.	108	21	4

*   Figures from the Judge-list 1968
* * Figures from the annual report
--   No annual report available; firm not included in our sample
+
   According to the 'Anti-Report', Counter Information Service, London 1971

TABLE IV

26 largest companies of the United States in 1970

	Rank Fortune	Number of countries in which subsidiaries and affiliates [7]	Number of EC-countries in which subsidiaries and affiliates [2]
1. General Motors Corporation	1	21	4
2. Standard Oil Co. (New Jersey)	2	25	5
3. Ford Motor Company	3	30	5
4. General Electric	4	32	4
5. International Business Machines (IBM) Inc.	5	14	5
6. Mobil Oil Corporation	6	62	3
7. Chrysler Corporation	7	26	2
8. International Telephine Telegraph Corporation	8	40	5
9. Texaco Inc.	9	30	4
10. Western Electric	10	--	--
11. Gulf Oil Corporation	11	61	3
12. U.S. Steel	12	10	2
13. Westinghouse Electric Corp.	13	12	2
14. Standard Oil Company of California	14	26	4
15. Ling-Temco-Vought [9]	15	x	x
16. Standard Oil Company (Indiana)	16		
17. Boeing [9]	17	24	5
18. E.I. Du Pont de Nemours & Co.	18	20	5
19. Shell Oil [9] [15]	19	1 **	0
20. General Telephone & Electronics Corporation	20	15 *	x
21. RCA Corporation	21	18	5
22. The Goodyear Tire & Rubber Company	22	22	4
23. Swift & Co.	23	10 *	0
24. Union Carbide Corporation	24	34	4
25. Procter & Gamble Co., the	25	24	4
26. Betlehem Steel Corporation	26	11 *	0

x   No information available from any sources
*   Figures from the Judge-list 1968
**   Figures from the annual report
--   No annual report available; firm not included in our sample

TABLE V

26 largest Japanese firms in 1970

	Rank Fortune	Number of countries in which subsidiaries and affiliates [7]	Number of EC-countries in which subsidiaries and affiliates [2]
1. Nippon Steel Corporation [9]	6	1	0
2. Hitachi [10]	9	1	0
3. Toyota Motor [12]	17	1	0
4. Matsushita Electric Industrial Co. Ltd. [9]	18	1	0
5. Mitsubishi Heavy Industries [12]	19	1	0
6. Nissan Motor Co. Ltd. [12]	23	2	0
7. Tokio Shibaura Electric Co.Ltd. [12]	26	2	0
8. Nippon Kokan K.K. [12]	35	1	0
9. Sumitomo Metal Industries Ltd. [12]	41	1	0
10. Kobe Steel Ltd. [12]	46	1	0
11. Mitsubishi Electric Corporation [12]	63	1	0
12. Kawasaki Steel Corporation [10]	64	1	0
13. Ishikawajima-Harima Heavy Industries [12]	67	2	0
14. Taiyo Fishery	78	--	--
15. Idemitsu Kosan	79	--	--
16. Toray Industries Inc. [12]	89	1	0
17. Honda Motor Co. Ltd, [12]	90	2	0
18. Nippon Electric Co. Ltd. [9]	93	4	0
19. Asahi Chemical Industry Co. [12]	95	1	0
20. Mitsubishi Chemical Industries Ltd. [12]	97	1	0
21. Komatsu [12]	101	1	0
22. Nippon Mining [12]	104	3	0
23. Kawasaki Heavy Industries	105	--	--
24. Toyo Kogyo [12]	109	1	0
25. Unitika	111	--	--
26. Kanegafuchi Chemical Industry Co. Ltd. [12]	116	1	0

-- No annual report available; firm not included in our sample.

TABLE VI

26 largest companies of other countries in 1970

	Nationality	Rank Fortune	Number of countries in which subsidiaries and affiliates [7]	Number of EC-countries in which subsidiaries and affiliates [2]
1. Nestlé Alimentana A.G.	Swiss	25	15	5
2. Broken Hill Propriety [9]	Australian	31	7 **	0
3. Ciba-Geigy A.G. [16]	Swiss	39	37 **	5
4. Alcan Aluminium	Canadian	51	34 **	5
5. A.G. Brown, Boveri & Co.	Swiss	53	17	5
6. Hoffmann - La Roche	Swiss	66	2 **	0
7. International Nickel [9]	Canadian	73	14 **	5
8. Volvo A.B.	Swedish	77	13 *	1
9. Massey-Ferguson Ltd.	Canadian	82	15 **	4
10. Svenska Kugellagerfabrik A.B.	Swedish	84	36	4
11. Canada Packers [10]	Canadian	86	6 **	1
12. Colonial Sugar Refining [9]	Australian	87	1 **	0
13. Allmänna Svenska Elektriska A.B.	Swedish	106	24	2
14. Saab-Scania [10]	Swedish	113	4	1
15. Distillers Corporation-Seagrams	Canadian	119	x	3
16. Steel Co. of Canada [9]	Canadian	128	5 **	1
17. Sandoz A.G.	Swiss	130	37	5
18. L.M. Ericsson Telephone	Swedish	131	28 *	3
19. Gränges	Swedish	132	15 [17]	3
20. Northern Electric	Canadian	150	--	--
21. De Beers Consolidated Mines [9]	South-African	151	x	x
22. Alusuisse (Schweizerische Aluminium A.G.)	Swiss	153	16	5
23. Gebrüder Sulzer A.G.	Swiss	165	21	3
24. Domtar [13]	Canadian	169	2 **	0
25. Moore	Canadian	183	--	--
26. Svenska Tandsticks A.B.	Swedish	187	27	4

*	Figures from the Judge-list 1968
**	Figures from the annual report
--	No annual report available; firm not included in our sample
x	No information available from any source

1.3. Product-group

After having established a definite list of companies to be included in our
sample we decided to order these according to the products they produce:

1. electro-technique
2. food & tabacco
3. heavy machinery
4. automobile
5. rubber products
6. chemical
7. petro-chemical
8. iron & steel
9. nonferrous metals
10. conglomerates
11. other products

The source used for categorizing the companies was again the Fortune directory.
The product first named in Fortune was regarded as the most important one and
decisive for the category in which the firm was placed. Problems arose with
American companies, since the Fortune directory on American firms did not give
a list of products for each company. To categorize these we used different sources,
but mainly the annual report. It was therefore important to have a clear and
restricted definition of conglomerate.

For a definition of conglomerate we used one which stresses the aspect of non-
related diversification. Thus a conglomerate is "typically an aggregation of
functionally unrelated or incoherent enterprises". [18]

This definition is far more restricted than the definition which stresses the
market aspect and defines conglomerate as a business "that operates in a series
of different markets, each of which it encounters different competitors and
different conditions of demand and supply". [19]

With our sample of large firms nearly all of them would have been categorized
as conglomerates, had we used this last definition. Now only LTV, Swift, ITT and
Guest Keen & Nettlefolds fell into that category. Difference between petro-
chemical and chemical was not made because the products differ necessarily.

In this case we argued that difference in origin of the products was important
enough to allow for a special category "petro-chemical" in which the oil companies
were singled out from chemical industries.

Since the size of firm matters mostly in relation to its direct competitors,
we ranked the firms in the same product-group (thus in that product-group in
which their main activities are concentrated) according to their sales,
(see table VII).

TABLE VII

Industrial firms in the sample according to size, per product.

1. Electro technique	3. Heavy Machinery
1. General Electric Company (New York)	1. The Boeing Company
2. International Business Machine Corporation	2. Mitsubishi Heavy Industries Ltd.
3. Westinghouse Electric Corporation	3. Mannesmann AG
4. Philips	4. AG Brown Boveri & Cie.
5. General Telephone & Electronics Corporation	5. Gute Hoffnungshütte AG
6. Hitachi Ltd.	6. Ishikawajima - Harima Heavy Industries Co. Ltd.
7. RCA Corporation	7. British Insulated Callender's Cables
8. Siemens AG	8. Massey Ferguson Ltd.
9. Matsushita Electric Industrial Co. Ltd.	9. AB Svenska Kugellagerfabriken
10. AEG-Telefunken	10. Tube Investment Ltd.
11. Tokyo Shibaura Electric Co. Ltd.	11. Komatsy Ltd.
12. The General Electric Company Ltd. (Londen)	12. Gebrüder Sulzer AG
13. Compagnie Générale d'Electricité	
14. Robert Bosch GmbH	
15. Mitsubishi Electric Corporation	
16. Hawker Siddeley Group Ltd.	
17. Thomson Brandt	
18. Nippon Electric Co. Ltd.	
19. Thorn Electrical Industries Ltd.	
20. Allmänna Svenska Elektrika AB	
21. L.M. Ericsson Telephone Co.	
2. Food and Tobacco	
1. Unilever	
2. The Procter & Gamble Company	
3. Nestlé Alimentana S.A. Unilac Inc.	
4. British-American Tobacco Company Ltd.	
5. Imperial Tobacco Group Ltd.	
6. Ranks Hovis McDougall Ltd.	
7. The Colonial Sugar Refining Company Ltd.	
8. Unigate Ltd.	
9. The Union International Company Ltd.	

4. Automobiles	6. Chemical
1. General Motors	1. E.I. Du Pont De Nemours & Co. Ltd.
2. Ford Motor Company	2. Imperial Chemical Industries Ltd.
3. Chrysler Corporation	3. Farbwerke Hoechst AG
4. Volkswagenwerk AG	4. Union Carbide Corporation
5. Daimler-Benz AG	5. Badische Analin & Soda Fabrik AG
6. Fiat Sp.A	6. Montedison Sp.A
7. Toyota Motor	7. Farbenfabriken Bayer AG
8. Régie Nationale des Usines Renault	8. AKZO N.V.
9. British Leyland Motor Corporation Ltd.	9. Rhône Poulenc SA
10. Nissan Motor Co. Ltd.	10. Ciba Geigy AG
11. Citroën	11. Courtaulds Ltd.
12. Peugeot Automobiles S.A.	12. F. Hoffmann-La Roche & Co. AG
13. A.B. Volvo	13. Toray Industries, Inc.
14. Honda Motor Co. Ltd.	14. Asahi Chemical Industry Co. Ltd.
15. Tokyo Kogyo Co. Ltd.	15. Mitsubishi
16. Saab-Scania Aktiebolag	16. Sandoz AG

5. Rubber Products	7. Petrochemical
1. Goodyear Tire & Rubber	1. Standard Oil Company (New Jersey)
2. Dunlop Co. Ltd., the	2. Royal Dutch/Shell Group
3. Pirelli Sp.A.	3. Mobil Oil
4. Compagnie Générale des Etablissements Michelin	4. British Petroleum Company Ltd.
	5. Texaco Inc.
	6. Gulf Oil Corporation
	7. Standard Oil of California
	8. Standard Oil Company (Indiana)
	9. Compagnie Française des Pétroles
	10. Shell Oil (New York)
	11. Ente Nazionale Idrocarburi
	12. Entreprise de Recherches et d'Activités Pétrolières
	13. Petrofina

8. Iron and Steel	10. Conglomerates
1. United States Steel Corporation	1. International Telephone and Telegraph Corporation
2. Nippon Steel Corporation	2. Ling-Temco-Vought Inc.
3. British Steel Corporation	3. Swift & Company
4. August Thyssen Hütte AG	4. Guest, Keen and Nettlefolds Ltd.
5. Bethlehem Steel Corporation	
6. Broken Hill Proprietary Company Ltd.	
7. Nippon Kokan K.K.	
8. Fried. Krupp Hüttenwerke AG	
9. Sumitomo Metal Industries Ltd.	
10. Kobe Steel Ltd.	
11. Hoesch AG	
12. ARBED	
13. Rheinstahl AG	
14. Kawasaki Steel Corporation	
15. Wendel Sideror	
16. Italsider Sp.A	
17. Usinor	
18. Cockerill-Ougrée-Providence et Espérance-Landoz Cockerill N.V.	
19. Steel Company of Canada Ltd., the	

9. Nonferrous Metals	11. Various
1. Pechiney	1. National Coal Board
2. Metallgesellschaft AG	2. Saint-Gobain/Pont-à-Mousson
3. Alcan Aluminium Ltd.	3. Reed International Ltd.
4. Ugine Kuhlmann	4. Coats Patons Ltd.
5. International Nickel Company Ltd. the	5. Canada Packers Ltd.
6. Rio Tinto-Zinc Corporation, the	6. The Bowater Paper Corporation Ltd.
7. Consolidated Tin Smelters Ltd.	7. Kanegafuchi Chemical Industry Co. Ltd.
8. Nippon Mining Co. Ltd.	8. Gränges AB
9. Alusuisse, Schweizerische Aluminium AG	9. Svenska Tandsticks AB
	10. De Beers Consolidated Mines Ltd.
	11. Domtar Ltd.

2. BANKS

2.1. Selection of the banks

Banks were selected in the same way as industrial firms. That is, for the
categories B, C, D and E the 8 largest banks were selected, whereas for A
13 banks were selected (see table VII to XI).

The criterium for size was not, as with the industrial firms, sales. We
used in accordance with Fortune's "fifty largest commercial banks outside
the U.S." and "the 50 largest commercial banking companies" assets as an
indicator for size. Of course the disadvantage of using assets as an
indicator for the size of banks, is the same as with industrial firms.
However, if the banks are ranked according to deposits, the order does not
change very much. Deposits will not be used as an indicator for size since
it would bias our selection in favour of deposit banks.[20]

In the case of British banks only 5 of them were selected. Smaller banks
did not appear in the Fortune-list, neither in the Banker's Almanac.[21]
Besides, two of the top 5 banks were a result of a merger in 1969; Barclays
Bank Ltd. and Barclays Bank DCO formed Barclays Bank. Standard Bank and
Chartered Bank formed Standard and Chartered Banking Group.

2.2. Internationality of the banks

In banking business distinction is made between branches, representative
offices and correspondents. Branches and representative offices of a bank
were regarded as subsidiaries or affiliates, but correspondents were not,
since they cannot be regarded as part of the bank.

Information on branches and representative offices abroad was collected from
the annual report or from the Banker's Almanac. The numbers given in the
last two rows of table VII to XI are based on existing branches, representative
offices and affiliates in banking business, not on interests the bank may have
in industrial firms.

TABLE VIII

12 largest banks of EC-countries plus AMRO in 1970

	Nationality	Rank Fortune	Number of countries in which branch or affiliate [7]	Number of EC-countries in which branch or affiliate [2]
1. Banque Nationale de Paris	French	3	30'	4'
2. Banca Nazionale del Lavoro	Italian	4	13	4
3. Credit Lyonnais [8]	French	5	15'	3'
4. Deutsche Bank	German	6	10	3
5. Westdeutsche Landesbank Girozentrale [8]	German	8	3	1
6. Banca Commerciale	Italian	14	7	3
7. Société Générale	French	15	20	3
8. Dresdner Bank	German	20	12	3
9. Banco di Roma	Italian	22	10	3
10. Credito Italiana	Italian	24	7'	3'
11. Commerzbank	German	29	38	4
12. Algemene Bank Nederland	Dutch	38	24	3
13. Amsterdam-Rotterdam Bank [22]	Dutch	48	2	2

Figures from the Bankers' Almanac

TABLE IX

5 largest banks of the United Kingdom in 1970

	Rank Fortune	Number of countries in which branch or affiliate 7)	Number of EC-countries in which branch or affiliate 2)
1. Barclays Bank	1	25	3
2. National Westminster Bank	2	110'	5'
3. Midland Bank	16	100'	3
4. Lloyds Bank	21	7-	3
5. Standard & Chartered Banking Group	35	44	3

' Figures from the Bankers' Almanac

- The annual report did not give exact information on foreign subsidiaries and affiliates. The number given is a conservative estimate.

TABLE X

8 largest banks of the U.S. in 1970

	Rank Fortune	Number of countries in which branch or affiliate	Number of EC-countries in which branch or affiliate
1. Bank America (S. Franc.)	1	60	5
2. First National City Corp. (N.Y.)	2	50'	5'
3. Chase Manhattan Corp. (N.Y.)	3	40	5
4. Manufacturers Hanover Corp. (N.Y.)	4	18	4
5. J.P. Morgan (N.Y.)	5	14'	4'
6. Western Bancorporation (L.A.)	6	7	1
7. Chemical New York Corp. (N.Y.)	7	14	1
8. Bankers Trust New York Corp, (N.Y.)	8	24	4

' Figures from the Bankers' Almanac

For reasons explained in chapter 2 we combined Bank America Corporation and
Bank of America NT and SA; First National Cirty Corporation and First National
City Bank; The Chase Manhattan Corporation and The Chase Manhattan Bank NA.;
Manufacturers Hanover Corporation and Manufacturers Hanover Trust Company;
J.P. Morgan and Co. Incorporated and Morgan Guaranty Trust of New York;
Chemical New York Corporation and Chemical Bank; Bankers Trust New York
Corporation and Bankers Trust Company. The Western Bancorporation is an
investment trust and not a bank.

TABLE XI

8 largest Japanese banks in 1970

	Rank Fortune	Number of countries in which branch or affiliate [7]	Number of EC-countries in which branch or affiliate [2]
1. Fuji Bank	10	6	1
2. Sumitomo Bank [10]	11	12	3
3. Mitsubishi Bank	12	7	2
4. Sanwa Bank	13	8	2
5. Industrial Bank of Japan	18	4	1
6. Bank of Tokyo	23	32	5
7. Tokai Bank	25	5	1
8. Mitsui Bank	27	7	0

TABLE XII

8 largest banks from other countries in 1970

n	Nationality	Rank Fortune	Number of Countries in which branch or affiliate [7]	Number of EC-countries in which branch or affiliate [2]
1. Royal Bank of Canada	Canadian	7	30	3
2. Canadian Imperial Bank of Commerce [9]	Canadian	9	13	2
3. Bank of Montreal [9]	Canadian	17	14	4
4. Union Bank of Switzerland [9]	Swiss	26	1	1
5. Swiss Bank Corp.	Swiss	31	14	1
6. Swiss Credit Bank [9]	Swiss	32	13	0
7. Bank of Nova Scotia	Canadian	33	18	3
8. Toronto Dominion Bank	Canadian	39	--	--

-- No annual report or other source available; firm not included in the sample

Footnotes to "Selection of the firms".

1) The term EC-country is used for a member-country of the European Communities
   (ESCS, EEC, Euratom) in 1970.
2) Belgium and Luxembourg are regarded as one country, not only because
   Luxembourg is extreemly small, but also because there exist a tight
   economic union between the two countries.
3) Yearbook of International Organizations 1968 (12th ed.) edited by the
   Union of International Associations, Brussels 1969, p. 1195-1196.
4) In an oral communication Judge admitted that for this reason his lists
   are not very reliable.
5) Yearbook of International Organizations 1970/1971 (13th ed.) edited for
   the Union of International Associations by R.A. Hall, Brussels 1971,
   p. 1029. The introduction is G.P. Speeckaert's.
7) The country, in which the company is incorporated counts for one as well.
8) State-owned or controlled.
9) The Annual Report of 1971 was used.
10) The Annual Report of 1971 was used.
11) Gutehoffnungshütte has, according to the Judge-lists, affiliates in 19
    countries. In the Annual Report, however, none of these were mentioned.
12) No annual report could be obtained; instead EXTEL information sheets
    were used, which, unfortunately, do not include the outside directors.
13) The Annual Report of 1973 was used.
14) All affiliates in the Common Market belong to Unilever N.V.
15) Shell Oil is part of the Shell-group.
16) Ciba A.G. and J.R. Geigy A.G. merged in October 1970. In the Judge-list
    they are still regarded as seperate.
17) This figure is given for Trafikaktiebolaget Grängesbergoxelösund
    (the Grängesberg Co.).
18) Quoted from Hearings on Economic Concentration, Part I, Conglomerates and
    other Aspects, Washington 1964 by H.W. de Jong, Ondernemingsconcentraties,
    Stenfert Kroese, Leiden, 1971, p. 170.
19) Idem.
20) The selection is biased nevertheless, because the English 'merchant banks'
    and French 'merchant banks' are small according to both deposits and assets.
    They are not included in our sample, although they are very important in
    linking the industries to financial institutions.

268

21) <u>Banker's Almanac and Yearbook 1969-1970</u>, T. Skinner & Co., London 1970.

22) According to our criteria the Amsterdam-Rotterdam Bank should not be included. We decided to do so, to make a better comparison possible with the 'Dutch' network given in the study on political and economic elites in the Netherlands, (Graven naar Macht, 1975).